GeroPsychology
European Perspectives for an Aging World

Dedicated to the memory of
Paul B. Baltes

GeroPsychology

European Perspectives for an Aging World

Edited by
Rocío Fernández-Ballesteros

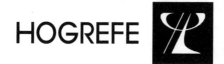

HOGREFE

Library of Congress Cataloging in Publication

is available via the Library of Congress Marc Database under the
LC Control Number 2007928886.

Library and Archives Canada Cataloguing in Publication

Geropsychology: European perspectives for an aging world / Rocío Fernández
Ballesteros, editor.
Includes bibliographical references.
ISBN 978-0-88937-340-2
1. Aging—Psychological aspects. 2. Older people—Psychology. 3. Older people—
Mental health. 4. Aging—Psychological aspects—Research—Europe. I. Fernández
Ballesteros, Rocío

RC451.4.A5.G472	2007	618.97'689	C2007-903236-2

© 2007 by Hogrefe & Huber Publishers

PUBLISHING OFFICES
USA: Hogrefe & Huber Publishers, 875 Massachusetts Avenue, 7th Floor,
            Cambridge, MA 02139
            Phone (866) 823-4726, Fax (617) 354-6875; E-mail info@hhpub.com
EUROPE: Hogrefe & Huber Publishers, Rohnsweg 25, 37085 Göttingen, Germany
            Phone +49 551 49609-0, Fax +49 551 49609-88, E-mail hh@hhpub.com

SALES & DISTRIBUTION
USA: Hogrefe & Huber Publishers, Customer Services Department,
            30 Amberwood Parkway, Ashland, OH 44805
            Phone (800) 228-3749, Fax (419) 281-6883, E-mail custserv@hhpub.com
EUROPE: Hogrefe & Huber Publishers, Rohnsweg 25, 37085 Göttingen, Germany
            Phone +49 551 49609-0, Fax +49 551 49609-88, E-mail hh@hhpub.com

OTHER OFFICES
CANADA: Hogrefe & Huber Publishers, 1543 Bayview Avenue, Toronto,
            Ontario M4G 3B5
SWITZERLAND:Hogrefe & Huber Publishers, Länggass-Strasse 76, CH-3000 Bern 9

Hogrefe & Huber Publishers. Incorporated and registered in the State of Washington,
USA, and in Göttingen, Lower Saxony, Germany.

Printed and bound in the USA
ISBN: 978-0-88937-340-2

Foreword

This is a wonderful and timely book and, being a lifespan psychologist myself, I want to recommend it to all who are interested in psychology's answer to the new challenges presented to Europe and our discipline by the growing share of elderly in our communities. Why? The editor and her colleagues have brought together facts and figures on the current situation of scientific research and academic teaching on aging, and have assembled authors from around Europe who write authoritatively about what we know and how this knowledge was achieved in various basic and applied topics of aging. This combination is unique and without competition.

When it comes to the daily experiences with aging, the Europeans in a sense count among the world champions. In many countries the share of people in the age range 0 to 14 compared to those 65 years and older is about the same, and in a few countries, such as Italy, the oldest even form a higher percentage. This is the combined result of extended life expectancies and low fertility rates, with the consequence of a growing burden for the adult age groups that have to take care for those younger and older. The question is whether we as a society are prepared to deal with around 75 million Europeans aged 65 and older, and this figure, which refers to 2004, is projected to grow rapidly.

These and other facts led the United Nations to develop the 2002 International Plan of Action on Ageing, requiring specific measures to achieve a better understanding of aging concerning psychosocial development, options for health promotion, and the design of supportive environments. European science looks back on a long tradition of research in such fields, but is the state of the art enough in term of substantive knowledge and scientific training to develop and implement social policies and programs?

To help answer these questions the European Federation of Psychologists' Associations (EFPA) was asked by its Spanish member organization to form a task force of renowned specialists in the field who would analyze the situation in Europe concerning research and teaching in "Geropsychology." We found a group of energetic and knowledgeable scientists who, under the leadership of Rocio Fernandez-Ballesteros, herself the winner of EFPA's prestigious Aristotle Award in 2005, have worked on this project for three years. As member of the executive committee with the portfolio for science, I was their liaison with EFPA.

This book is the result of this task force's work, and it is impressive. For the first time we know as comprehensively as possible that there is indeed a lot of research, but that it mainly covers only a few topics, with impairment of cognitive competencies most frequent and prevention of aging-related ailments, unfortunately, usually at the bottom. Here is much room for improvement. In addition, we have a big divide between East and West in Europe, with countries of the latter region (but not all) much more productive thus far in research and dissemination of knowledge on psychological aging. In part this reflects the urgency of the challenges in this region, but actually the disparity originates more in a relative lack of international collaboration and networking in the East. This situation particularly needs improvement, and hopefully this book will be instrumental in achieving this, especially given the fact that there is a great tradition of multisite, multitopic cross-national studies in Europe.

The factual priorities of research are mirrored in the situation of academic teaching and training. The bulk of established programs refer to development and aging in general and to psychopathology and assessment, and even this somewhat one-sided focus is not represented in all European countries. Other issues of pressing urgency, such as the necessity for lifelong learning and the activation of new and alternate work roles in later periods of the life-span, are very much underrepresented. Given the changes in the demographic composition of the populations in Europe, psychology is urged to establish the ground for a new culture of aging, including opportunities for fulfilling, productive activities for the later years – and all this to the advantage of all generations and cohorts.

What is most in need of change is the situation of post-graduate training and specialization – in only a few countries do we have specialized study programs for geropsychology, and also very few professors within this specific field.

Here I have to refer to EFPA again. We developed the EuroPsy standard for the comprehensive training of psychologists (www.efpa.be), and this model allows for the addition of fields of specialization achieved subsequent to the MA or equivalent. Thus far the specializations envisioned relate for instance to psychology concerning work and organizations or clinical issues. I deem it very important to think about geropsychology as another field of specialization that would signify psychologists' qualified competence to work on psychological aging issues, such as intervention, education, and clinical work. The many chapters of the book devoted to current knowledge in the field give a representative overview on such topics, and moreover they introduce readers into the world of renowned European researchers in the field.

What should be the next step? If I see it correctly it would be joint efforts to increase research collaboration across Europe and to implement advanced training, probably accomplished best by multi-site teams and utilizing new forms such as virtual graduate schools. I am confident that EFPA will, and can, contribute to such endeavors.

Rainer K. Silbereisen
EFPA Executive Committee Member

List of Contributors

Paul B. Baltes†
Max Planck Institute for Human Development, Berlin, Germany
Department of Psychology, University of Virginia, USA

Stig Berg
Institute of Gerontology, School of Health Sciences, Jönköping University, Sweden

M. Dolores Calero
Department Personality and Psychological Assessment and Treatment, University of Granada, Spain

Gian Vittorio Caprara
Department of Psychology, University of Rome "La Sapienza," Rome, Italy

Mariagiovanna Caprara
Department of Psychology, University of Rome "La Sapienza," Rome, Italy

Svein Olav Daatland
Norwegian Social Research, Oslo, Norway

Anna Dahl
Institute of Gerontology, School of Health Sciences, Jönköping University, Sweden

Anastasia Efklides
School of Psychology, Aristotle University of Thessaloniki, Greece

Rocío Fernández-Ballesteros
Department of Psychobiology and Health, Autonoma University of Madrid, Spain

Alexandra M. Freund
Department of Psychology, University of Zurich, Switzerland

Susanne Iwarsson
Department of Health Sciences, University of Lund, Sweden

Andreas Kruse
Institute of Gerontology, University of Heidelberg, Germany

Ute Kunzmann
Center for Lifelong Learning and Institutional Development, Jacobs University of Bremen, Germany

Ursula Lehr
Institute of Gerontology, University of Heidelberg, Germany

Despina Moraitou
School of Psychology, Aristotle University of Thessaloniki, Greece

Sven Nilsson
Institute of Gerontology, School of Health Sciences, Jönköping University, Sweden

Constança Paúl
UNIFAI/ICBAS, University of Porto, Portugal

Herminia Peraita
Department of Basic Psychology, UNED (National Distance University), Spain

Martin Pinquart
Department of Developmental Psychology, University of Jena, Germany

Susanna Re
Institute of Gerontology, University of Heidelberg, Germany

Rainer K. Silbereisen
Department of Developmental Psychology and Center for Applied Developmental Science, University of Jena, Germany

Patrizia Steca
Faculty of Psychology, University of Milan "Bicocca," Italy

Lluis Tárraga
ACE Foundation, Catalan Institute of Applied Neurosciences, Barcelona, Spain

Per Torpdahl
Geropsychiatric Department, University Hospital in Aarhus, Denmark

Hans-Werner Wahl
Department of Psychological Aging Research, University of Heidelberg, Germany

Joachim Wilbers
Project Care, Frankfurt, Germany

María Dolores Zamarrón
Department of Psychobiology and Health, Autonoma University of Madrid, Spain

Table of Contents

Foreword
Rainer K. Silbereisen   V

List of Contributors   VI

1. GeroPsychology. Demographic, Sociopolitical, and Historical Background
Rocío Fernández-Ballesteros, Martin Pinquart, and Per Torpdahl   1

2. Main Trends in Geropsychology in Europe: Research, Training, and Practice
Martin Pinquart   15

3. Age Identifications
Svein Olaf Daatland   31

4. Person-Environment Relations
Hans-Werner Wahl and Susanne Iwarsson   49

5. Semantic Memory in Healthy Aging
Herminia Peraita   67

6. Affect and Emotions
Despina Moraitou and Anastasia Efklides   82

7. Personality and Self-Beliefs
Mariagiovanna Caprara, Patrizia Steca, and Gian Vittorio Caprara   103

**8. Old-Old People: Major Recent Findings and the European Contribution
to the State of the Art**
Constança Paúl   128

9. Cognitive Plasticity and Cognitive Impairment
Rocío Fernández-Ballesteros, María Dolores Zamarrón,
M. Dolores Calero, and Lluis Tárraga 145

10. Cognitive Decline and Dementia
Stig Berg, Anna Dahl, and Sven Nilsson 165

11. Demographic Change, the Need for Care, and the Role of the Elderly
Ursula Lehr, Susanna Re, and Joachim Wilbers 183

12. Quality of Life, Life Satisfaction, and Positive Aging
Rocío Fernández-Ballesteros, Andreas Kruse, María Dolores Zamarrón,
and Mariagiovanna Caprara 197

13. Wisdom: Adult Development and Emotional-Motivational Dynamics
Ute Kunzmann 224

14. Toward a Theory of Successful Aging: Selection, Optimization, and Compensation
Alexandra M. Freund and Paul B. Baltes. 239

1. Geropsychology

Demographic, Sociopolitical, and Historical Background

Rocío Fernández-Ballesteros, Martin Pinquart, and Per Torpdahl

Introduction

In demographic terms, Europe is the oldest continent in the world. In 2004 in Western Europe (EU-15 plus Switzerland and Norway) there were 66 million inhabitants over 65, and if we take Eastern Europe (EU-10) into account, the total European (EU-25) elderly population was around 75 million.

Although 50-year projections are somewhat uncertain, on the basis of increasing life expectancy and the decline in fertility over the last 25 years, and in line with the United Nations demographic projections for the year 2050, it is predicted that half a century from now Europe will have about 300 millions inhabitants over 60 (UN, 2002).

On the basis of these sociodemographic data, several sociopolitical decisions have been taken by the United Nations (UN, 2002), the World Health Organization (WHO, 2002), and the UN Economic Commission for Europe (UNECE, 2003). In fact, the II International Plan of Action on Ageing (MIPAA, UN, 2002) and its strategy for Europe (UNECE, 2003), the Research Agenda on Ageing for the 21st Century (developed by the International Association of Gerontology in collaboration with the United Nations; UN-IAG, 2003; Andrews, et al. 2006), and the policy framework for developing healthy and active aging (WHO, 2002) were all discussed and approved by the year 2002. The general objective of all of these documents is to cope with the challenge of aging; moreover, in all international recommendations for scientific or political action, psychology and psychologists are strongly involved in and committed to the field of aging, age, and the aged (Birren, 1996).

Taking into consideration the demographic situation and data and the research findings, the European Federation of Psychologists Associations (EFPA), at its 2003 general assembly in Vienna, approved setting up a Task Force on Geropsychology with the objectives, among others, of examining the relevant contexts and issues to which psychologists (with their scientific knowledge and professional competences) can contribute to the enhancement of elders' quality of life and well-being, of deciding which European universities and research centers will develop official research programs on the psychological study of aging, and of identifying and organizing the profile of European research.

The task force has been working since 2004 using two main strategies: (1) Internet search on geropsychological research, training, and practice, and (2) survey of key persons suggested by all EFPA organizations throughout Europe working on geropsychology (see Chapter 2). This book presents data on those strategies. However, before presenting some data from this work, we will provide some demographic data at the root of scientific interest in the study of aging.

Europe: The World's Oldest Continent

Table 1 shows two indicators of population aging for the 25 European countries and for EU-15 and the new EU-10: percentage of inhabitants over 65 and ratio of youngest (0–14) to oldest (65 +) for the year 2003 (European Council, 2004). As it can be seen, there are considerable differences among countries in these indicators. For example, in

Table 1. Percentage of older and younger European population in Western and Eastern European countries

European Countries	% Population per age	
	< 15	65+
Western Countries:	17	16
Austria	17	15
Belgium	18	17
Denmark	19	15
Finland	18	15
France	19	16
Germany	16	16
Greece	15	17
Ireland	21	11
Italy	14	19
Luxembourg	19	14
Netherlands	19	14
Portugal	16	16
Spain	15	17
Sweden	18	17
UK	19	16
Eastern Countries:	18	13
Cyprus	22	10
Czech Rep.	16	14
Estonia	18	15
Hungary	17	15
Latvia	17	15
Lithuania	19	14
Malta	20	12
Poland	19	12
Slovakia	19	11
Slovenia	16	14

Italy almost one in five inhabitants (19.2%) is over 65, while in Ireland the figure is around 1 in 10 (11.1%). Taking into consideration the proportion of youngest to oldest, it is in Italy where we find the fewest children per older inhabitant (14/19), while in Ireland there are almost two children per older adult (21/11). There are also countries with a high percentage of inhabitants over 65 and a relatively good balance of youngest and oldest. For example, Sweden has 18% of over-65s and 17% children.

If we compare Western and Eastern Europe, on the basis of the 15-member EU and the 10 nations that joined in 2005 (includes Malta), Western Europe is significantly older than Eastern Europe; on average one in six citizens in Western Europe are older than 65, and there are more older citizens than children, while in Eastern Europe (considering EU members only), one in seven citizens are over 65, and there are more children than older adults. Looking at projections made by the United Nations (2000), by the year 2050, 30% of Western Europe's population will be over 65, while 12% will be over 80.

As is well known, population aging depends on the ratio of fertility to mortality, or its derivative, life expectancy at birth (migration is a third type of population data, which we do not consider here; see Diez-Nicolás, 2004). **Figure 1** shows the evolution of fertility in European countries (in terms of number of children per woman in reproductive age range); in most of them fertility is declining strongly, but in others the pattern is the opposite (e.g., in Scandinavian countries, where demographic transition took place earlier). However, we can say that fertility is declining in all Eastern and most Western European countries, though on average Western countries have higher fertility rates than Eastern ones, several of which fall short of the replacement rate.

Life expectancy at birth was increasing all over the world throughout the 20th century, during which it almost doubled in European countries. **Figure 2** shows life expectancy in 25 European countries with data for most of the EU-15 and EU-10.

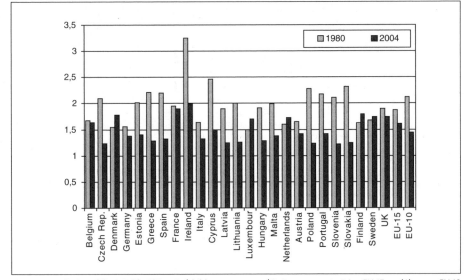

Figure 1. Evolution of the total fertility rate (children per women) in European countries, EU-15, and the new EU-10 (1980–2004; European Council, 2004)

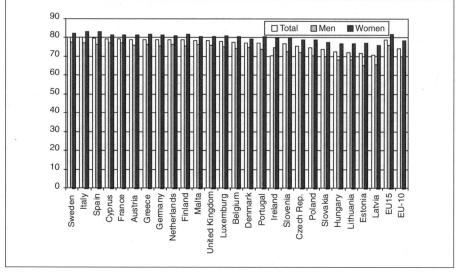

Figure 2. Life expectancy at birth in European countries, EU-15, and the new EU-10 (European Council, 2004)

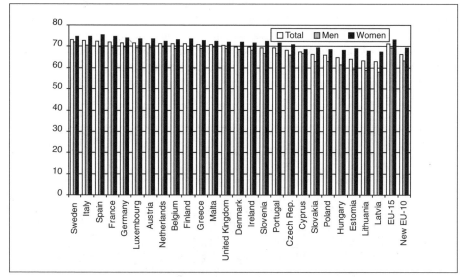

Figure 3. Disability-free life expectancy at birth in European countries, EU-15, and the new EU-10, year 2003 (European Commission, 2005)

As it can be observed, total life expectancy runs from 80.1 years in Sweden to 70.9 years in Latvia. The highest life expectancy for men is also in Sweden (77.7), while the lowest is in Estonia (65.3); highest life expectancy for women is 83.3 years (Spain) and lowest is 76 years (Latvia). In conclusion, it can be said that there is almost 5 years difference in life expectancy between Western and Eastern European countries.

Although living longer is important – since it is an indicator of human development – the most important concern is whether people are living in good or poor health. Disability Free Life Expectancy (DFLE) are measures of the remaining years a person of a specific age is expected to live in a healthy condition (European Commission, 2005).

Figure 3 shows that DFLE for 25 European countries have similar profiles to those of life expectancy. Europeans can expect (at birth) a mean of some 7 years of disability (approximately 6 years for men and almost 8 years for women). Highest total DFLE is in Sweden, at 73.3, and lowest is in Latvia, at 62.8.

In summary, increasing life expectancy can be considered an indicator of giving more "years to life" but it is highly important to give "life to years;" thus, the most important finding is that evolution over time (1998 to 2003) shows an increasing DFLE (EC, 2005). How psychology as a science and as a profession can work toward increasing disability free life expectancy is one of the key issues in geropsychology.

Sociopolitical Influences on Geropsychology Research and Profession

Population aging is not only a trend in the European region but a worldwide phenomenon. The silent demographic revolution occurred during the 20th century and is the expression of human intelligence and social development but is also a challenge for science and society. At the same time that aging is an opportunity for individuals and societies, aging is associated with risk of illness and disability, causing pain and suffering to the individual and his or her family, and it is linked to high social and health costs. The United Nations called for a First World Assembly on Ageing at Vienna in 1982 and adopted the First International Plan of Action on Ageing, which guided the course of thinking and action on aging over the last decades of the 20th century. Twenty years later, in 2002, at the Madrid Second World Assembly, the Second International Plan of Action on Ageing (MIPAA) was approved (UN, 2002). At the same time, specific recommendations for the European Region (UNECE, 2002) as well as a Research Agenda on Ageing for the 21st Century were decided by the joint effort of the International Association of Gerontology and the UN Program on Ageing (2003).

As has been pointed out by Andrews et al. (2006), the link between policy, research, and professional work is usually not explicitly known and sometimes missing. However, in the case of aging, documents addressing policies and professional and research needs and requirements are explicitly known and have been published and disseminated. Nevertheless, these documents are not usually distributed (or may even be neglected) by target research teams and professional bodies (COP, 2002). Let us present an overview of the MIPAA general recommendations, noting some of the relevant psychology issues.

Figure 4 shows how the MIPAA is organized through three priority directions: (1) Aging and development, (2) Advancing health and well-being, and (3) Ensuring enabling and supportive environments. Each priority direction has a set of Issues divided into objectives and recommendations. Let us give some examples from the *Research Agenda on Ageing for the 21st Century* (IAG-EU, 2003) about the involvement of psychology and psychologists in these three priority directions.

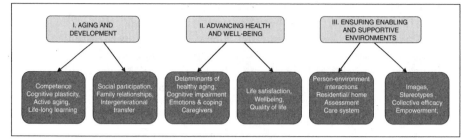

Figure 4. MIPAA priority directions and psychology issues

1. *Aging and development.* The main idea behind this priority direction is that older persons must be full participants in the development process and also share its benefits. This is a very general objective requiring much more research on cognitive resources in old age (cognitive plasticity), concepts and determinants of active aging, and the extent to which there are potential developments and competences over the life cycle. In addition, life-long learning, access to knowledge, education, and training are required to enlarge and increase human development and human capital. This priority direction also emphasizes the importance of the study of the psychosocial determinants of participation and integration, family relationships, and intergenerational transfer and solidarity, all relevant issues in social psychology.

2. *Advancing health and well-being into old age.* Good health is a precondition for psychological well-being and quality of life. In fact, as has been stated, at the population level, the most important indicator for improving living conditions in old age is healthy life expectancy. The WHO defines health as the state of complete physical, mental, and social well-being, not merely the absence of disease. The research agenda emphasizes the importance of defining and delimiting the scope of healthy aging, including individual behavioral habits and psychosocial determinants of healthy aging (cognitive functioning, emotions, and coping), and physical and mental health. Finally, life satisfaction, well-being, and, partially, quality of life, are subjective constructs, therefore the research agenda emphasizes the importance of the development of measures, harmonization of them between countries, and their description across age.

3. *Ensuring enabling and supportive environments.* The promotion of an enabling environment for social development was one of the central goals of the MIPAA in obtaining commitments to strengthen policies and programs to create inclusive, cohesive societies for all ages. The research agenda emphasizes the importance of studying person-environment interactions, residential, home, and care contexts, as well as situations of elder abuse. Finally, linking priority directions III and I, the study of images of aging, ageism, as well as how to empower elders in order to promote their participation in society and increase their self and collective efficacy are critical research arenas.

These examples illustrate how sociopolitical plans, such as the Second International Plan of Actions on Ageing, can lead research and how, necessarily, they are influencing professional practice through national political programs and actions.

European Contributions to Geropsychology: Past and Present

The aging of the European population calls for more basic and applied research on geropsychology. European aging research can build upon on a long history. There are prominent European traditions in aging research and in the psychology of aging in particular. Ideas about the aging process can be traced back to Greek and Roman philosophers, such as Democritus (460–370 B.C.), Epicurus (341–271 B.C.), Plato (427–327 B.C.), Aristotle (384–322 B.C.), and Cicero (106–42 B.C.). For example, Plato emphasized that the feeling of being old is dependent on the person's view of young and old people, and that living a righteous life would be a precondition of aging peacefully. In addition, Cicero discussed the need for memory training in older adults and encouraged older adults to make themselves useful in various advisory, intellectual, and administrative functions. These thoughts are still reflected in recent models in the field of geropsychology (for more information on the early history of geropsychology, see, for example, Birren & Schroots, 2001).

The beginning of empirical research on psychological aspects of aging can be traced back to the work of the Belgium statistician Adolphe Quêtelet (1796–1874; Quêtelet, 1835) on age-differences in mental performance, morality, suicide, delinquency, and other aspects of behavior. The assessment of mental performance, reaction time, and other measures in over 9,300 visitors to the International Health Exhibition of London from age 5 to 80 by the British physician and natural scientist Sir Francis Galton (1822–1911; Galton, 1983) marked the beginning of *empirical* psychological life-span research. Later, Galton set up an experimental laboratory and assessed age-differences in sensory thresholds. Although his work was cross-sectional, Galton had already suggested longitudinal studies for analyzing human development and aging.

In the first half of the 20th century, a growing number of researchers from different European countries started research on geropsychology, although there were not yet research institutes on aging with large or even interdisciplinary research programs (the first institute on aging research was founded in 1928 at Stanford University in the United States). For example, Paul Ranschburg (1870–1945), a Hungarian neurologist, studied the pathology of cognitive function and memory in older persons (Ranschburg, 1912). In Russia, Ivan Pavlov (1894–1936) analyzed age-differences in the learning abilities of dogs and found that older dogs built conditioned reflexes more slowly (Pavlov, 1926). In Germany, Weiss (1927) tested the performance of 500 ticket collectors of the German railway who had to find out the shortest way between two destinations. Although Weiss had expected to find a negative association between age and performance, he could not find such a result. One year later, Giese (1928) published a study on self-perceptions of aging. He asked readers of German newspapers to identify signs of getting old. Age at the first perception of signs of aging varied between 18 and 82. Not surprisingly, respondents most often associated aging with physical changes. In 1919, the first report on psychotherapy with older adults was published by the German psychoanalyst Karl Abraham (1919/1927). He held an optimistic view on the treatment of older adults and suggested that the age at which the older adult started psychotherapy was less important than the age of the patient at the time the psychological problem began.

In 1933, Charlotte Bühler (1893–1974) published her book on the life course at the University of Vienna, which was the second textbook on life-span development. In her book, Bühler analyzed life courses of 200 scientists, artists, technicians, and politicians, and included the results of 50 biographical interviews with residents of nursing homes in Vienna. Similar to U.S. researchers of that time period, her model of the life course was strongly tied to biological models of growth and decline, and she associated old age with regression.

The first scientific gerontological journal was founded in 1938 in Germany (*Zeitschrift für Altersforschung*). Although this journal originally had a strong biological and medical focus, from the beginning there were individual papers on psychological topics (e.g., on age-differences in mental performance and the inner mental world; Bracken, 1939).

In the prewar period, the center of psychological aging research shifted from Europe to the United States. Many European researchers emigrated to the United States, such as Erik Erikson, whose book *Childhood and Society* (1950) encouraged research in life-span psychology and geropsychology, and Charlotte Bühler.

Whereas geropsychology expanded rapidly in the United States after World War II (Riegel, 1973, 1977), it took time to rebuild and expand aging research in Europe, for example, due to the destroyed scientific infrastructures, different priorities of the fatherless young generation, and the emigration of many scientists, all of which resulted in a widening gap between geropsychological research in Europe and the United States. Nonetheless, in 1946 a research group on physical and mental abilities of older workers was founded at the University of Cambridge in the UK (e.g., Welford, 1958), and in the 1950s psychological aging studies started in France (Pacaud, 1953), The Netherlands (Van Zooneveld, 1958), Finland (Karsten, 1959), and other European countries.

In recent decades there has been a considerable increase in aging-related research in Europe. We used the PsycInfo electronic database for a bibliometrical analysis of change in the numbers and percentages of European studies in the field of geropsychology over the last 60 years. We first identified publications that included the search terms (*ageing* or *aging* or *late life* or *old age* or *geriatric* or *gerontol**). We next analyzed the subgroup of studies with at least one author coming from a European country. On average, 21.6% of the identified studies were authored or coauthored by a European researcher, as compared to 46.4% of studies authored by researchers from the United States. About 1% of the studies were coauthored by researchers from Europe and the United States.

As shown in **Figure 5**, in the first years of the 21st century, the number of publications on aging-related topics is now more than 35 times higher than it was in the late 1940s (551 vs. 19,342). The number of publications began to rise in the 1960s, and the increase further accelerated in the 1980s. An even steeper rise was observed for European publications: For example, between 2001 and 2005, the percentage of European publications was more than 360 times higher than it was in the late 1940s (15 vs. 5,517). Whereas in the late 1940s and in the 1950s, between 1% and 2.7% of the aging-related publications came from Europe, the percentage increased to about 12% in the late 1970s and early 1980s, and to 28.5% in the first half of the current decade (2001–2005). In 2005, about 31.8% of all related publications had at least one author from Europe.

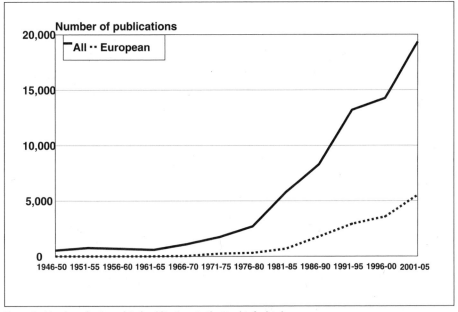

Figure 5. Number of aging-related publications in the PsychInfo database

A bibliometrical analysis of aging-related publications from different European countries is reported by Pinquart (this volume).

Going back to Galton (1883), longitudinal studies rather than cross-sectional studies have been recommended for studying aging, as, for example, age-differences in cross-sectional studies are confounded with cohort differences and because interindividual differences in intraindividual change of psychological variables can only be identified with a longitudinal study design. We included the search term *longitudinal* into our analysis and analyzed the change in the number of studies that referred to longitudinal work. In most cases, these papers reported results from a longitudinal study on aging. In a few cases, they summarized available data from previous longitudinal studies or compared longitudinal and other research designs from a methodological view. As shown in **Figure 6**, the number of papers on longitudinal aging studies has dramatically increased since the late 1970s, and is now more than 130 times higher than it was in the 1940s and 1950s. Note that the absolute numbers overestimate change in the number of longitudinal studies as usually more than one paper is published from each longitudinal study.

Similarly, the percentage of papers on aging-related topics from European authors has increased. For example, only one individual longitudinal study was available from European authors between 1946 and 1965 (4.5% of the available papers on longitudinal research of that time period). However, the percentage of European papers that employed a longitudinal research methodology has increased from 12.9% (1966–1969; mainly based on the Bonn Longitudinal Study on Aging) to 39.5% (2000–2005).

In international research, cognitive aging and psychopathology in old age are the

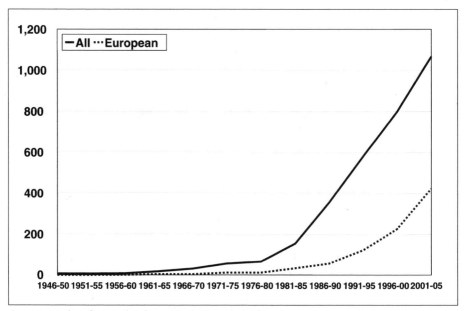

Figure 6. Number of aging-related papers in the PsycInfo database that used a longitudinal study design or that referred to longitudinal research methods

most prominent topics with more than 20,000 papers each, followed by developmental issues (about 12,300 papers), psychological assessment (8,800 papers), environmental issues (e.g., adaptation of the environment to age-associated change in abilities) and gender issues (5,200 publications each), death, dying, and bereavement (about 4,100 studies), work and retirement (3,950 publications), clinical interventions (psychotherapy and counseling; about 3,450 papers), social relationships in old age (about 3,400 publications), caregiving (about 2,000 studies), aging and ethnicity (about 1,950 papers), prevention and health promotion (about 1,800 publications), nursing homes (about 1,550 studies), chronic illness (about 950 papers), ageism and elder abuse (about 750 publications), and longevity (about 500 studies). As shown in Figures 8a and 8b, identical topics are most prevalent in international and European research. However, the percentage of publications from European researchers was above average (> 21.6%) for psychopathology (e.g., depression, anxiety, dementia; 30.9%), cognitive aging (29.7%), psychological assessment (26.3%), caregiving (23.6%), and aging in nursing homes (23.4%), and average for death, dying, and bereavement (21.2%). The percentage of European publications was below average with regard to longevity (18.3%), prevention and health promotion (18.1%), developmental issues (16.9%), gender issues (16.3%), ageism and elder abuse (15.6%), social relations (14.2%), chronic illness/long-term care (12.7%), and ethnic differences (5.9%). The very low percentage of European publications on ethnic issues reflects the lower ethnic heterogeneity in most European countries when compared to the United States and Canada, and the fact that most working migrants who came to Western Europe after the 1950s have not yet reached old age. In addition, ethnic conflicts that happened in the former

Yugoslavia and in parts of the former Soviet Union did not lead to published research on their impact on older adults.

Although the Internet search slightly underestimates the number and percentage of European studies (as, for example, books and chapters in languages other than English are not listed in the electronic database), it shows that geropsychological topics have gained importance in European research, and in international research in general. Geropsychology in Europe is growing relatively fast and is narrowing the gap with the United States.

Despite that fact that the number of 0–14-year-old Europeans is almost identical to the number of older adults aged 65 and above, and that in the whole world there are about 3.8 times more people who are 0–14 years old than 65 years and above (United Nations, 2005), there were almost 6 times more studies on children and adolescents in the PsycInfo database than on older adults. Given the higher percentage of older adults in Europe, the number of European studies on children and adolescents was only 4.2 times higher than the number of studies on old age. Nonetheless, these data indicate a need for a further increase in aging-related research in Europe and around the world.

Looking at the increasing numbers of older adults it is obvious that there is a growing need for expertise and, therefore, it is necessary to discuss in which way we can recruit psychologists to the field of geropsychology and what kind of competencies they should have.

A while ago the European Federation of Psychologists' Association (EFPA) developed some European standards for education and training in professional psychology called EuroPsy. The argument was that it should be a basis for free mobility and automatic recognition based on some common standards.

Right now there is an ongoing pilot project in six EU member states (Finland, Germany, Hungary, Italy, Spain, and the UK) conducting a EuroPsy certification and registration for a EuroPsy Professional Card containing relevant information on the psychologist's education and training.

The EuroPsy requirements for qualification for independent practice are as follows:
1. Completion of education and training in psychology at a recognized university level of at least 6 years' duration, including:
   a. A university degree in psychology, which has a duration equivalent to at least 5 years of full-time study (300 ECTS),
   b. At least 1 year of supervised practice (included in or added to the university degree program), and
   c. Commitment in writing to the ethical code of psychologists in the country of practice and the European Metacode of ethics for psychologists.

It could be argued that there should also be some common standards for the specialist in geropsychology for dealing with the demands of working with older adults. Standards or guidelines refer to statements that suggest or recommend specific professional behavior, endeavors, or conduct for psychologists. The specific goals of these guidelines are to provide practitioners with a frame of reference for engaging in clinical work with older adults. Basic information and further references and guidelines can be organized into six sections (attitudes, general knowledge, clinical issues, assessment, intervention, and education).

Because the United States has the most advanced infrastructure for teaching and research in geropsychology as well as strong national organizations, such as the Gerontological Society of America and the American Psychological Association with Division 20 on Adult Development and Aging, and because detailed suggestions and recommendations for teaching and applying geropsychology have been developed in the United States, several of their recommendations may be easily applied to Europe, such as suggestions on effective forms of psychological interventions for psychological disorders, which are based on best (international) empirical evidence. Nonetheless, although European scientists and practitioners could learn from U.S. experiences in establishing, teaching, and applying geropsychology, recommendations from the United States would have to be adapted to specific national conditions, and not all recommendations could be applied to every European country. For example, recommendations for integrating aging topics in the training of undergraduates could be applied to all countries that offer undergraduate courses in the field of psychology, whereas those related to PhD programs would not be relevant for countries that could not (yet) offer these programs. Note that even in the United States, the first PhD specialty training program in clinical geropsychology was only launched in 2004 (Qualls et al., 2005).

About This Book

Geropsychology: European Perspectives for an Aging World provides an overview of current European research and practice in the field of aging, age, and the aged (Birren & Schroots, 2001), most of them linked with MIPAA priority directions and research recommendations (UN, 2002; UN-IAG, 2003; Andrews et al., 2006).

Emerging from the EFPA Task Force on GeroPsychology, the first two chapters deal with introductory issues: demographic, sociopolitical, and historical bases, as well as the main trends in research, training, and practice. The second block (Chapters 3 and 4) refers to basic issues related to the subjective concept of age and person-environment relationships. The third block (Chapters 5, 6, 7, and 8) contains chapters devoted to healthy aging, including semantic memory, affect and emotion, and personality and the self, while Chapter 8 is devoted to the "oldest old," given their demographic significance in Europe. The fourth block (Chapters 9, 10, and 11) looks at cognitive decline, cognitive impairment and dementia, and the need for care in Europe. Finally, Chapters 12, 13, and 14 deal with issues of positive geropsychology such as quality of life, life satisfaction, wisdom, and successful aging.

Most of the chapters include an overview of European research in a particular field. It should be stressed that both the topics covered and authors represent a small, but outstanding, sample of the field of research on aging in Europe.

References

Abraham, K. (1927, orig. 1919). The applicability of psycho-analytic treatment to patients at an advanced age. In D. Bryan & A. Strachey (Eds.), *Selected papers on psychoanalysis* (pp. 312–317). New York: Brunner/Mazel.

Andrews, G.R., Sidorenko, A., Gutman, J., Gray, V.N., Anisimov, V., Bezrukov, V. et al. (2006). Research on ageing: Priorities for the European region. *Advances in Gerontology, 18,* 7–14.

Birren, J.E., & Schroots, J.J. (2001). History of geropsychology. In J.E. Birren & K.W. Schaie (Eds.), *Handbook of the psychology of aging* (pp. 3–28). San Diego, CA: Academic Press.

Bracken, H. v. (1939). Die Altersveränderungen der geistigen Leistungsfähigkeit und der seelischen Innenwelt [Age-associated changes of cognitive performance and the inner mental world]. *Zeitschrift für Alternsforschung, 1,* 256–266.

Bühler, C. (1933). *Der menschliche Lebenslauf als psychologisches Problem* [Human life course as a psychological problem]. Leipzig, Germany: Hirzel.

Colegio Oficial de Psicólogos (2002). *Psychology, psychologists, and ageing.* Madrid, Spain: COP.

Díez-Nicolás, J. (2004). Implications of population decline for the European Union (2000–2050). In A. Narquina (Ed.), *Environmental challenges in the Mediterranean (2000–2005).* The Netherlands: Kluwer Academic Pub.

Erikson, E. (1950). *Childhood and society.* New York: Norton & Co.

European Commission. (2005). *Health in Europe. Data 1998–2003.* Brussels, Belgium: European Communities.

European Commission. (2005). *Population in Europe 2004.* Brussels, Belgium: European Communities.

European Council. (2004). *Population. Europe-wide comparative review.* Brussels, Belgium: European Council.

Fernández-Ballesteros, R., & Caprara, M. (2003). Psychology of aging in Europe. *European Psychologist, 8,* 129–130.

Galton, F. (1883). *Inquiries into human faculty and its development.* London: Macmillan.

Giese, F. (1928). *Erlebnisformen des Alterns: Umfrageergebnisse über Merkmale persönlichen Verfalls* [Perceptions of aging: Survey results about characteristics of personal decline]. Halle, Germany: Markhold.

International Longevity Center-UK and the Merk Company Foundation (2006). *The state of ageing and health in Europe.* London: ILC & Merk Co.

Karsten, A. (1959). Adjustment to old age in industry. *Vita Humana, 2,* 87–101.

Qualls, S.H., Segal, D.L., Benight, C.C., & Kenny, M.P. (2005). Geropsychology training in a specialist geropsychology doctoral program. *Gerontology and Geriatrics Education, 25*(4), 21–40.

Quêtelet, A. (1835). *Sur l'homme et le développement de ses facultés* [On man and the development of his faculties]. Paris: Bachelier.

Pacaud, S. (1953). Le vieillissement des aptitudes; déclin des aptitudes en fonction de l'age et due niveau d'instruction [The decline of abilities as a function of age and level of instruction]. *Biotypologie, 14,* 65–94.

Pavlov, I.P. (1927, original 1926). *Conditioned reflexes.* London: Oxford University Press.

Ranschburg, P. (1912). *Das kranke Gedächtnis* [The ill memory]. Leipzig, Germany: Barth.

Riegel, K.F. (1973). On the history of psychological gerontology. In C. Eisdorfer & M.P. Lawton (Eds.), *The psychology of adult development and aging* (pp. 37–68). Washington, DC: American Psychological Association.

Riegel, K.F. (1977). History of psychological gerontology. In J.E. Birren & K.W. Schaie (Eds.), *Handbook of psychology of aging* (pp. 70–102). New York: van Nostrand-Reinhold.

UNECE. (2003). *Ageing populations. Opportunities and challenges for Europe and North America*. Geneva: United Nations.

United Nations. (2002). *Madrid international plan of action on ageing*. New York: Author.

United Nations and the International Association of Gerontology. (2003). *Research agenda on ageing for the 21st century*. Vancouver, Canada: IAG.

United Nations Department of Economic and Social Affairs. (2005). *World population perspectives: The 2004 revision* (Volume III). New York: United Nations.

Van Zooneveld, R.J. (1958). An orientation study of the memory of old people. *Geriatrics, 13*, 532–534.

Weiss, E. (1927). Leistung und Lebensalter [Performance and age]. *Industrielle Psychotechnik, 4*, 227–245.

Welford, A.T. (1958). *Aging and human skills*. London: Oxford University Press.

World Health Organization. (2002). *Active ageing. A policy framework*. Geneva, Switzerland: WHO.

2. Main Trends in Geropsychology in Europe

Research, Training, and Practice

Martin Pinquart

Europe is the continent with the oldest population in the world. By 2025, about one-third of Europe's population will be aged 60 or over with greatest increase being among its oldest citizens (75+ years) (WHO, 2002). At the United Nations Second World Assembly on Ageing in Madrid in 2002, the health and well-being of older people was recognized as one of the most pressing and universal social issues of our time (Antonucci, Okorodulu, & Akiyama, 2002). Thus, psychological research is needed on the development of physical and mental health in late life, and on interventions that promote psychological and physical health of older adults. In addition, psychologists have to be increasingly prepared for working with older adults. This requires the integration of aging-related topics into psychology courses, but also the addition of special courses on geropsychology or psychogerontology to curricula in the field of psychology and gerontology (DeVries, 2005). Finally, as the "graying of society" has consequences for different fields of application of psychology (e.g., work, leisure, health care), psychologists who have been trained in aging-related topics are needed for each of these fields.

Based on these considerations, the European Federation of Psychologists' Associations (EFPA) launched a Task Force on Geropsychology. A main goal of the Task Force was to get an overview of teaching, research, and practice of geropsychology in Europe. For doing that, a questionnaire was developed that could be sent to key persons from all European countries. In order to identify key persons from the field of geropsychology, the EFPA Head Office asked all EFPA members to nominate one or more key persons. With the help of the EFPA, we received the names of key persons from 10 out of 31 EFPA members (from Austria, Belgium, Czech Republic, Denmark, Finland, Israel, Iceland, Norway, Sweden, and Spain). The national organizations of three countries nominated more than one key person (Denmark: 2, Finland: 4, and Spain: 3), who sent us a joint response (Finland, Spain), or answered parts of the questionnaire on teaching/research and application, respectively (Denmark). In order to identify additional key persons (also from non-EFPA members), we checked electronic databases (Ageline, PsycInfo) for publications in the field of geropsychology from other European countries. As almost no entries were available from many Eastern European countries and as some e-mail addresses of authors in the databases were outdated, we also checked the web-pages of the main universities of these countries for courses in geropsychology and for colleagues who teach these courses. Unfortunately, from these web pages information was often only available in their native language or there seemed to be no courses in geropsychology. Finally, we contacted the national gerontological associations for key persons in the field of geropsy-chology. In sum, we tried to contact psychologists or institutes from all European countries. If we did not get an answer, and reminder letters remained unanswered, we tried to identify alternative persons, if available.

Finally, we received answers from 30 countries (Austria, Belgium, Bulgaria, Belarus, Bosnia-Herzegovina, the Czech Republic, Denmark, Estonia, Finland, France, Germany, Great Britain, Greece, Hungary, Iceland, Israel, Italy, Lithuania, Luxembourg, Macedonia, the Netherlands, Norway, Portugal, Romania, Russia, Serbia, Spain, Sweden, Switzerland, and Turkey). Thus, information was gathered from all larger Western European countries, except Ireland, Malta, and Cyprus. However, no information was available from Albania, Poland, Slovakia, and from many successors of the former Yugoslavia and of the former Soviet Union, in most cases reflecting the fact that we were not able to identify any psychologists who research or teach in the field of aging.

The results of the questionnaire study on geropsychology in Europe will be presented in three parts, starting with research on psychology and aging.

Research in Geropsychology

The key persons were asked about the most important topics of research on geropsychology (psychology and aging) in their country. Based on an Internet search of important international topics of research in geropsychology, they were given a list of 17 topics to rate (4 = most important topic[s], 3 = important topic, 2 = some research, but less important topic, 1 = no research on that topic). In addition, the respondents were free to add further topics. As shown in **Figure 1**, the most important topics of research in geropsychology were dementia and general cognitive development. Psychological aspects of caregiving, affective disorders, successful aging, social development and intergenerational relationships, chronic illness and long-term care, psychological assessment, and work and retirement played a less important role, but were among the most important topics of research in some countries. Other topics, such as personality, death/dying/bereavement, prevention and health promotion, environmental issues, age-stereotypes/ageism, and psychotherapy and counseling of older clients were less important, and were not subjects of research in 25 to 55% of the countries under investigation.

The most important institutions of geropsychological research were universities (67%) and other state-run institutions (43%; more than one answer was possible). Private research institutions were generally of secondary importance, and did not play any role in 40% of the countries. Main sources of funding were foundations (70%), followed by the government (30%), and universities (23%). Research sponsored by industry was only mentioned by five key persons (17%).

The countries differed considerably in the amount of research on geropsychological topics. According to the key persons, there was no research on psychology of aging in Belarus, and Serbia, and a very small amount of research in Bosnia-Herzegovina and Macedonia (**Table 1**). Similarly, with the exception of Ireland, few (if any) research

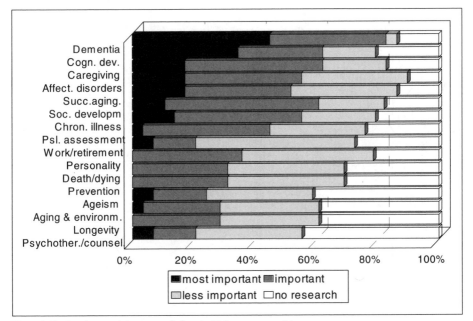

Figure 1. Topics of research in geropsychology in 30 European countries.

activities in that field can be expected in those countries for which no information on geropsychology was available. However, the questionnaires showed broad research programs in geropsychology in most Western and Northern European countries, and in Germany, Sweden, Austria, Israel, and Portugal in particular.

With regard to our question on whether geropsychologists from their country would work on multidisciplinary studies on aging, 77% of the key persons reported such studies in the field of life span development, 73% in the field of mental health or psychiatry, but only 17% in the field of physical health and epidemiology. Psychologists participated in multidisciplinary studies in the fields of neurology, psychophysiology, and biology of aging in only one country each.

Some 63% of the key persons reported that researchers in their countries participate in international research networks in the field of geropsychology. Although 76% of the key persons from Western European countries reported participation in such networks, only 40% of the key persons from Eastern European countries gave an affirmative answer (Czech Republic, Estonia, Lithuania, and Russia). We further asked for a listing of the countries in the research network. International research networks most often included cooperation with West European countries (45 reports), the United States (15), and Canada (13). However, key persons reported research networks with colleagues from (other) Eastern European countries in only three cases.

Many of the European cross-national studies are or have been founded by the Framework Programmes of the European Union. For example, the European Study on Adult Well-Being (ESAW) was conducted during 2002 and 2003 in Austria, Italy, Luxembourg, the Netherlands, UK, and Sweden (Ferring et al., 2004). The project

Table 1. Topics of geropsychological research in 30 European countries

Country/Topic	Dementia	Cognitive development	Caregiving	Affective disorder	Successful aging	Social development	Chronic illness/LTC	Psychological assessment	Work	Personality	Death & dying	Prevention	Ageism	Aging & environment	Longevity	Psychotherapy
Austria	4	4	4	3	4	3	4	4	2	2	4	3	2	3	3	4
Belgium	3	4	3	2	3	3	2	3	2	2	2	2	2	2	1	2
Belarus	1	1	1	1	1	1	1	1	1	1	1	1	1	1	1	1
Bosnia-H.	1	1	1	2	1	4	1	1	1	1	1	2	1	1	1	1
Bulgaria	3	3	3	3	2	3	3	3	2	3	3	2	2	3	3	2
Czech R.	4	2	3	4	3	3	3	1	3	2	3	2	3	2	2	2
Denmark	4	3	2	2	2	2	2	2	2	2	2	2	1	2	3	2
Estonia	2	1	4	2	4	3	1	2	3	3	1	1	4	3	1	1
Finland	4	4	1	3	3	2	2	3	4	3	2	2	2	4	2	2
France	4	3	2	3	2	1	2	2	2	2	2	3	1	2	2	2
Germany	4	4	3	2	4	3	3	2	2	3	3	2	2	3	3	3
UK	4	4	3	2	3	2	4	2	2	3	4	3	2	2	3	2
Greece	3	3	2	2	2	3	1	3	1	2	1	1	1	1	1	1
Hungary	3	4	3	4	1	1	3	2	2	3	3	2	2	2	2	2
Iceland	3	1	3	2	2	2	2	3	2	1	1	1	2	1	1	1
Israel	3	2	3	4	3	4	3	2	2	3	3	3	3	2	3	2
Italy	4	4	1	3	3	3	2	3	3	3	1	3	1	1	3	1

Table 1. Topics of geropsychological research in 30 European countries (continued)

Country/Topic	Dementia	Cognitive development	Caregiving	Affective disorder	Successful aging	Social development	Chronic illness/LTC	Psychological assessment	Work	Personality	Death & dying	Prevention	Ageism	Aging & environment	Longevity	Psychotherapy
Lithuania	3	3	2	3	2	3	3	1	1	3	3	2	1	3	1	1
Luxembourg	4	2	4	2	4	3	4	2	1	2	3	2	1	1	1	1
Macedonia	1	1	2	1	2	1	1	1	1	2	1	1	1	1	1	1
Netherlands	4	4	3	4	4	3	3	3	2	2	2	3	2	2	2	3
Norway	4	3	4	4	2	3	3	3	2	2	3	3	2	2	2	4
Portugal	3	3	4	3	4	3	4	3	4	1	3	1	3	3	1	1
Romania	3	3	2	2	3	1	1	2	2	1	1	1	1	1	2	1
Russia	3	2	3	3	2	3	2	2	2	3	2	2	3	2	2	3
Serbia-M.	1	1	1	1	1	1	1	1	1	1	1	1	1	1	1	1
Spain	4	3	3	3	3	2	3	3	3	2	2	3	3	2	2	2
Sweden	4	4	3	3	3	2	3	3	2	2	2	3	2	3	3	3
Switzerland	4	4	3	3	3	4	3	2	2	2	4	1	3	2	2	1
Turkey	3	2	2	2	2	1	3	1	1	1	1	1	1	1	1	1

Note. 1 = no research on that topic, 2 = some research/less important topic, 3 = important topic, 4 = most important topic(s). LTC = long-term care

MOBILATE (Enhancing Mobility in Later Life: Personal Coping, Environmental Resources, and Technical Support) assessed older adults' day-to-day mobility and the interplay between their personal resources and resources of their physical and social environment. Participants of that study came from Finland, Germany, Hungary, Italy, and the Netherlands, and selected results have been published by Mollenkopf, Marcellini, Ruoppila, Széman, Tacken, and Wahl (2004). The ENABLE-AGE study (Enabling Autonomy, Participation, and Well-being in Old Age) assessed the role of the home environment as a determinant for healthy aging in Germany, Hungary, Latvia, and the UK (Iwarsson, Wahl, & Nygren, 2005). In addition, researchers from Germany, Israel, Norway, Spain, and the UK cooperated in the OASIS study (Old Age and Autonomy: The Role of Service Systems and Intergenerational Family Solidarity), which focused on the association between social support and older adults' quality of life (Motel-Klingebiel, von Kondratowitz, & Tesch-Römer, 2004). Furthermore, clinical psychologists and neuropsychologists participated in the DIADEM study on timely recognition of dementia in Europe, which was completed in Belgium, France, Ireland, Italy, the Netherlands, Portugal, Spain, and the UK (Iliffe, De Lepeleire, & Van Hout, 2005). In addition, the EXCELSA Cross-European Longitudinal Study on Ageing investigated the interplay of environmental, sociodemographic, psychosocial, health, biological factors, and lifestyle in older adults from Austria, Finland, Germany, Italy, the Netherlands, Poland, Portugal, and Spain (Fernández-Ballesteros et al., 2004). Because aging includes biological, psychological, and social changes, most cross-national research projects on aging were interdisciplinary, and psychologists from one country may have worked with sociologists or psychiatrists from other countries. Finally, important European contributions on quality of life in older adults are summarized in the chapter by Fernández-Ballesteros, Kruse, Zamarrón, and Caprara in this volume.

With regard to large national studies, Seematter-Bagnoud and Santos-Eggimann (2006) recently summarized 39 European population-based studies on older adults (≥ 50 years). Thirty-one of them included data collection on cognitive aging and/or psychological well-being (studies from Denmark, Finland, France, Germany, Italy, the Netherlands, the UK, Sweden, and Switzerland). In their overview on 37 longitudinal psychological aging studies, Schaie and Hofer (2001) included 14 European studies including the Berlin Aging Study, the Bonn Longitudinal Study of Aging (Germany), the Gender Study of Unlike-Sex Dizygote Twins (Sweden), the Groningen Longitudinal Aging Study (the Netherlands), the Gerontological and Geriatric Population Studies in Göteborg (Sweden), the German Interdisciplinary Longitudinal Study of Adult Development, the Kungsholmen Project (Sweden), the Amsterdam Longitudinal Aging Study (Netherlands), the Lund 80+ Study (Sweden), the Maastricht Aging Study (the Netherlands), the Manchester and Newcastle Longitudinal Studies of Aging (UK), the Nordic Research on Aging (Denmark, Sweden, and Finland), the Octogenarian Twin Study (Sweden), and the Swedish Adoption/Twin Study of Aging. For example, the Swedish Adoption/Twin Study of Aging was the first to show that individual differences in cognitive abilities are under substantial genetic control in middle and late adulthood, but that genetic variance decreased longitudinally for the cognitive factor (e.g., Finkel, Pedersen, Plomin, & McClearn, 1998).

Several well-known theories in the field of geropsychology and life span psychology have been developed in Europe. For example, starting in the 1980s, Paul Baltes and colleagues developed the psychological model of selective optimization with compensation, which focuses on the management of the dynamics between gains and losses (e.g., Baltes, 1997). As another example, Jutta Heckhausen, with Richard Schultz from the United States, developed a life span theory of control (e.g., Heckhausen & Schulz, 1993), in which they combined the distinction between primary control (effort to change the environment) and secondary control (psychological adaptation to given environmental conditions) with the concepts of selection and compensation, resulting in four control strategies. These models have been widely applied to aspects of aging, such as the prioritization of tasks and coping with age-associated losses and chronic illness. The dissemination of these models in international research, and in the United States in particular, was probably supported by the fact that both scientists have collaborated with colleagues from the United States, and have been or are still working in the United States.

Because many key persons had difficulties with estimating the numbers of aging-related publications from their countries, we first used the electronic PsycInfo database for computing the number of aging-related publications in the English language for each country (search terms were: *geriatric* or *gerontol** or *ageing* or *aging* or *elderly* or *old age* or *late life* or *very old*). The data were retrieved on July 14th, 2006. This analysis gives a rough estimation of publication activities, although some relevant journals or papers may not have been listed in the database and part of the publications came from psychiatrists, sociologists, social workers, or related professions. Unfortunately, no information on the authors' profession was available in the database for narrowing the search. Nonetheless, this analysis shows very large national differences in the numbers of aging-related publications. The largest number of aging-related publications came from the UK (1,567), which, in part, reflects the fact that English is the native language of British researchers. In addition, more than 1,200 publications were listed from Sweden, Germany, the Netherlands, and Italy. Between 560 and 760 publications were available from Israel, France, and Finland, and between 200 and 350 from Spain, Switzerland, Ireland, Belgium, Denmark, and Norway (**Figure 2**). The observed differences reflect, in part, related differences in the size of the countries and in the numbers of psychologists and other scientists working in the field of aging. However, differences in the size of the countries could not explain the small numbers of publications from many Eastern European countries. Here, low numbers probably reflect low levels of research activities and language-related barriers, respectively.

A further impression of language-related barriers comes from the answers to our question on where the European psychologists publish their work, and whether it is mainly published in their native language or in English: In 47% of the countries, most research is published in national journals in their native language, and another 16% and 14% of geropsychological research is published in monographs in their native language or is available only in unpublished research reports, respectively. For example, the key persons from Belarus, Bosnia-Herzegovina, Lithuania, Macedonia, Serbia, and Russia reported that no publications on geropsychology from their countries are available in international journals. Only 27% of all respondents reported that most research is pub-

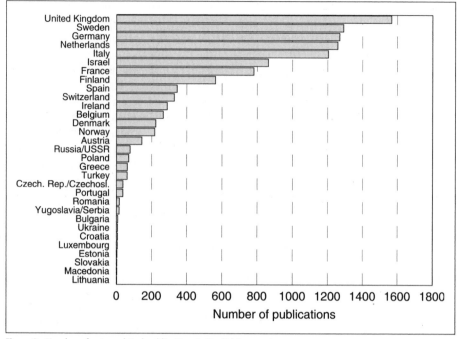

Figure 2. Number of aging-related publications in English by country

lished in English language journals (Belgium, Finland, Germany, Israel, the Netherlands, Norway, Sweden, and the UK).

The key persons were further asked for the number of aging-related publications in
their national language(s) that have been published during the previous five years.
Language-related barriers were most obvious with regard to Bulgaria, Russia, and Estonia. For example, according to the key person, 87 papers have been published in the
Bulgarian language as compared to six English papers from Bulgarian authors. Similarly, Russian scientists have published 70 Russian papers in the previous five years as
compared to 13 English papers, and Estonian researchers have published 50 papers in
their native language(s) as compared to six English papers. For the other East European
countries, low numbers of publications mainly reflect low levels of research activities
on aging-related topics.

Teaching Geropsychology

With regard to teaching clinical geropsychology, the American Psychological Association
has suggested guidelines that can easily be adapted to other fields of geropsychology and
to geropsychology in Europe (APA, 2000). First, aging-related topics should be a component of training of all students in the field of psychology (general exposure). Thus, related
topics have to be integrated into psychology courses on diverse topics, such as clinical

psychology (psychological health in old age, assessing older clients, psychotherapy and counseling with older adults), general psychology (e.g., aging-related changes in perception or cognition), neuropsychology (e.g., associations between age-associated changes of the brain and behavioral changes), human development (life span development), personality (continuity and change of personality), social psychology and family psychology (e.g., change in social relations across the life span, intergenerational relations of older adults), health psychology (e.g., health promotion in old age), as well as industrial and organizational psychology (e.g., motivation and performance of older workers, retirement transitions). As only very limited time may be available for age-related topics in these courses, introductory courses in geropsychology may be a better choice if scientists from the field of geropsychology are in the faculty. Second, special courses or even complete programs at the undergraduate and graduate level are needed for students who want to work with older adults in the future. Ideally, these courses should involve some practical experience. Third, advanced training, such as a postgraduate program, is necessary for psychologists who want to become experts in the field of aging. Finally, geropsychology should be an important topic in the training of other professions, such as gerontologists, social workers, or nurses.

The questionnaire study on geropsychology in Europe was mainly focused on the training of psychologists. We, first, presented a list of eight topics for teaching geropsychology based on an internet search on aging-related topics and on published recommmendations about knowledge and skills required of psychologists working with older adults (Molinari et al., 2003). The key persons were asked whether these areas are regular topics of training for students in the field of psychology (4 = at all institutes or departments, 3 = at most institutes or departments, 2 = only at few institutes or departments, 1 = no). In addition, the respondents were free to include additional topics that were important in their countries. As shown in **Figure 3**, the most frequent

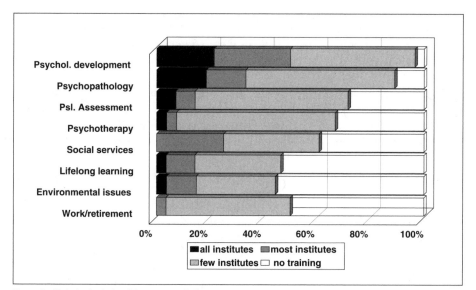

Figure 3. Main topics in teaching geropsychology

topic of training was life span development and psychological development in old age, which was taught at all institutes in six of the 30 countries, and was not a topic of training for psychologists in only one of the countries (Portugal). Aspects of psychopathology, such as depression or dementia in old age, were the second most frequent topics, followed by psychological assessment of older adults, psychotherapy and counseling of older clients, social services for older adults, life-long learning, environmental issues, and psychological aspects of work and retirement. However, the last three topics were not subjects of teaching in half of the participating countries. Very few key persons added topics for teaching to our list. Two of them mentioned cognitive aging (which is otherwise included in seminars and lectures on life span development in general), the aging personality (1 mention), physical health in old age and its relationship with psychological development (1), quality of life in the elderly (1), and death and death anxiety (1).

We also asked the key persons for an estimation of the average number of hours of training (lectures, seminars) in these fields. We analyzed the teaching hours only for those countries in which the topic was at least taught in some institutes or departments. On average, developmental issues were estimated to fill 22 h (1–150 h), life-long learning 8 h (1–16 h), mental illness in old age 7 h (1–20 h), psychological assessment and environmental issues 6 h (1–18 h), psychotherapy/counseling of older adults 5 h (1–10 h), and work and retirement, as well as social services for older adults 4 h each (2–20 h and 1–10 h, respectively).

When we average the frequency of teaching geropsychology across the eight most important topics, respondents from Sweden, Norway, and Austria reported that all topic were taught at all or most psychological institutes. Respondents from the Czech Republic, Luxembourg, Germany, Italy, the Netherlands, Belgium, and Lithuania reported that these topics were taught, on average, at some or most psychological institutes. In addition, key persons from Spain, Bulgaria, Romania, Switzerland, and Bosnia-Herzegovina reported that, on average, these topics were taught at few institutes. The lowest levels of teaching aging-related topics were reported in Belarus, Serbia-Montenegro, Turkey, Finland, Portugal, and Israel. In these countries, aging-related topics only played a role in courses on developmental psychology at few institutes, and sometimes in courses on psychopathology or social services.

According to the key persons, postgraduate programs on geropsychology or gerontology were available in 47% of the countries under investigation (Austria, Bulgaria, the Czech Republic, Denmark, France, Germany, Greece, Israel, the Netherlands, Norway, Spain, Switzerland, Sweden, and the UK). In 63% of these programs, training is mainly academic, and in 37% mainly professional.

In our questionnaire study, 30% of the key persons reported that geropsychology is a regular topic of postgraduate training in clinical psychology or psychotherapy. These programs are mainly professional (77%) rather than academic (23%). However, the number of hours of seminars or lectures on gerontopsychology vary considerably between the countries, ranging from about 15 (Austria, Germany, Spain) to 500 (Luxembourg; $M = 127$). In postgraduate training that included age-related topics, programs provided information on assessment of older adults (63%), psychotherapy with older adults (63%), and psychological disorders in old age (50%). Prevention of mental health problems of older adults (12.5%), and evaluation of interventions with older adults (12.5%) played a much smaller role in these programs.

In a few cases, geropsychology was also a topic in psychological postgraduate programs other than clinical psychology and psychotherapy. This is the case in postgraduate programs on neuropsychology (10%), cognitive psychology (7%), developmental psychology (3%), and community psychology (3%), with 15 to 60 h of training in aging-related topics. Here, programs provide information about environment-behavior transactions of older adults, caregiver interventions, epidemiology of cognitive problems in old age, clinical research with older adults, and program evaluations.

We also asked for an estimation of the number of dissertations in the field of geropsychology that were completed in the last 5 years. On average, the respondents reported that 15 dissertations, or 3 per year, were completed. The largest number of geropsychological dissertations were reported in Spain (50), Germany (50), the Netherlands (50), Sweden (50), and Israel (30). The numbers were lower for France (20), Switzerland (20), Belgium (15), Norway (15), Portugal (10), Finland (5), the Czech Republic (5), Russia (5), Bulgaria (3), Denmark (2), Austria (1), Greece (1), Hungary (1), and Iceland (1). Unfortunately, no information on that question was available from the UK and Italy.

The number of full professors in the field of geropsychology in European countries is quite low. According to our key persons, there were, on average only 2.3 full professors per country (with the highest number of 20 in France) or a total of 69 persons. Again, information was lacking from the UK and Italy.

Although the role of geropsychology in study programs in the field of psychology was the main topic of our questionnaire study, we want to briefly summarize information on the role of geropsychology in gerontology programs. In 2000, Meyer surveyed gerontology study courses in Central, Western, and Southern Europe, and found the training situation very heterogeneous. Of the European full-time study programs in gerontology, 80% are found at Western European universities. Of the 58 European gerontology study programs that were reviewed, 23 were offered in the UK, 9 in France, 6 each in Spain and Germany, 3 in Switzerland, 2 each in Belgium, the Netherlands, and Ireland, and 1 each in Finland, Italy, Malta, and Austria. Seven of the courses qualified at an undergraduate level, 40 were postgraduate programs with a Master's degree as the most common degree, and 11 were postvocational programs. Geropsychology courses were part of 84% of the gerontology programs, with the most frequent topics being mental health or psychopathology, psychological development, social relations in old age (including relationships between older adults and their formal and informal supporters), cognitive psychology, and interventions (e.g., memory training). However, only few programs had a main focus on geropsychology or life span development (University of Erlangen-Nürnberg/Germany; University of Grenoble/France, University of London/Birkbeck College; University of Lyon/France, University of Nijmegen/the Netherlands). No under- or postgraduate courses were available at that time in Denmark, Greece, Italy, Luxembourg, Norway, and Portugal.

In 1999, a consortium of 18 European universities started to develop a new European master's program in gerontology (EuMaG; Heijke, 2004), and in 2006, universities and/or gerontological associations from 24 European countries collaborated in the program (www.eumag.org). The administrative center for program development is located at the University of Amsterdam (Heijke, 2004). In that master's program, psychogerontology is one of five core modules. The module was developed at the Institute of Gerontology at the University of Heidelberg, Germany, and other countries collaborate in teaching this module. It focuses on basic concepts and theories related to cognitive aging, personality, adaptation, and social integration. Selected topics are successful aging, coping strategies, dementia, and depression. Additional information on that program is available online at www.eumag.org.

Application of Geropsychology

In the final section of the questionnaire, we wanted to know the main fields of application of geropsychology, perceived needs for future application, and the number of psychologists who work mainly in the field of aging. The key persons were asked to identify the three most important fields of application of geropsychology in their country. Geropsychology was most often applied in the clinical field (70% of the countries under investigation). This was reported by key persons from Austria, Bosnia-Herzegovina, Bulgaria, the Czech Republic, Denmark, Finland, France, Germany, the UK, Hungary, Iceland, Israel, Italy, Lithuania, the Netherlands, Norway, Russia, Spain, Sweden, Switzerland, and Turkey. About 60% of the key persons reported the social field as one of the three most important applications of geropsychology in their country (Austria, Bosnia-Herzegovina, Bulgaria, the Czech Republic, Denmark, Estonia, France, Germany, Israel, Italy, Lithuania, Macedonia, Norway, Portugal, Romania, Russia, Spain, and Sweden). Applying geropsychology in prevention of health problems and health promotion were also reported by 40% of the respondents (Estonia, France, Germany, the UK, Macedonia, the Netherlands, Norway, Portugal, Spain, Sweden, Switzerland, and Turkey). In addition, adult education as a main topic of application was mentioned by 33% of the key persons (Austria, Bulgaria, Denmark, Finland, Hungary, Italy, Lithuania, the Netherlands, Russia, and Switzerland). However, only 17% of the key persons reported geropsychology being widely applied in the field of work and retirement (Estonia, Finland, Israel, Portugal, and Romania).

The question on how many clinical psychologists with a main focus on geropsychology were active in their countries was obviously difficult to answer, and six key persons could not provide this information. In the other countries, the estimations of the number of psychologists varied considerably, from 0 (Belarus, Bosnia-Herzegovina, Estonia, Serbia, Turkey) to 1,500 in France ($M = 146$, $SD = 348$; median = 10).

Finally, we also asked (with an open question) in which field geropsychology has not yet been applied in their country, but should be applied in the future. Here prevention and promotion of healthy aging were most often mentioned (33%), followed by work/retirement (27%), education and the social field (20%), psychotherapy (7%), liaison with primary somatic units (7%), caregiving (7%), traffic psychology (3%), successful aging (3%), and health economics (3%).

Discussion and Conclusions

When analyzing the reports of the key persons from 30 European countries, we have to be aware that some information was more easily available, and that it was probably easier to summarize data on research, teaching, and application of geropsychology from smaller countries, from those with a better scientific infrastructure, and from those with general guidelines for studying psychology that are obligatory for all departments and institutes that train psychologists. For example, for the German-speaking countries, an electronic database that summarizes German publications in the field of psychology (Psyndex) was used for estimating the numbers of geropsychological publications in German language and for analyzing main research topics. As another example, a colleague from Ireland who has published in the field of geropsychology reported not being able to fill out our questionnaire because of the heterogeneity of teaching and research between Irish psychology departments. In addition, whereas some colleagues had contacted geropsychologists from other universities of their country before filling out our questionnaire, others may have invested less effort. In order to increase the validity of the reports, we used the electronic database PsychInfo and a standardized search strategy for estimating numbers of publications from each country. In addition, we used reports from the Framework Programmes of the European Commission for adding further information on the participation of psychologists in international research networks. Nonetheless, the information from the key persons seemed to be, in general, quite accurate.

With the exception of Ireland (see **Figure 2**), there seemed to be very little research on the psychology of aging (if any) in the European countries from which no key person was available, so our averaged data may somewhat overestimate activities in research, teaching, and the application of geropsychology in Europe.

Despite these limitations, several conclusions can be drawn from the present work. First, with regard to research, we conclude that there are many important contributions by Western European researchers to geropsychology, such as the longitudinal studies on aging. However, much more effort is needed to establish research programs on geropsychology in Eastern Europe. Here, psychology departments and individual researchers could benefit from international cooperation with researchers from Western Europe and from the United States, who have a lot of experience in that field (e.g., by exchange of scientists, cross-national studies). For the new members of the European Union, some joint research projects with Western European countries could be funded with the help of Framework Programmes of the European Union.

The number of full professors in the field of geropsychology in many European countries is still very low compared to U.S. standards. For example, in the field of developmental psychology, many psychology departments in the United States have full professors of child development, adolescent development, and adult development and aging. In Europe, there is usually only one full professor (or none) for the whole life span, who is, in most cases, a specialist in childhood or adolescence. Thus, a higher number of full professors in the field of geropsychology would be recommended for increasing research and teaching psychology of aging in Europe.

In addition, more research should be published in the English language in international/European journals rather than in native languages. The new European Journal of Aging may help to increase the number of European publications on geropsychology, although up to now papers from Eastern Europe are (still) lacking in that journal. In addition, European and international journals should offer some editorial support for colleagues who are not (yet) fluent in English.

Second, conclusions regarding teaching geropsychology have to take into account the heterogeneity of present conditions of Eastern and Western European countries, from an occasional inclusion of a few aging-related topics in some countries to well-established graduate programs in geropsychology in others. As a basic recommendation, aging-related topics have to be included in the training of all undergraduates in the field of psychology. This should be, at least, the case in lectures and seminars on developmental psychology, and in the applied field (e.g., assessment and evidence-based interventions with older adults in programs on clinical psychology; age-associated change in performance and motivation as well as retirement transitions in programs on industrial and organizational psychology; life-long learning in seminars on educational psychology, etc.). A recently published volume by Whitbourne and Cavanaugh (2003) gives many good suggestions on how to integrate aging-related topics into teaching undergraduates, and a special issue of *Gerontology and Geriatrics Education* offers recommendations for training in clinical geropsychology in graduate and postgraduate programs (Hinrichsen & Zweig, 2005)

With regard to the application of geropsychology in the clinical field, our data show that few clinical psychologists work exclusively or mainly with older clients. Given the age-associated decline in mobility, special practices of clinical geropsychologists may only make sense in urban areas with a high density of older inhabitants. Thus, it is more important to integrate geropsychology in the graduate and postgraduate training of *all* clinical psychologists than to offer a postgraduate training for clinical geropsychologists in particular (although a number of such specialists would be needed for working in geriatric or psychiatric hospitals and in urban ambulant psychotherapeutic practices for older adults). In fact, as geropsychology was a regular topic of postgraduate training in clinical psychology or psychotherapy in only 30% of the European countries under investigation, and as many psychotherapists are, therefore, not well prepared for working with older clients, more effort is needed to integrate aging-related topics into their postgraduate training. Postgraduate courses should provide knowledge on differentiation between normal aging (e.g., age-associated cognitive decline) and pathological aging (e.g., dementia, depression), on psychological disorders in old age (e.g., Alzheimer's disease), on assessment of older clients (e.g., the Geriatric Depression Scale, the Mini Mental State Examination), and on evidence-based interventions (e.g., adaptation of cognitive-behavioral depression therapy to work with older patients). Important knowledge on these topics is summarized in two handbooks (Duffy, 1999; Lomranz, 1998).

Postgraduate training in geropsychology cannot be established in all European countries, as small countries have only one, or very few, psychology departments, and as only a limited numbers of specialists would be needed in these countries. Here the best solution is opening the national programs of Western European countries to postgraduate students from smaller countries, similar to the model of the EuMaG. Training a minimum number of specialists in the field of geropsychology from all European countries would also help to increase the number of related courses in these countries for future students.

Third, with regard to the application of geropsychology, a stronger focus on prevention and promotion of healthy aging is needed. Given the fact that the graying of society is associated with a dramatic increase in health care costs and, that up to now, few geropsychologists do prevention work, psychologists should play a larger role in the promotion of healthy life styles in middle and late adulthood (e.g., Hermanova, 1995; Levkoff & Berkman, 1995). Similarly, declining birth rates indicate an increasing importance of older workers. Thus, European psychologists should play a greater role in overcoming negative stereotypes of employers about older workers, and in helping older workers with mastering changing demands at the work place and with compensating age-associated declines (e.g., Armstrong-Stassen & Templer, 2005).

References

Antonucci, T., Okorodulu, C., & Akiyama, H. (2002). Well-being among older adults on different continents. *Journal of Social Issues, 58*, 617–626.

American Psychological Association (2000). *Training guidelines for practice in clinical geropsychology*. Washington, DC: APA Division 12, Section II (Clinical Psychology).

Armstrong-Stassen, M., & Templer, A. (2005). Adapting training for older employees: The Canadian response to an aging workforce. *Journal of Management Development, 24*, 57–67.

Baltes, P.B. (1997). On the incomplete architecture of human ontogeny: Selection, optimization, and compensation as foundation of developmental theory. *American Psychologist, 52*, 366–380.

DeVries, H.M. (2005). Clinical geropsychology training in generalist doctoral programs. *Gerontology and Geriatrics Education, 25*(4), 5–20.

Duffy, M. (Ed.). (1999). *Handbook of counseling and psychotherapy with older adults*. Hoboken, NJ: Wiley.

Fernández-Ballesteros, R., Zamarrón, D., Rudinger, G., Schroots, J.F., Hekkonen, E., Drusini, A. et al. (2004). Assessing competence: The European Survey on Aging Protocol (ESAP). *Gerontology, 50*, 330–347.

Ferring, D., Balducci, C., Burholt, V., Wenger, C., Thissen, F., Weber, G. et al. (2004). Life satisfaction of older people in six European countries: Findings from the European Study on Adult Well-Being. *European Journal of Ageing, 1*, 15–25.

Finkel, D., Pedersen, N.L., Plomin, G.E., & McClearn, G.E. (1998). Longitudinal and cross-sectional twin data on cognitive abilities in adulthood: The Swedish Adoption/Twin Study of Aging. *Developmental Psychology, 34*, 1400–1413.

Heckhausen, J., & Schulz, R. (1993). Optimization by selection and compensation: Balancing primary and secondary control in lifespan development. *International Journal of Behavior Development, 16*, 287–303.

Heijke, L. (2004). The European master's program in gerontology. *European Journal of Ageing, 1*, 106–108.

Hermanova, H. (1995). Healthy aging in Europe in the 1990s and implications for education and training in the care of the elderly. *Educational Gerontology, 21*, 1–14.

Hinrichsen, G.A., & Zweig, R.A. (2005). Models of training in clinical geropsychology. *Gerontology and Geriatrics Education, 25*(4), 1–4.

Iliffe, S., De Lepeleire, J., & Van Hout, H. (2005). Understanding obstacles to the recognition of and response to dementia in different European countries: A modified focus group approach using multinational, multidisciplinary expert groups. *Aging and Mental Health, 9*, 1–6.

Iwarsson, S., Wahl, H.-W., & Nygren, C. (2005). Challenges of cross-national housing research with older people: Lessons from the ENABLE-AGE project. *European Journal of Ageing, 1*, 79–88.

Levkoff, S., & Berkman, B. (1995). Health promotion/disease prevention: New directions for geriatric education. *Educational Gerontology, 22*, 93–104.

Lomranz, J. (Ed.). (1998). *Handbook of aging and mental health: An integrative approach*. New York: Plenum.

Meyer, M. (2000). *Studium der Gerontologie in Europa: Ausbildungsprogram und Professionalisierungsstrategien – Gegenwärtiger Stand und zukünftige Entwicklungen* [Studying gerontology in Europe: Training programs and strategies of professionalization: Present state and future developments]. Aachen, Germany: Shaker.

Mollenkopf, H., Marcellini, F., Ruoppila, I., Széman, Z., Tacken, M., & Wahl, H.-W. (2004). Social and behavioral science perspectives on out-of-home mobility in late life: Findings from the European project MOBILATE. *European Journal of Ageing, 1*, 45–53.

Molinari, V., Karel, M., Jones, S., Zeiss A., Cooley, S.G., Wray, L. et al. (2003). Recommendations about the knowledge and skills required of psychologists working with older adults. *Professional Psychology: Research and Practice, 24*, 435–443.

Motel-Klingebiel, A., von Kondratowitz, H.-J., & Tesch-Römer, C. (2004). Social inequality in the later life: Cross-national comparison of quality of life. *European Journal of Ageing, 1*, 6–14.

Schaie, K.W., & Hofer, S. (2001). Longitudinal studies in aging research. In J.E. Birren & K.W. Schaie (Eds.), *Handbook of the psychology of aging* (5th ed., pp. 53–77). San Diego, CA: Academic Press.

Seematter-Bagnoud, L., & Santos-Eggimann, B. (2006). Population-based cohorts of the 50s and over: A summary of worldwide previous and ongoing studies for research on health in aging. *European Journal of Ageing, 3*, 41–49.

Whitbourne, S.K., & Cavanaugh, J.C. (2003). *Integrating aging topics into psychology: A practical guide for teaching*. Washington, DC: American Psychological Association.

WHO (2002). *Active aging: A policy framework*. Geneva, Switzerland: World Health Organization.

3. Age Identifications

Svein Olav Daatland

Introduction

Bodily signs of aging trigger unpleasant feelings in most of us. We start each day by examining ourselves in the mirror, and we continue by mirroring ourselves in the eyes of others. We are not able to escape our appearances and the social judgments they provoke. Early in life we welcome the signs of added years, but we soon – in fact, surprisingly soon – see the extra years as threats rather than rewards. We may try to make ourselves blind to the visible signs of "aging," we may try to avoid being categorized as "older" by others, and we may attempt to hide ourselves behind creams, exercises, or even plastic surgery. However, age is a very visible cue, and it's hard to pass it off as something else.

There's a cultural element in this. The Austrian author Stefan Zweig wrote in his autobiography *The World of Yesterday* about how young people in Vienna in his childhood, toward the end of the 19th century, aspired to appear and be recognized as "settled" as early as possible. They tried to look older then they were in response to a conservative and settled culture that they felt would last forever. How wrong they were.

Becoming "old" may not have been an ideal even then, and is even less so today. Maybe there is more to today's discontent with aging than a reaction to being labeled as old and outdated by an ageist culture. Perhaps there is a more general, possibly even a universal, displeasure in observing how the body changes and promises decay to come? A feeling of becoming a stranger to one's body, and then, so to speak, a stranger to one's external self? To the extent that there is a core self that is established early in life, one may experience a growing discrepancy between appearances and self-identity with increasing age, even a feeling of being betrayed by one's body. The aging body may be perceived as a stranger, and as a false cover over an internal and forever fresh inner self. The "external me" may crack and crumble, but the "internal me" is felt as good as ever on the inside; is it then "forever young" (without aging) or rather "forever me" (without age)?

Observations like these have been the source for two well-known theories about the aging self: "the ageless self" hypothesis by Kaufman (1986), and "the mask of aging" hypothesis by Featherstone and Hepworth (1990). The first gravitates toward the "forever me" interpretation, suggesting that age is irrelevant for identity; that aging is an outside matter, while you are forever your true (authentic) self on the inside. The second hypothesis (mask of aging) leans toward the "forever young" interpretation, in which a youthful self – established early in life – eventually finds itself trapped and hid by an aging body. They both address the controversies between internal and external representations of the self, between fixed and fluid identities, and between continuity and change over the life course. These questions are central theoretical controversies for psychology and sociology in general, and for social gerontology in particular (Biggs, 2004, 2005).

Age is an important factor in social perception, but has received far less attention than gender and race (Montepare & Zebrowitz 1998). We know less, therefore, about age identities than about gendered and ethnic identities. Age may, however, be as powerful a cue and identity marker as sex and ethnicity, and because age-related differences are prevalent and normally easily observable, they appear in many domains, of which some are both socially and politically salient. Access to quite a few social positions and rights are, for example, regulated according to age.

The subjective perception of age and aging is an underresearched area even in gerontology. The gerontological tradition is dominated by a top-down, objectivized perspective, where age and aging is observed and evaluated from the outside and by professionals (Daatland, 2002). Why not study how age and aging is experienced from the inside? Those that have done so tend to find that most adults see themselves as younger than their age, and they would like to be even younger (see, for example, Zola, 1962; Kastenbaum, Derbin, Sabatini, & Artt, 1972; Montepare & Lachman, 1989; Montepare, 1996; Goldsmith & Heiens, 1992; Öberg & Tornstam, 2001; Westerhof, Barrett, & Steverink, 2003). We know little about why this is so, what it means, and what the causes and consequences are. These questions are, therefore, explored in the present chapter: How is age and aging perceived from the inside? What age identities do people hold? What are the causes and consequences of these perceptions and identifications? The contrast between universal and cultural explanations is part of this discussion. Are the subjective representations of age and aging best seen as reactions to aging as a threat to universal human needs, or are they better understood as a culturally induced defense against ageism and social declassification?

We shall return to these questions after an empirical tour in the landscape of subjective age and aging. *Subjective aging* refers to the personal experiences of age-related changes. When and how are such changes felt? Do they follow the "master narrative" of aging as loss and decline, or are they perceived as both multidimensional and multidirectional? *Subjective age* refers to the age identities held by the person, in this case how old the person feels (*feel age*) and would like to be (*ideal age*). Why are most people attracted to younger age identities?

Background

There are several reasons why we need to know more about these questions. First, and most generally, is the insight from social interactionism that people respond to the meanings they construct more than to some objective order. W.I. Thomas phrased this elegantly in his theorem: "If men define situations as real, they are real in their consequences." Robert Merton (1968) carried this insight further with the self-fulfilling prophecy concept. Perceptions of age and aging are part of our socially constructed world, and as such are guiding our identifications and motivations; probably more so than actual (chronological) age (Featherstone & Hepworth, 2005).

A second reason is illustrated by the studies of self-stereotyping in old age. We are sensitive to age differences even as small children, and we gradually internalize age stereotypes as part of the socialization process. Rothermund and Brandstädter (2003) suggest that age stereotypes may become incorporated into our self-views through some form of "social contamination." This process may induce the development of younger self-images as a self-protective strategy. The age stereotypes that, in modern societies, are negative toward older ages, are eventually turned against oneself when one grows older and produce passivity, poorer health, and even higher mortality, according to Levy and colleagues (Levy, 2003; Levy, Slade, & Kasl, 2002; Levy, Slade, Kunkel, & Kasl, 2002).

A third, and related, reason for exploring the subjective sides of aging refers to the nature–nurture paradigm. To what extent are self-perceptions of age and aging a response to biology, to culture, or both? Is aging and old age a sociocultural stigma that people try to protect themselves against, as Groucho (not Karl) Marx does when he refuses to become a member of a club that allows someone like him as a member. Are perceptions of aging more likely influenced by a universal fear of illness and death?

A fourth reason that we need more knowledge about age perceptions is the need to clarify age and the self as theoretical constructs. Paradoxically, gerontology has always struggled with the age concept, and has tended to treat (chronological) age as a "black box" without clarifying age-related concepts such as health and social roles. Observed differences between age groups have been attributed to declining health, to retirement, and to other externals such as the loss of a spouse or a friend, and the aim of research has been to reduce the observed age difference to such factors. A more holistic perspective, where age is allowed a quality of its own, is left to philosophers or to philosophizing psychoanalysts such as Jung and Erikson. A similar story goes for the self-concept, where the impact of age has been played down relative to sex, ethnicity, class, and the like. But age is, in fact, an all-inclusive, and constantly changing entity with many dimensions that we all need to adapt to, and might, therefore, also be a powerful perspective for the investigation of the self-concept, both as an active "I" and a reflective "me." For example: Do I like myself as this or that age? How do others see me? What does this or that age expect of me and allow me to do?

The empirical questions that guide this chapter are, then, simply how people experience aging, what their subjective age identities are, and what the causes and consequences of these self-definitions are. The theoretical ambition reaches further toward a better understanding of age and the self as phenomena and constructs, which will be touched upon more briefly – and speculatively – in the concluding section.

Data and Measurements

The main data source for the chapter is the first wave of the Norwegian Life Course, Ageing, and Generation Study (NorLAG), which was carried out by Norwegian Social

Research (NOVA). Personal interviews (n = 5,559), supplemented by postal question-naires (n = 4,169), were collected in 2002–2003 among people aged 40–79 (mean age = 57.6), living in their own homes in 30 communities all over Norway. The sample is stratified by local context and is a fair representation of the country. The questions about subjective age and aging were part of the postal questionnaire, hence, the data presented refer to the n = 4,169 sample. Response rates for the personal interview was 67.4%, of which 74.6% also responded to the drop-off questionnaire.

There is, to my knowledge, no established research tradition or research instruments as far as subjective aging is concerned. One of the more ambitious attempts was done within the German Aging Study, which measured 47 positive and negative aging ex-periences in different domains such as health, social contacts, personality, etc. (Steve-rink, Westerhof, Bode, & Dittmann-Kohli, 2001). All statements started with the phrase "To me aging means . . ." or ended with the phrase ". . . has nothing to do with my age." Respondents could confirm or disconfirm the statements by indicating if they found them completely or mostly true or untrue. A series of factor analyses resulted in a three-factor solution, indicating physical decline (for example, "aging means that my health declines"), personal growth (". . . that I continue to make plans"), and social loss (". . . that I feel lonely more often") as dimensions of subjective aging. These three categories more or less reflect the tripartite division of aging by gerontologists into biological, psychological, and social aging, which are also readily differentiated by laypersons, and even among children, according to Montepare (1996).

The approach used here was simpler. As the respondents ranged in age from 40 to 80, they were first prepared with a phrase stating that "no matter what age one is, one is older than earlier in life." The respondent was then asked to agree or disagree (slight-ly or strongly) with four statements about age changes "until this date." Two of the statements indicated positive change ("a positive influence on my life," "higher self-acceptance"), two indicated negative change ("have to give up things," "changes I don't like"). The respondent was next asked to indicate changes for the better or worse in "the latest 10 years" for more concrete capabilities like physical fitness, memory for names, work ability, and work motivation. The selection of indicators was done on their face validity and were not strictly theory-informed.

Subjective age studies have a far stronger tradition. Measurements have been both indirect and direct, categorical and continuous. A review article by Barak and Stern (1986) identified five types of scales and concepts: (1) *identity age*, where respondents are asked to identify with age categories such as adult, middle aged, old, etc.; (2) *comparative age* is another categorical measurement, asking the informants to state whether they feel older or younger than their actual age; (3) feel age is measured simply by stating in years how old one feels; (4) *cognitive age* includes feel age together with other subjective ages such as *look age, do age, think age* (Kastenbaum et al., 1972), but may be combined with a categorical approach where persons are asked to state which age decade they identify with (20s, 30s, 40s, etc.); and finally, (5) *stereotype age*, which is an indirect approach with the use of a semantic differential to describe age groups, followed by an indication of how they fit oneself (George, Mutran, & Pennypacker, 1980).

There are advantages and disadvantages with either of these approaches, and they tap different dimensions of age identity. Some of the measures refer to the ages of "me" (feel age, look age), others to the ages of "I" (do age, think age). The NorLAG study employed the most direct approach, simply asking people to state how old they felt (in years), and how old they would like to be if they had a choice. Hence, the data here refer to feel age and ideal age, and the differences between each of the two and actual age.

We shall add some descriptive findings from a second data set, the Norwegian Monitor Study in 2005, as this covers the whole adult population aged 18 and over (postal questionnaire, $n = 3,849$, 70% response rate). The analytical section will, however, be restricted to the NorLAG material and the 40–79 age bracket, as the Monitor study includes too few of the relevant variables for analytical purposes. The Monitor study uses the same instruments as NorLAG to measure feel age and ideal age, but includes also an assessment of look age, as indicated by how old the respondents believe they are perceived by others.

Descriptives

Subjective Aging

In line with Steverink et al. (2001), we shall organize the findings on subjective aging along a number of assumptions. We first assume that aging refers to processes that occur over most of the life course, not only in older years, and that people may, therefore, recognize aging rather early in life. Quite a few, for example, may be concerned about loss or graying of hair long before they reach 40. Some may see midlife as a watershed beyond which they are no longer young, if not yet old (Schwaiger, 2006).

A second set of assumptions see aging as a multidimensional phenomenon. Age changes may, therefore, have different timing and rhythm along different dimensions. A third assumption adds multidirectionality to that of multidimensionality, implying that (observed and perceived) aging may have both negative (decline) and positive (growth) trajectories. Steverink et al. (2001) distinguish between weak and strong multidirectionality, but found support for the weak variant only, indicating that people do indeed perceive both positive and negative changes with age, but even the positive changes have a negative (decline) trajectory. Strong multidirectionality also indicates the presence of positive trajectories in late life.

The fourth and final assumption refers to the role of age as an explanatory factor. Does age indeed come out as a "black box" in the analyses, or does actual age have an impact on subjective aging beyond the effect of age-related losses in health and other resources? We are also interested in the extent to which aging is perceived differently by women and men, and in rural and urban settings, which are questions we return to in the analytical section.

The descriptive findings on subjective aging are given in **Figures 1 and 2**, and indicate support for multidimensionality, multidirectionality, and early awareness of aging. Both positive and negative changes are reported; there is even an indication of strong multidirectionality, as self-acceptance is perceived to increase with age all through these age groups, and mostly for the very oldest, those aged 70–79 (**Figure 1**).

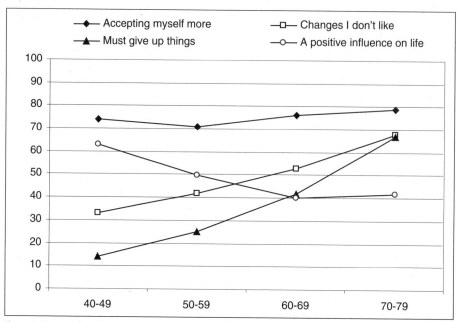

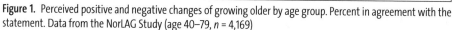

Figure 1. Perceived positive and negative changes of growing older by age group. Percent in agreement with the statement. Data from the NorLAG Study (age 40–79, n = 4,169)

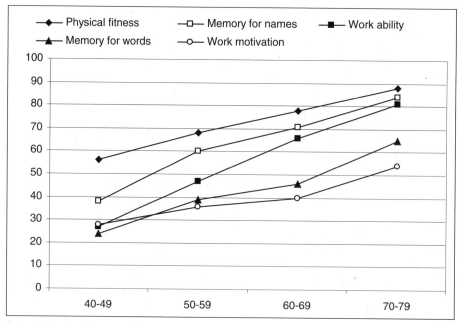

Figure 2. Perceived changes to the worse the last ten years by age group. Percent stating changes to the worse for each ability. Data from the NorLAG Study (age 40–79, n = 4,169)

Negative changes are, however, far more prominent, and are already reported by a substantial minority in the 40s and increase with age. Perceptions also vary within each age group. Some report "no change" in either direction, indicating that age means little or nothing for the characteristic in question. Respondents from all age groups report both positive and negative changes of getting older on all four characteristics presented in **Figure 1**, but the balance grows increasingly negative with age, except for self-acceptance. There is a negative majority for "changes I don't like" as early as age 60, but not until age 70 for "having to give up things." Quite a few seem to be provoked by the idea of getting older ("changes I don't like") before they perceive more concrete signs of this in the form of losses ("having to give up things").

Negative changes are even more evident in **Figure 2**, which presents the perceived changes over the past 10 years in more concrete physical and mental capabilities such as memory for names and physical fitness. Early recognition of aging is here seen in the high rates of people who in their 40s already report a loss of physical fitness (56%) and a poorer memory for names (38%). Most of the others report "no change" in these capacities, hence, there are very few indeed (less than 10%) who experience positive changes in any of these capacities. There is, therefore, only evidence of weak multidirectionality as far as these abilities are concerned, which is, to some extent, explained by the selected abilities being those that were assumed to decline with age. If traits and characteristics like generosity and empathy had been included, they might have shown a more positive gradient, in line with the popular stereotype of older people as being "warm, but incompetent" (Montepare & Zebrowitz 1998). Multidimensionality is also evident in the results of a factor analysis of the nine characteristics in **Figures 1 and 2** (not shown here), which produces a three-factor solution fairly similar to that found by Steverink et al. (2001), but here representing physical decline, cognitive decline, and personal growth, the latter mainly represented by increased self-acceptance.

It is hardly surprising that subjective (experienced) aging is mostly negative, and more and more so the older one gets. Less self-evident is the varying rhythm and timing among persons and dimensions on the one hand, and the presence of some positive trajectories on the other. It is also interesting to find an awareness of *negative* age changes as early as in the 40s and of *positive* changes (self-acceptance) as late as the late 70s. The latter may be taken as support for psychological developmental theories about a maturation of the personality in later life, as suggested for example by Jung (1930), Erikson (1986), Seim (1989), and Biggs (1999).

How strongly these experiences are shaped by age or by age-related losses in health and other resources is a theme for the analytical section. Let us first look closer at the descriptive findings about subjective age.

Age Identities

Research on subjective age and age identities have a much stronger tradition than research on subjective aging, but have produced little in terms of theories. The field is, then, reasonably well documented, but poorly understood, and the documentation is strongly biased toward the western world. We need not only more theorizing, but also better data. Most earlier studies have been carried out on small and local samples, the great majority from the United States, and few of them include middle-aged and younger persons. Those that do, tend to conclude that teenagers feel older than their age, young adults in the 20s are OK as they are, while a growing number seem to already feel uncomfortable with their age in the early 30s (Montepare & Lachman, 1989; Goldsmith & Heiens, 1992).

Among the more robust findings of earlier studies are that people from early midlife onward tend to feel younger than their age, and would like to be even younger. There is less consensus about why this is so, and what the causes and consequences are, beyond a correlation with (actual) age, health, and personal control beliefs. The distance between subjective and actual age tends to increase with age, while good health and personal control tend to make you feel younger, but also less dissatisfied with your current age. Good health, then, tends to *increase* the gap between feel age and actual age, and to *reduce* the gap between ideal age and actual age. Patterns like these have been fairly consistent over time as far back as the 1950s and 1960s. Since they are also rather general from country to country (within the western sphere), they might also point in the direction of equally general explanations.

The strength of the two Norwegian data sets is that they refer to large, national samples with a broad age representation. **Figure 3** illustrates how age is emerging as a burden for a substantial number of Norwegians as early as in the 20s. As early as 30, more than half feel younger than their age, and would like to be even younger. By the age of 40 and 50 and beyond, around three out of four feel younger than their age, while

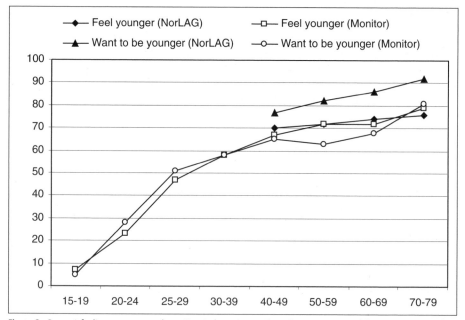

Figure 3. Percent feeling younger, and wanting to be younger, than their current age (plus-minus one year) by age. Data from the NorLAG Study (age 40–79, *n* = 4,169), and the Norwegian Monitor Study (age 18+, *n* = 3,849)

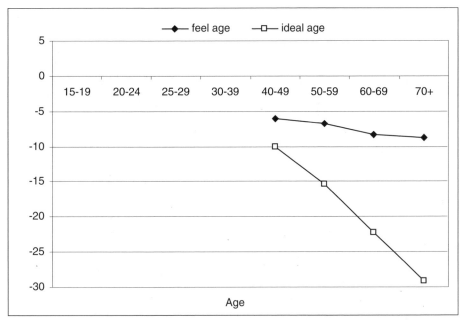

Figure 4. How much younger than their chronological age the respondents feel (feel age) and want to be (ideal age). Average number of years by age group. Data from the NorLAG Study (age 40–79, n = 4,169)

four out of five would like to be even younger. The Norwegian data, thus, accommodate reasonably well to the "general norm" of earlier studies.

How the gap between subjective and actual age increases with age is illustrated in more detail in **Figures 4 and 5**. Feel age varies from 6 years below actual age in the 40s to nearly 9 years lower in the 70s according to the NorLAG study. The corresponding gap for ideal age is 10 to 30 years (!) younger (**Figure 4**). Taken literally, the NorLAG respondents perceive the ideal age to be somewhere between 35 and 45. No gender differences could be observed for feel age, but women seem to be more satisfied with their age then men, or more precisely, they seem to be less dissatisfied with their age than men are. The average man between 40 and 79 would like to be around 20 years younger than his age, the average woman "only" 15 years younger.

The Norwegian Monitor data allow us to follow the trends for the whole adult life course (**Figure 5**). The cross-over between actual and subjective age appears before age 30. Norwegian teenagers and young adults identify with their actual age or feel slightly older, but by age 30, the majority feel and want to be younger. Hence, middle and later life are far from being the ideal years of life, which is hardly surprising. Less evident, perhaps, is that the burden of age is already felt with the emerging of adulthood.

The main findings are in line with those from other European studies, like Öberg and Tornstam (2001) for Sweden; Uotinen, Suutama, and Ruoppila (2003) for Finland; Westerhof et al. (2003) for Germany; and Montepare (1996) and Gana, Alaphilippe, and Bailly (2004) for France. There is, to my knowledge, no truly comparative study in this area, but comparative exercises by Westerhof et al. (2003), Westerhof & Barrett

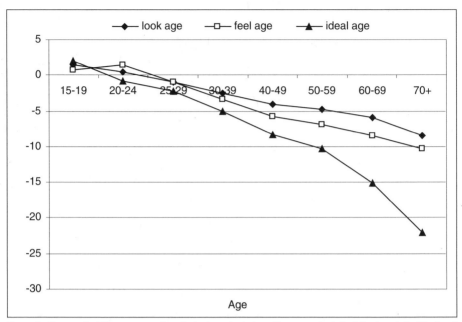

Figure 5. How much older or younger than their chronological age the respondents look (look age), feel (feel age) and want to be (ideal age). Average number of years by age group. Data from the Norwegian Monitor Study (age 18+, *n* = 3,849).

(2005), and Uotinen (1998) conclude that the subjective age profile is somewhat lower in the U.S. than in Europe (Germany and Finland). They attribute this to a stronger youth-orientation in the U.S. and, hence, to a cultural influence.

Causes and Consequences

How can we explain these patterns, and what are their implications? For one thing, we need to recognize that several phenomena and mechanisms are involved, which may need separate explanations. Although the majority feel younger than their age, and want to be even younger, the correlation between the two is no more than *r* = 0.20, hence, they refer to rather different phenomena. There are also moderate correlations between subjective aging and subjective age. All these indicators express a negative attitude to getting older, be it in the form of resistance, defiance, denial, or protection, and whether they are attempts to escape from the expected threats of later life or a defensive reaction to social declassification.

We have already suggested several types of explanations for such reactions, referring partly to structural, social, psychological, and existential factors. Most concretely, aging and old age may have low attraction simply because they imply a loss of access to attractive roles and goods, but why are these reactions also appearing early in life, when the structural conditions are in the process of becoming more favorable (Logan,

Ward, & Spitze, 1992)? A more social explanation sees the resistance to aging as a self-protective strategy in an ageist society that stereotypes and devalues later life and older people, but again, why should the reactions appear so early? Are they then better described as a reaction to a loss of youth than as a fear of old age? More psychological explanations such as a need for continuity of self may also be involved, as may more existential needs and fears.

We are not able to test these possibilities directly, but may throw some light on them by exploring the extent to which subjective age and aging are responses to (actual) age itself, or are better understood as reactions to age-related losses in personal resources and social roles. For this purpose we have run a series of multiple regressions with subjective age and aging as dependent variables. Age, gender, and personal resources such as health, self-esteem, mastery, and education are included as explanatory variables, together with social roles (working or retired, married or single) that are assumed to function as age cues (see, for example, Hagestad, 1990). A contextual indicator (community size) is added on the assumption that age and aging may be seen and experienced differently in urban (large) and rural (small) settings. Age and education are treated as categorical variables because they are likely to have a non-linear relationship to subjective age and aging. The youngest (40–49 years) are then the reference group for those in their 50s, 60s, and 70s respectively, while those with only primary school education are a reference for those with high school and university education. Health, mastery, and self-esteem are represented as standard scores (z-scores) in order to make it easier to compare the effects of these factors. Health is otherwise indicated by scores on the Short Form 12 scale, developed from the larger SF-36 version by Gandek et al. (1998). Mastery is an indicator for "personal control over desirable outcomes," and is measured by the mastery scale of Pearlin and Schooler (1978), while self-esteem is indicated by the scores on the Rosenberg (1965) 10-item self-esteem scale.

Subjective Aging

Logistic regressions were run for each of the nine indicators of subjective aging listed in **Figures 1 and 2**, with, all in all, parallel findings, so only four of them are shown here in order to save space (**Table 1**). The major finding is that actual age emerges as the main explanatory factor on all dimensions, even after control for resources, roles, and context. Health affects subjective aging in the expected direction in the sense that good (physical and mental) health tend to be associated with less negative experiences of aging. Self-acceptance is a deviating case with no effect of health, possibly indicating that both good and bad experiences may add to your self-acceptance, which is indeed suggested by a positive correlation of self-acceptance with both positive and negative aging experiences, although most strongly with the positive (not shown here). The beneficial impact of psychological resources such as mastery and self-esteem is also evident in the analysis (**Table 1**). High scores on these resources tend to add to the positive experiences of aging, and to reduce the negative experiences. Social roles seem to have little effect on perceived aging, as was also found by Westerhof and Barrett

Table 1. Logistic regression for personal experiences of aging in selected dimensions. Odds ratios. Data from the NorLAG Study (age 40–79, n = 4169).

	Must give up things		Accept myself more		Poorer memory for names		Poorer work ability	
	1	2	1	2	1	2	1	2
Age and gender								
50–59	**2.029**	**1.814**	0.888	0.888	**2.420**	**2.437**	**2.364**	**2.348**
60–69	**4.249**	**3.394**	1.160	1.228	**3.917**	**3.825**	**5.385**	**3.817**
70–79	**12.452**	**9.388**	1.353	**1.520**	**9.152**	**8.784**	**12.257**	**6.246**
Women	**0.782**	**0.590**	1.159	**1.189**	1.121	1.089	1.054	**0.837**
Resources and roles								
Physical health		**0.623**		0.948		**0.905**		**0.436**
Mental health		**0.847**		0.983		0.965		**0.743**
Mastery		**0.630**		**1.130**		0.919		**0.883**
Self-esteem		0.960		1.095[a]		**0.835**		**0.803**
High school		0.868		0.837		**1.222**		1.154
University		0.806		**0.710**		**1.506**		**1.429**
Retired		0.972		0.935		1.042		**2.045**
Single		1.007		0.958		**0.727**		0.847
Rural		1.021		0.979		1.141		**1.389**
CONSTANT		**0.275**		**3.196**		**0.499**		**0.342**
Nagelkerke R^2	0.204	0.329	0.007	0.018	0.152	0.178	0.205	0.395
(n)		(4002)		(4003)		(4014)		(4008)

Significant scores in **bold**. [a]p = 0.052.
Reference group for age is those aged 40–49, and for education those with primary school only. Women, retired, and single are dichotomous variables and contrasted to men, active workers, and married respectively. Rural is indicated by the size of the community, in five categories from larger (urban) to smaller (rural). Health, mastery, and self-esteem is indicated by standard scores (z-scores), and measured as explained in the text.

(2005), but in contrast to what was reported by Logan et al. (1992). The retired do, however, experience a larger loss of work ability than those still at work, which is reasonable. This is also the case for people in rural compared to urban areas, possibly reflecting the presence of more manual labor in the rural areas.

The explanatory power of age is reduced, in particular for the oldest age group, when the age-related losses in resources are included in the analysis. This is primarily so for the feeling of "having to give up things" and experiencing a "poorer work ability." Age is still the major explanatory factor for perceived aging in the full model. The odds for having experienced a poorer memory for names, a poorer work ability, and "having to give up things" is six to nine times higher for respondents aged 70–79 compared to respondents aged 40–49 – after controlling for differences in health and personal resources. Perceived self-acceptance is also a deviating case in the sense that the effect of age *increases* (around 10%) when resources are added to the analyses, implying that the positive association between age and self-acceptance is partly masked by a decline in mastery and self-esteem with increasing age.

Women seem to have less negative, and more positive, experiences with aging than men, while education seems to be a risk more than a resource as far as subjective aging is concerned. Respondents with a university degree tend to report more loss in memory and work ability than those with primary education only. They also report less positive effect of aging on self-acceptance (**Table 1**), perhaps in response to some form of relative deprivation (frustrated expectations, see, for example, Michalos, 1985) or a tendency to compare themselves with younger people.

Age Identities

Ordinary linear regressions were run for *age identities*, as measured by how much younger (than actual age) the respondents feel and how much younger they would like to be (**Table 2**). The first (feel age–actual age) is labeled subjective age perception (SAP), and the second (ideal age–actual age) as chronological age satisfaction (CAS), as suggested by Uotinen et al. (2003). Actual age is again found to be the most powerful factor. Personal resources play a role too, in the sense that good health, and high self-esteem and mastery scores contribute to feeling younger on the one hand, and to being more satisfied with one's current age on the other.

A less obvious finding is that women seem to be less dissatisfied with their age than men. There is no gender difference in SAP, but women have a difference between ideal and actual age that is 4.7 years less than that of men, as indicated by the unstandardized (B) regression coefficient in **Table 2**. Women also tend to report less negative age changes than men do, as already stated, and in contrast to the "double burden" image of aging for women suggested by Susan Sontag and others (referred in Schwaiger, 2006). Education seems to be a mixed blessing as far as perceived age is concerned. The highly educated are more satisfied with their current age, but they feel relatively older than those with less education, again possibly in response to higher expectations and to having selected a younger reference (comparison) group than the less educated.

Negative (and positive) experiences of aging may have an impact on age identities. We have, therefore, added the four indicators of subjective aging (from **Table 1**) to the explanatory model for SAP and CAS (in **Table 2**). The findings of this analysis (not shown here) indicate that the negative experiences of aging tend to make you feel somewhat older, and to make you somewhat less satisfied with your current age, as would be expected. The other relationships (to age, health, etc.), already commented on, are also valid in the expanded model.

Three Hypotheses

A major, and general, finding through all the analyses is how (chronological) age comes through as a major explanatory factor beyond what results from age-related losses in health, personal resources, and social roles. Why this is so, and what it is about

Table 2. Ordinary linear regression for "subjective age perception" (feel age–actual age) and "chronological age satisfaction" (ideal age–actual age). Unstandardized (B) and standardized (β) coefficients. Data from the NorLAG Study (age 40–79, n = 4,169).

	Subjective age perception		Chronological age satisfaction	
	B	β	B	β
Age and gender				
50–59	−0.997	−0.055	−4.557	−0.148
60–69	−2.144	−0.110	−9.771	−0.295
70–79	−2.601	−0.116	−15.636	−0.410
Women	−0.153	−0.009	4.737	0.168
Resources and roles				
Physical health (z-scores)	−0.877	−0.103	0.368	0.025
Mental health (z-scores)	−0.592	−0.068	0.290	0.020
Mastery (z-scores)	−0.597	−0.072	0.789	0.056
Self-esteem (z-scores)	−0.676	−0.082	0.636	0.045
High school education	0.391	0.024	0.746	0.026
University education	0.975	0.053	2.697	0.086
Retired	−0.728	−0.042	−1.405	−0.048
Single	−1.466	−0.078	−0.683	−0.021
Rural	−0.357	−0.019	−1.417	−0.045
R^2		0.061		0.274
(n)		(3813)		(3827)

Significant scores in **bold**. For details, see comments to Table 2.

"age" that makes this difference, is harder to explain. Is it simply a matter of measurement bias? Does the age factor still contain some more subtle indications of poor health than we have been able to capture in our measurements, thus, leaving the age factor still contaminated with health differences? Maybe so, but hardly to the extent that the age effect should disappear. The sheer size of the age effect makes this improbable. Chronological age, which by quite a few gerontologists is seen as an "empty category," without explanatory power in and of itself, becomes potent and full of meaning, and subsequently a meaning that most people try to protect themselves against beginning rather early in life.

We have no information about what meanings the informants themselves associate with the various age and aging indicators and react so negatively to. This should be a theme for future studies. Let me here simply suggest three types of hypotheses to explain the younger age identities, which together, or each by themselves, may be productive. The first is sociocultural, the second is psychobiological, and the third psychosocial.

– *The cultural explanation* sees the younger age identity as a protection against stigma and social stereotyping. The more youthful age identity that Uotinen (1998) and

Westerhof et al. (2003) found for the U.S. compared to Finland and Germany respectively, was interpreted in this direction, but otherwise stable patterns across time and space over the last 40–50 years indicate that more general, even universal, mechanisms may be in play, at least as a supplement to the cultural explanation. Also indicating a more general explanation is that the attraction of a younger age identity appears so early in life and, thus, is hard to see as a response to negative images of old age as such. It may more likely be a reaction to a loss of youth and the youth-related hopes of opportunities to come. The realities of a settled life can hardly compete with such dreams. It is also, in a way, self-evident to feel younger than your actual age, because this is where you come from and what you know. You can hardly know what the fifties are like on your first day in this decade, when you have 10 years as forty-and-something immediately behind you. And finally, feeling somewhat younger may primarily, and simply, be in response to negative stereotypes of aging and later life that is not only a child of modernity, but may have universal roots. What you feel younger than is the stereotypical idea of that age, and feeling younger (than this idea) is then simply a way of balancing out the stereotype. If so, there is no illusion in this, rather a correction of negative and stereotypical myths about aging. Feeling younger is in this case an indication of realism and not some form of false consciousness, and should be promoted rather than ridiculed. Feeling younger than your actual age has, in fact, been found to be good for your health and quality of life (or the other way around; the direction of causality is not self-evident). This is found in quite a few studies and is substantiated (but not shown) here. The larger gap between ideal and actual age is another matter, and is associated with poor health and a low quality of life.

– *The psychobiological hypothesis* assumes that aging and the passing of time provoke anxiety and defensive reactions against the threat of death and lost attachments. People will then tend to prevent, even deny, aging. A variant of this idea is found in the so-called "terror management theory," where "terror" refers to the fear of death (Solomon, Greenberg, & Pyszczynski, 2004). This hypothesis is hard to reconcile with the generality of the reported trends, which are already apparent when images of death must be assumed to be very vague and far from consciousness. Moreover, the "terror" of a death to come may be assumed to be stronger in midlife than in old age, and should have produced more denial of aging in the 50s and 60s than in the 70s, when people tend to come to terms with the idea of a finite life.

– *The psychosocial hypothesis* leans toward social identity theory, and sees the younger age identity as a need for continuity and protection of self against internal (bodily aging) and external (stigma) threats, perhaps even as a form of nostalgia, and a longing back to the "true self" that was established and recognized in early adulthood. Both the hypothesis of the "ageless self" by Kaufman (1986), and the "mask of aging hypothesis" by Featherstone and Hepworth (1990), are related to this way of thinking.

The mechanisms that may be assumed to underlie these hypotheses are several, from the management of anxiety, to the protection of status, and the preservation of self-esteem. These and other ideas need to be developed further and tested empirically. A preliminary conclusion is that age has a powerful impact on social judgments and self-perceptions. This is seen also in the celebrations of milestones such as turning 30, 50, or 70. "Round" years like these are perceived as symbolic turning points of the life course, and more so than any "institutionalized age" such as the official retirement age.

Concluding Remarks and Future Perspectives

We are indeed sensitive to age, both to our own age and that of others. This sensitivity is probably a universal response to the internal and external changes that are associated with aging. Our bodies are changing and so are our roles in family and society, and our status in the eyes of others and ourselves. We may try to protect a sense of true and stable self behind these changes, and feel "forever young" or "without age" behind the bodily or societal caricatures that are imposed on us. An alternative scenario and strategy is that of change, to develop a more "mature" self and personality, integrated, but still different from one's younger self, as suggested by Erikson's theory of ego development (1986) and Biggs's (1999) ideas about the "mature imagination."

I would, therefore, suggest a more general image, that of an "age-sensitive self" (Daatland, 2006), which is confronted by internal and external changes with increasing age, and struggles to maintain continuity, meaning, and self-respect. "The ageless self" may be one way of adapting to these challenges, another strategy may be to hide behind a "mask of aging," but there are also other and maybe more productive strategies that involve the possibility of change rather than a preservation of "what is," which at any rate is increasingly difficult as one grows older.

We need to know more about the protective strategies of the self in response to age and aging, their strengths and weaknesses, and under what conditions they are beneficial or harmful. Data like those presented here can help us part of the way, but need be guided by more explicit theorizing and expanded by more in-depth data.

References

Barak, B., & Stern, B. (1986). Subjective age correlates: A research note. *The Gerontologist, 26*, 571–578.

Biggs, S. (1999). *The mature imagination.* Buckingham, UK: Open University Press.

Biggs, S. (2004). New ageism: Age imperialism, personal experience, and aging policy. In S.O. Daatland & S. Biggs (Eds.), *Ageing and diversity. Multiple pathways and cultural migrations* (pp. 95–106). Bristol: Policy Press.

Biggs, S. (2005). Beyond appearances: Perspectives on identity in later life and some implications for method. *Journal of Gerontology, Social Sciences, 60B*, S118–S128.

Daatland, S.O. (2002). Time to pay back? Is there something for psychology and sociology in gerontology? In L. Andersson (Ed.), *Cultural gerontology* (pp. 1–11). Westport, CT: Auburn House.

Daatland, S.O. (2006, November). *The age-sensitive self.* Paper presented at the 59th GSA Annual Conference, Dallas.

Erikson, E.H. (1986). *The life cycle completed.* New York: Norton.

Featherstone, M., & Hepworth, M. (1990). Images of aging. In J. Bond & P. Coleman (Eds.), *Ageing in society. An introduction to social gerontology* (pp. 250–275). London: Sage.

Featherstone, M., & Hepworth, M. (2005). Images of aging. Cultural representations of later life. In M.L. Johnson (Ed.), *The Cambridge handbook of age and aging* (pp. 354–362). Cambridge, UK: Cambridge University Press.

Gana, K., Alaphilippe, D., & Bailly, N. (2004). Positive illusions and mental and physical health in later life. *Aging and Mental Health, 8,* 3–12.

Gandek, B., Ware, J.E., Aronsen, N.K., Apolone, G., Bjorner, J.B., Brazier, J.E. et al. (1998). Cross-validation of item selection and scoring of the SF-12 Health Survey in nine countries. Results from the IQOLA project. *Journal of Clinical Epidemiology, 11,* 1171–1178.

George, L.K., Mutran, E.J., & Pennypacker, M.R. (1980). The meaning and measurement of age identity. *Experimental Aging Research, 6,* 283–298.

Goldsmith, R.E., & Heiens, R.A. (1992). Subjective age: A test of five hypotheses. *The Gerontologist, 32,* 312–317.

Hagestad, G. (1990). Social perspectives on the life course. In R.H. Binstock & L.K. George (Eds.), *Handbook of aging and the social sciences* (pp. 151–163). New York: Academic Press.

Jung, C.G. (1930). *Die Lebenswende. Gesamte Werke* [Life turning point. Collected works] (Vol. 8). Olten, Switzerland: Walter Verlag.

Kastenbaum, R., Derbin, V., Sabatini, P., & Artt, S. (1972). The ages of me – Toward personal and interpersonal definitions of functional aging. *Aging and Human Development, 3,* 197–211.

Kaufman, S.R. (1986). *The ageless self. Sources of meaning in late life.* Madison, WI: University of Wisconsin Press.

Levy, B.R. (2003). Mind matters: Cognitive and physical effects of aging self-stereotypes. *Journal of Gerontology, Psychological Sciences, 58B,* P203–P211.

Levy, B.R., Slade, M.D., & Kasl, S.V. (2002). Longitudinal benefit of positive self-perceptions of aging and functional health. *Journal of Gerontology, Psychological Sciences, 57B,* P409–P417.

Levy, B.R., Slade, M.D., Kunkel, S.R., & Kasl, S.V. (2002). Longevity increased by positive self-perceptions of aging. *Journal of Personality and Social Psychology, 83,* 261–270.

Logan, J.R., Ward, R., & Spitze, G. (1992). As old as you feel: Age identity in middle and later life. *Social Forces, 71,* 451–467.

Merton, R.K. (1968). The self-fulfilling prophecy. In R.K. Merton, *Social theory and social structure* (pp. 475–490). New York: The Free Press.

Michalos, A.C. (1985). Multiple discrepancies theory (MDT). *Social Indicators Research, 16,* 347–414.

Montepare, J.M. (1996). An assessment of adults' perceptions of their psychological, physical, and social ages. *Journal of Clinical Geropsychology, 2,* 117–128.

Montepare, J.M., & Lachman, M.E. (1989). You're only as old as you feel: Self-perceptions of age, fears of aging, and life satisfaction from adolescence to old age. *Psychology and Aging, 4,* 73–78.

Montepare, J.M., & Zebrowitz, L.A. (1998). Person perception comes of age: The salience and significance of age in social judgments. *Advances in Experimental Social Psychology, 30,* 93–161.

Öberg, P., & Tornstam, L. (2001). Youthfulness and fitness – Identity ideals for all ages? *Journal of Aging and Identity, 6,* 15–29.

Pearlin, L.J., & Schooler, C. (1978). The structure of coping. *Journal of Health and Social Behavior, 19,* 2–21.

Rosenberg, M. (1965). *Society and the adolescent self-image*. Princeton, NJ: Princeton University Press.

Rothermund, K., & Brandstädter, J. (2003). Age stereotypes and self-views in later life: Evaluating rival assumptions. *International Journal of Behavioral Development, 27*, 549–554.

Schwaiger, L. (2006). To be forever young? Toward reframing corporeal subjectivity in maturity. *International Journal of Ageing and Later Life, 1*, 11–41.

Seim, S. (1989). *Teenagers become adult and elderly*. Oslo, Norway: Norwegian Institute of Gerontology, Report 5-1989.

Solomon, S., Greenberg, J., & Pyszczynski, T. (2004). The cultural animal: Twenty years of terror management theory and research. In J. Greenberg, S.L. Koole, & T. Pyszczynski (Eds.). *Handbook of experimental existential psychology* (pp. 13–34). New York: Guilford.

Steverink, N., Westerhof, G.J., Bode, C., & Dittmann-Kohli, F. (2001). The personal experience of aging, individual resources, and subjective well-being. *Journal of Gerontology, Psychological Sciences, 56B*, P364–P373.

Uotinen, V. (1998). Age identification: A comparison between Finnish and North-American cultures. *International Journal of Aging and Human Development, 46*, 109–124.

Uotinen, V., Suutama, T., & Ruoppila, I. (2003). Age identification in the framework of successful aging: A study of older Finnish people. *International Journal of Aging and Human Development, 56*, 173–195.

Westerhof, G., Barrett, A., & Steverink, N. (2003). Forever young? A comparison of age identities in the United States and Germany. *Research on Aging, 25*, 366–383.

Westerhof, G.J., & Barrett, A.E. (2005). Age identity and subjective well-being: A comparison of the United States and Germany. *Journal of Gerontology, Social Sciences, 60B*, S129–S136.

Zola, I.K. (1962). Feelings about age among older people. *Journal of Gerontology, 17*, 65–68.

4. Person-Environment Relations

Hans-Werner Wahl and Susanne Iwarsson

Importance of Person-Environment Relations in Aging

A diversity of converging arguments supports the assumption that the environment matters as people age. The *time budget and action range argument* refers to the fact that the home environment has been identified as a major context for aging persons, because aging persons, particularly those in very old age beyond the age of 80 or 85 years, spend, on average, most of their daytime hours in their home or rather near to their home (Baltes, Maas, Wilms, & Borchelt, 1999). Next, the *living at the same place argument* is important. Typically, older people have lived a long time in the same physical location, which leads to strong cognitive and affective ties of the old person to his or her environment (Oswald & Wahl, 2005). The *competence argument* acknowledges that old age is a period in life in which loss in competencies significantly enhances the "press" and the constraints of the physical environments (Lawton, 1999). Particularly the oldest old are at a higher risk of requiring personal assistance, living alone, having lower income, being socially isolated, living in homes in need of repair, and in neighborhoods with a tendency toward decline. Also, loss in functioning is a driving force behind declining out-of-home mobility as a major resource for quality of life. The link between the physical environment and aging outcomes can, therefore, be expected to be particularly powerful for the very old, who also are at greater risk for chronic diseases and functional vulnerabilities that impact on everyday living. In other words, the everyday difficulties imposed by age-related functional decline such as mobility problems, sensory loss, or cognitive impairment significantly shape the dynamics of persons and environments. Age-related loss of competencies is also among the major reasons for residential decisions and relocation to sheltered environments, a critical life event on the individual level, as well as a challenge for societies and communities in terms of offering high quality planned housing and institutions to a substantial portion of their population. In terms of application and intervention, an understanding of person-environment (p-e) relations in old age is important because in cases of substantially decreased competence, such as in dementia-related disorders, improvement of the physical environment may become the only "therapeutic" alternative (Cohen & Weisman, 1991). The *need argument* refers to the notion that, rather independent of frailty, there continues to be a strong desire among older people to "age in place." Finally, the *cohort dynamics argument* underscores that ongoing changes in the person-physical environment system tell us much about the changing *Zeitgeist* in the culture of aging at large. For instance, there are new housing options such as various multigenerational living arrangements and assisted housing solutions all over Europe, which can be seen as the material reflection of a new culture of aging. It is also worth noting in this context that trends in terms of improved quality, provision, and increased use of assistive technology or home adaptation play a substantial role for the observed increase in functioning of older people over time (Spillman, 2004). Given this prominence of environments for aging processes and outcomes, research questions in this array certainly belong to the core challenges of gerontology.

Need for an Interdisciplinary Approach in Environmental Gerontology: Geropsychology, Occupational Therapy, and More

Striving toward a better understanding of the role of the environment as people age, frequently coined environmental gerontology, has been a core topic within gerontology since the 1950s (Wahl & Gitlin, 2007). On the one hand, because key players in this field of inquiry such as F. Carp, E. Kahana, M.P. Lawton, and R. Scheidt are psychologists (see Wahl & Weisman, 2003), geropsychology (GP) offered a major input to the scholarly treatment of p-e relations. On the other hand, disciplines such as occupational therapy (OT) entered the field based on practical, professional experiences and a growing body of theoretical contributions (e.g., Kielhofner, 2002), subsequently followed by conceptual input, methodological expertise, as well as new research findings (Iwarsson, 2004).

As a result of these developments, a major aim of this chapter is to transcend the psychological perspective on p-e relations in old age, emphasizing synergies between GP and OT. The chapter draws from an intensive collaboration between GP and OT developed in the context of the interdisciplinary project, "Enabling Autonomy, Participation, and Well-Being in Old Age: The Home Environment as a Determinant for Healthy Ageing" (ENABLE-AGE), which was funded by the European Commission (EC) from 2002 to 2004 (QLRT-2001–00334; Iwarsson, Nygren, Oswald, Wahl, & Tomsone, 2006).

Why is collaboration between GP and OT a promising, though still underused, pathway for the treatment of p-e relations in later life? In both fields, emphasis is put on the physical environment as a neglected sphere in human aging research, and balances or imbalances of person capabilities and physical environment demands are major targets of both approaches, though the theoretical traditions differ. For example, key concepts of GP such as adaptation or p-e fit have put strong emphasis on the older persons' psychological architecture interacting with the physical surrounding, e.g., cognitive functioning, personality, and environmental needs (Lawton, 1999). In contrast, key terms based on OT approaches, such as accessibility (Iwarsson & Ståhl, 2003; Steinfeld & Tauke, 2002) and activity, focus more on functional limitations in relation to the environment, resulting in engagement in meaningful activities (Kielhofner, 2002). That is, in addition to the GP focus on p-e relations, OT scholars engaged in environmental gerontology emphasize the importance of p-e-activity transactions (Iwarsson, 2004), and major attention is paid to how tasks and activities of daily life are influenced by personal and environmental aspects. Specifically, environmental interventions such as home modifications, development of new housing alternatives, and redesign of public outdoor areas or public transport are tools used to support and maintain quality of life in old age.

In conclusion, the simultaneous consideration of research from GP and OT adds to a better understanding of p-e relations. Of course, additional fields such as technology, social science, and physical planning are needed for p-e research and we also include these in our next section addressing basic trends of p-e research in Europe.

Basic Trends in Person-Environment Research in Old Age in Europe

In order to identify trends in European p-e research related to aging since around 1990, we use a template differentiating between contents and levels of analysis (see **Table 1**). In terms of *contents*, we first address research concerned with the role of the home environment for aging, be it private home environments, senior housing, or institutional settings. Second, we consider research related to out-of-home environments such as studies treating neighborhood issues, the use of outdoor spaces, public facilities, and outdoor mobility at large. Third, we will focus on physical environments in terms of products and technology, in particular assistive technology. We will also consider different *levels of analysis*, making a distinction between research on p-e relations on the micro to meso level (e.g., home environment or neighborhood research) as compared to the meso to macro level (e.g., urban as compared to rural environments).

Applying this scheme to the European aging research landscape, with respect to *home environments*, the private household has been a major target of research, with emphasis on objective as well as perceived aspects. Such research has been strong in Sweden (e.g., Fänge & Iwarsson, 2005a), Germany (e.g., Oswald & Wahl, 2005; Wahl, Oswald, & Zimprich, 1999), and Great Britain (e.g., Burholt & Naylor, 2005; Peace, 1993; Sixsmith & Sixsmith, 1991). Slangen-de Kort's (1999) research in the Netherlands on how older adults solve problems related to their home environments also deserves mentioning. The ENABLE-AGE Project has provided a major extension of this work by collecting person and home environment data in Germany, Great Britain, Hungary, Latvia, and Sweden (Haak, Dahlin-Ivanoff, Fänge, Sixsmith, & Iwarsson, 2006; Iwarsson et al., 2006; Nygren et al., 2007; Oswald et al., 2007). European research on home environments has also put major emphasis on sheltered housing facilities. For example, Saup (2003) provided a longitudinal study on aging in sheltered

Table 1. A differentiation of contents and levels of analysis in environmental gerontology research

Level of analysis	Contents of the physical environment		
Micro – Meso Meso – Macro	Home environments	Outdoor environments	Products and technology

housing in Germany with measurement waves before and several times after relocation, while Peace and Holland (2001) addressed meaning aspects of sheltered living facilities and inclusive housing in England. Also, research in institutional settings has found ongoing attention, with issues as diverse as exploring the role of institutional environment for dependence in Germany (Baltes & Wahl, 1992), addressing the relation between individual (such as activity, satisfaction, functional abilities, social relationships) and environmental characteristics (such as noise, safety conditions) in Spain (Fernandez-Ballesteros, Montorio, & Izal, 1998), and assessing the impact of specially designed institutional environments for the course and outcome of dementia such as work in Italy (Bianchetti, Benvenuti, Ghisla, Frisoni, & Trabucchi, 1997) or in Sweden (Elmstahl, Annerstedt, & Ahlund, 1997).

A major European aging research strand has also been concerned with the role of *out-of-home environments* as people age. One example is the project Enhancing Outdoor Mobility in Later Life – Personal Coping, Environmental Resources and Technical Support (MOBILATE), conducted in urban and rural regions in Finland, Germany, Italy, and the Netherlands (Mollenkopf, Marcellini, Ruoppila, Széman, & Tacken, 2005). In 2006, another major EC-funded project, Life Quality of Senior Citizens in Relation to Mobility Conditions (SIZE), which focused on the situation in eight European countries, was finalized (http://www.size-project.at/). In Sweden, OT research has reached acknowledged integration with traffic planning, resulting in methodological as well as applied research in collaboration with older people themselves and different community actors (e.g., Valdemarsson, Jernryd, & Iwarsson, 2005). In addition, the role of neighborhoods has found attention by scholars such as Scharf and colleagues, focusing on deprived neighborhoods in Great Britain (e.g., Scharf, Phillipson, & Smith, 2005); Deeg and colleagues (e.g., Deeg & Thomése, 2005), focusing on the role of diverse sociostructural quality of neighborhoods in the Netherlands; and the work of Oswald, Hieber, Wahl, and Mollenkopf (2005), focusing on the role of p-e fit issues in city districts in Germany.

With respect to the domain of the physical environment we label *products and technology*, early in the 1990s European aging research received substantial promotion by the EC's COST A5 program (COST A5, 1997). Many technology-oriented research projects addressing issues as diverse as dementia, stroke, smart homes, online assessment of vital functions, or vision and hearing loss have been conducted (see e.g., Mollenkopf, Mix, Gäng, & Kwon, 2001). It should be noted that during the 1990s European scholars (e.g., Bouma & Graafmans, 1992) "invented" the field of gerontechnology, making efforts to reduce the fragmentation within the research in this field. By long tradition, provision of assistive technology constitutes a core intervention within OT practice, and during recent years the body of research in this domain has grown considerably. Typically, based on the notion of p-e-activity transaction (Iwarsson, 2004), OT research involving products and technology deals with assistive technology related to everyday activities. Recent contributions focus on user needs and satisfaction and the psychology of day-to-day use of assistive devices in Belgium (Roelands, von Oost, Buysse, & Depoorter, 2002), the Northern countries (e.g., Brandt, Iwarsson, & Ståhl, 2004; Hedberg-Kristensson, Dahlin-Ivanoff, & Iwarsson, 2006), as well as cross-country comparative research (Löfqvist, Nygren, Széman, & Iwarsson, 2005). Another array addressing the issue of aging and technology concerns older Europeans' use of information and communication technology (e.g., Selwyn, Gorard, Furlong, & Madden, 2003), and in Sweden, Nygård and colleagues have published substantial research on technology use among persons with dementia (e.g., Margot-Cattin & Nygård, 2006). In terms of *level of analysis*, most of the p-e research in Europe tends to be located on the micro to meso level and conducted in urban settings. However, major research highlighting the distinction between urban and rural aging has been accomplished within the projects Older People in Europe's Rural Areas (OPERA; Scharf & Wenger, 2000) and MOBILATE (Mollenkopf et al., 2005). A special section in the *European Journal of Ageing* on "Ageing in Diverse Urban and Rural Settings" (2005) is a recent indication that a critical mass of research addressing the specifics of urban as compared to rural environments has successfully developed over the years.

In addition to the contributions of European scholars to environmental gerontology in terms of contents, major steps in the development of methodology have also been taken. Structured assessment tools have been developed addressing environmental gerontology key concepts such as usability (Fänge & Iwarsson, 2003), p-e fit in the home environment (Iwarsson, Nygren, & Slaug, 2005;), housing-related control beliefs (Oswald, Wahl, Martin, & Mollenkopf, 2003), as well as instruments targeting the ecology of institutional settings (Fernandez-Ballesteros et al., 1998) and assistive technology (Brandt et al., 2003). In addition, understanding of the interlinkages between important constructs such as residential satisfaction, meaning of home, usability, and housing-related control beliefs has been advanced (Oswald et al., 2007). Qualitative research methodology has also been furthered in the field of p-e issues in old age (e.g., Haak, Dahlin-Ivanoff, Fänge, Sixsmith, & Iwarsson, in press; Hovbrandt, Fridlund, & Carlsson, in press; Peace, 2005; Sixsmith & Sixsmith, 1991).

European Research on Person-Environment Relations in Aging: A Selection of Findings

Findings on Home Environments and Aging

Focus on the Objective Home Environment

A major finding concerned with the home environment addresses the classic issue of p-e fit. Iwarsson found in her research (e.g., Iwarsson, 2005) that accessibility, a construct considering the fit between functional limitations *and* objectively observed barriers in the home environment, is more important for functional ability than number of barriers. Wahl et al. (1999) found additional support for this assumption in a group of visually impaired elders, but also added complexity to p-e dynamics in the home environment. As was observed, p-e fit was particularly important for the exertion of instrumental activities of daily living (IADL), while no statistically meaningful relation was observed with respect to personal activities of daily living (PADL). The explanation given for this was that the objective environment becomes particularly important in more complex activities. Coping with the objective home environment is another basic challenge as people age. Slangen-de Kort (1999) found that personality dispositions seem to play a role here.

Focus on the Perceived Home Environment

European scholars have considered the role of the perceived home environment from a diversity of perspectives. In accordance with the North American literature, the construct of residential satisfaction has been the focus of several studies. Residential satisfaction is important because it adds to the explanation of life satisfaction (Oswald, Wahl, Mollenkopf, & Schilling, 2003), although a limitation for using this construct in statistical analysis is its usually low variance, that is, the majority of older persons are satisfied with their housing situation when asked in this general way. In addition, the well-known residential satisfaction paradox, i.e., a moderate to low correlation between objective home environment quality and (perceived) residential satisfaction, has gained further support. For instance, Fernandez-Ballesteros (2001) observed in a study with Spanish elders that perceived (subjective) home environment quality correlated only moderately ($r = -.36$) with objective need of repair.

Oswald and Wahl (2005) addressed the issue of meaning of home in a sample of German older adults without and with "environment-relevant" impairments (mobility loss, vision loss). Meaning of home was defined as a range of processes by which aging individuals form behavioral, cognitive, and affective ties to their home environments. Based on a mix of qualitative and quantitative methodology, meaning of home was found to be nurtured by five processes: (1) physical aspects, focusing on the experience of housing conditions; (2) behavioral aspects, related to the everyday behavior of the person at home and to ways of manipulating or rearranging items in the home; (3) cognitive aspects, representing especially biographical attachment to the home; (4) emotional aspects, expressing emotional attachment including the experience of privacy, safety, pleasure, and stimulation; and (5) social aspects, related to relationships with fellow lodgers, neighbors, or visitors. Healthy participants were more appreciative of the location, access, and amenity aspects of the home. Cognitive aspects were reported significantly more often among blind persons and those with mobility impairments as compared to persons without impairments. Similarly, the work of Burholt and colleagues (e.g., Burholt & Naylor, 2005), Peace (2005), and Sixsmith and Sixsmith (1991) in England added significantly to the insight that attachment to place is a focal area of growing older. Thus, attachment to place is a strong experience particularly in old and very old individuals, enhancing core elements of the aging person such as the self, identity, and quality of life.

Based on the notion of p-e-activity transactions, Fänge and Iwarsson developed a self-rated instrument intended to capture the concept *usability*, comprising three aspects: activity aspects, personal and social aspects, and physical environmental aspects (Fänge & Iwarsson, 2003). Based on several studies, they have demonstrated that usability is sensitive as a means to capture effects of housing adaptation (Fänge & Iwarsson, 2005b) and conceptually related to, but differentiated from, the objective housing aspect accessibility (Fänge & Iwarsson, 2003).

Findings on Out-of-Home Environments and Aging

Focus on Neighborhoods and Site of Living

A key study in this area was conducted by Scharf et al. (2005) in urban communities in England. The major concept driving this research was the multidimensional phenomenon of social exclusion, comprised of neighborhood exclusion, exclusion from material resources, social relations, civic activities, and basic services. Among 600 persons aged 60+ living in deprived neighborhoods, Scharf et al. found that a three-fold differentiation existed; 33% were not excluded on any of the five dimensions, whereas 31% experienced exclusion in one dimension and 36% exclusion in a cumulative manner. Substantial relations were observed with respect to ethnic origin, education, housing tenure, perceived health, and quality of life. A set of studies from Germany and the Netherlands centered on the concept of p-e fit or misfit between aging persons and neighborhood characteristics. Oswald, Hieber, Wahl, and Mollenkopf (2005) found that type of neighborhood correlated with p-e fit in the expected direction, i.e., higher fit was observed in more pleasant city districts, particularly in the domain of higher-order needs such as privacy, comfort, familiarity, and favored activities. Deeg and Thomése (2005) assumed that significant discrepancies between person and neighborhood characteristics such as high personal income in low quality neighborhoods may occur across the life course. They found that such person-neighborhood misfits reveal substantial relations with lowered mental and physical health.

Focus on the Description of Everyday Out-of-Home Behavior

Similar to home environments, a fundamental question is what kind of meaning older people relate to being mobile and able to use out-of-home environments. In a study on outdoor mobility in four European cities, older adults participating in case studies were asked what out-of-home mobility means to them. Statements like "Joy," "It's nourishing being with others," "You feel free to get around as you like," or "It's everything, it's life" demonstrate the high value placed on the ability to move about outside the home (Mollenkopf et al., 2005).

A major challenge of mobility research with older people is gaining a comprehensive picture of transport behavior, because traditionally there has been a strong focus on driving, which obviously is a limited view. The MOBILATE project (Mollenkopf et al., 2005) based on nearly 4,000 individuals aged 55+ in five countries put major emphasis on a broad understanding of mobility. Findings indicate that, besides good health, the availability of a car is a critical antecedent for out-of-home activity as well as for satisfaction with mobility. Also, private modes of transportation such as cars, bicycles, or walking are preferred. Public transport plays a role predominantly when no other alternatives are available, or when the public transport system is particularly well-organized with high frequency services and a dense network of stops. More than three quarters (77%) of the MOBILATE sample made at least one out-of-home trip during the two days before the interview; major motives were shopping, visiting friends and relatives, and going out for a stroll. Going by foot was the predominant mode of transport on these trips.

Focus on the Explanation and Modification of Everyday Out-of-Home Behavior

In terms of explaining interindividual differences in out-of-home behavior, the MOBI-LATE project provides a strong case for the consideration of a wide range of person as well as environmental variables. That is, health condition is only one, although an important person variable. In addition, Oswald, Wahl, and Kaspar (2005) found cognitive resources and control beliefs as major correlates of out-of-home behavior. On the environmental side, weather conditions, dangerous traffic conditions, and the availability of supportive transport systems such as low-floor buses all play a role in supporting or hindering outdoor mobility.

Another approach to explanation of differences in out-of-home mobility is to search for subgroups in terms of mobility patterns and then identify significant differences among such groups. This has been done by means of cluster analysis within the MOBI-LATE project (Mollenkopf, Kaspar, & Wahl, 2005), ending up in subgroups across a spectrum of the mobility rich and the mobility poor: The mobility poor tended to be older, female, lower in education, lower in availability of a private car, lower in mental functioning, and higher in external control beliefs.

Taking empirical results into societal planning processes, in Sweden, Ståhl and Iwarsson (2004) accomplished a demonstration project aiming to identify and prioritize concrete measures for implementing increased accessibility and safety in a residential area. Together with representatives for authorities and stakeholders, senior citizens in the study district took part in a prioritization process resulting in a program comprising the following general measures: separation of pedestrians and cyclists, lower speed limits, and better maintenance. Selected prioritized measures were wider sidewalks, curb cuts, and even surfaces of sidewalks. Most important, older people participating in this project found new ways to communicate with and influence responsible parties in society, and the authorities and stakeholders obtained new knowledge about the importance of small details in contrast to large infrastructure measures.

Findings on Products and Technology and Aging

Focus on Assistive Devices

The body of literature on use of assistive devices in old age is rapidly increasing. For example, in Denmark and Sweden OT researchers have investigated different aspects of need, use, and satisfaction with mobility devices. A recent retrospective longitudinal study in Sweden demonstrated that both the use of several mobility devices and the permanent use of such devices increased between 85 and 90 years of age (Dahlin-Ivanoff & Sonn, 2005). Based on a Danish study, Brandt and colleagues concluded that the majority of older powered-wheelchair users (Brandt et al., 2004) were satisfied with their mobility devices and used them frequently, while subgroups of users (women, users living alone, first-time users) were dissatisfied with their rollators (walkers). Nearly all powered-wheelchair users regarded their device as important and found that it gave them independence; the wheelchair made activity and participation possible. Going a bit deeper into how older people perceive use of mobility devices, Hedberg-Kristensson et al. (2006; Hedberg-Kristensson, Dahlin-Ivanoff, & Iwarsson, 2007) concluded that it took time and effort for older users to accept and find out how to use their mobility devices, and most users were not actively involved in the prescription process. Nevertheless, many users managed to integrate their mobility devices in their performance of daily activities and appreciated their devices, but there are major needs for quality improvement in the provision of mobility devices.

Focus on Gerontechnology Issues

The early volume on gerontology edited by Bouma and Graafmans (1992) had already underlined that a scope of research on technology and aging has been on stage across Europe since the late 1980s. As reported in this compilation of research, cognitive-psychological studies showed that the person-technology interface changes significantly as people age; examples rather critical of the use of technology decline in visual attention and dual-task performance. On the other hand, it is an important empirical insight that attitudes of aging persons toward new technology are far from negative or simply driven by calendar age. No support for a consistent relation between old age and technophobia was found. Wahl and Mollenkopf (2003) emphasized the need to differentiate among subgroups when it comes to technology acceptance. Four types were identified based on a sample of over 1,400 individuals aged 55+ from the study Everyday Technology for Senior Housing (http://www.sentha.tu-berlin.de/) as follows: (1) the positive advocates of technology; (2) the rationally adapting; (3) the sceptical and ambivalent; and (4) those critical and reserved with respect to technology. Usability of technology is a persisting problem as people age, in particular in the array of communication and entertainment technology as compared to household technology (Wahl & Mollenkopf, 2003). As demonstrated by Rudinger (1996) with respect to ticket machines as well as video cassette recorders, in order to enhance the use of technology and reduce negative age effects it is important to improve design and user interfaces.

Level of Analysis Issues

European research on p-e relations in aging has addressed linkages between the micro to meso as well as the meso to macro levels of analysis. For example, urban-rural comparisons have repeatedly shown disadvantages driven by this distinction on the level of individual behaviors of rural elders. In most European cities, older people can reach essential facilities mainly on foot or by public transportation. In rural areas, however, they often depend on a car or on other types of special transportation support; not only are shops and services less abundant, but public transportation is not sufficiently developed. This lack of infrastructure causes different patterns of IADL dependence among older persons living in rural areas compared to those living in urban districts (Iwarsson, 1998). The MOBILATE project mostly supported these kind of results; across countries the modes and possibilities of using out-of-home environments were more limited in rural areas (Mollenkopf et al., 2005).

A critical challenge of European gerontological research is to relate the macro context of different countries with the behavior of individuals or p-e constellations on the micro level (Iwarsson, Wahl, & Nygren, 2004; see Tesch-Römer & von Kondratowitz, 2006, for a comprehensive theoretical discussion of this problem). For instance, the MOBILATE Project showed that no single indicator of outdoor mobility was equally important in all regions studied with respect to quality of life. The only relevant aspect in at least half the regions was "satisfaction with the possibility to pursue leisure time activities." These findings show that as different as regional conditions are, so are the components of the social, built, and natural environments that contribute to older persons' satisfaction with life in general.

The ENABLE-AGE Project

Background and Conceptual Framework

The main objective of the ENABLE-AGE Project was to examine the home environment and its importance for major components of healthy aging (see also http//: www.enableage.arb.lu.se). The term healthy aging was used to address selected aspects of physical, mental and social health, which are assumed to be particularly relevant to housing. Among the core concepts chosen for the project were independence in daily activities and subjective well-being (Iwarsson et al., 2006). Community-residing, very old participants living alone were selected as the target group of this research, because this group has a pronounced risk of losing independence and becoming socially isolated. Very old individuals, particularly those living in single households, have been described as particularly sensitive to "environmental press" (Lawton, 1999), because of sensory, mobility, and cognitive declines. Data were gathered in urban regions in five European countries representing economically well-developed "old" European Union (EU) member states (Germany, UK, Sweden), as well as "new" member states that joined the EU in 2005 and are still in a period of major social and political transformation (Hungary, Latvia).

The ENABLE-AGE Project had several major targets. First, we were interested in relationships between objective and perceived housing in very old age. Second, relationships between objective and perceived housing and healthy aging outcomes, namely, independence in daily activities and well-being, served as the target for analysis. In addition, the ENABLE-AGE Project sought to advance methodological quality in the assessment of home environments and very old people. Third, the effects of diverse national backgrounds that differed in legislative systems, housing regulations, and socioeconomic living standards on these relationships were examined.

A functional definition of healthy aging was used in the ENABLE-AGE Project.

According to the ICF (WHO, 2001), there are multifaceted relationships among the components of body functions, activity and participation, and personal and environmental factors. Regarding the role of *objective housing*, the ecological theory of aging and the environmental docility hypothesis (Lawton, 1999), underlying many environmental gerontology studies (Wahl & Gitlin, 2007), was the main conceptual driving force. Individuals with low functional capacity are much more vulnerable to environmental demand than those with high capacity, and environmental details are critical to what they can manage in their everyday lives. The ecological theory and other classic p-e conceptions in GP and OT (e.g., Carp, 1987; Iwarsson, 2004) underscore the notion that it is the fit between personal competencies and needs and environmental conditions, rather than personal and environmental factors alone, that is key to understanding p-e relations as people age (Iwarsson, 2004, 2005). Regarding *perceived housing*, the ENABLE-AGE Project considered the meaning of home (Oswald & Wahl, 2005), its usability (Fänge & Iwarsson, 1999, 2003), and the concept of housing-related control beliefs (Oswald, Wahl, Martin & Mollenkopf, 2003). Finally, the ENABLE-AGE conceptual framework is based on the assumption that the macro context, particularly different legislations, housing regulations, and different socioeconomic standards in diverse European countries, deserves attention. For example, it can by assumed that socioeconomic condition differences among countries are linked with housing quality and concomitant outcomes. It could, however, also well be that the interplay between objective and perceived housing antecedents and healthy aging outcomes is so fundamental in nature that rather similar relations may be observed across a diversity of country backgrounds. In conclusion, the ENABLE-AGE explicitly merged OT (such as the WHO, 2001) and GP (such as the ecological theory of aging) perspectives. In addition, disciplines such as human geography, medicine, and sociology were also acknowledged.

Core Methodology Components of the ENABLE-AGE Project

The project included three study arms: (1) The ENABLE-AGE Survey Study; (2) the ENABLE-AGE In-Depth Study; (3) the ENABLE-AGE Update Review. *The ENABLE-AGE Survey Study*, from which selected findings will be summarized below, was based on a comprehensive questionnaire incorporating a wide range of well-proven self-report scales and observational formats, along with project-specific questions on housing and health. Data were collected at two occasions, spaced one year apart with a reduced assessment battery applied at follow-up. The *ENABLE-AGE In-Depth Study* focused on very old peoples' understandings of the meaning and experience of home in relation to health, well-being, and aging. The *ENABLE-AGE Update Review* gathered detailed documentation of building norms and guidelines in each country. In addition, national key policy topics related to housing older people were identified.

Because of differences in the population mean age and life expectancy between West/Central and East European countries, the use of the same age strata across countries was regarded as an inadequate approach, particularly for very old persons. For instance, given the life expectancies at birth in 2002 (study start) of 77 years of age (men) and 82 years of age (women) in Sweden as compared to 65 years of age (men) and 77 years of age (women) in Latvia, using the same age groups would have led, in Latvia, to a much more positively selected group of survivors as compared to Sweden (Iwarsson et al., 2004). In addition, given the fact that far fewer people in East European countries reach very old age, it would have been difficult to recruit sufficient numbers of participants in Latvia and Hungary. In order to adjust for such unbalanced positive selectivity, in Sweden, Germany, and the UK, the "younger" age groups comprised participants aged 81–84 years and the "older" 85–89 years. The corresponding age groups in Hungary and Latvia were selected as those aged 75–79 years and 80–84 years, respectively. In addition, only persons living alone in urban households were included (Iwarsson et al., 2004). The sample was stratified for gender with the aim of 25% men in each national sample. However, this was only partially achieved, particularly in the East European countries, because of the difficulties of recruiting very old men living alone. The final ENABLE-AGE Survey Study sample at baseline comprised 1,918 participants. Details of the national samples and of the methods used are provided in Nygren et al. (2007) and Oswald et al. (2007).

Selected Findings Based on the ENABLE-AGE Survey Study

A specific challenge in the p-e literature in aging is the explicit differentiation between environmental barriers and accessibility problems. Driven by the ecological theory of aging (Lawton, 1999) as well as the notion of p-e fit (Carp, 1987; Iwarsson, 2004), the term accessibility is seen as a relative concept since it expresses the relationship between the capacity of the person and the demands of the environment. Thus, accessibility is an important aspect of p-e-fit, comprising two components: the personal component describes the person's functional limitations and the environmental component describes physical environmental barriers.

An issue important for understanding the course and role of accessibility as people age is the detailed description of environmental barriers, recently addressed by Iwarsson, Nygren, Oswald, Wahl, and Tomsone (2006) based on Swedish, German, and Latvian ENABLE-AGE data. The findings revealed that environmental barriers were very common and in all three national samples the most prevalent environmental barriers were found in 77–98% of all dwellings investigated. Five out of the 20 most prevalent environmental barriers were found indoors, and they were all related to upper extremity skills. For example, "turning motion of wrist required" in kitchen/laundry room and in general in the dwelling (separate items for different parts of the home, $n = 2$), and "use requires hands" in kitchen/laundry room, hygiene room, and in general in the dwelling (separate items for different parts of the home, $n = 3$) were very prevalent in all three samples (83–98%). The analysis identifying the 20 single environmental barriers generating the "heaviest" accessibility problems at T1 in each of the three national samples demonstrated that four barriers were common; three were outdoors ("path and surfaces not level"; "high kerbs;" "no/too few seating places") and one was indoors ("wall-mounted cupboards in kitchen placed extremely high"). The results demonstrate in great detail the prevalence of environmental barriers and the magnitude of accessibility problems in housing. There were considerable similarities among the three national samples, showing that older people, to a large extent, live in houses with environmental barriers, especially in hygiene rooms and at entrances.

The purpose of a second study (Nygren et al., 2007) was to explore relationships between aspects of objective and perceived housing and to investigate whether cross-national comparable patterns exist across all five national ENABLE-AGE samples. The results demonstrated that it is not objective environmental barriers as such, but the p-e fit aspect accessibility that is related to perceived aspects of housing. For example, very old persons living in more accessible housing perceived their home as more useful and meaningful in relation to their routines and everyday activities and they perceived themselves as less externally controlled in relation to their housing. In addition, the relationships between objective and perceived aspects of housing were comparable across different countries. These relationships reflect the fundamental character of the home environment and aging-in-place issues, and they seem to be rather independent from the sociocultural background and socioeconomic conditions of different countries. Thus, objective and perceived aspects of housing have to be considered in order to understand the dynamics of aging in place.

The aim of a third study (Oswald et al., 2007) was to examine the relationship between aspects of objective and perceived housing and aspects of healthy aging, defined as independence in daily activities and subjective well-being. This research also examined the comparability of relationships between housing and healthy aging in the five countries involved in the ENABLE-AGE Project. Objective aspects of housing were again seen as a facet of p-e fit, referred to as accessibility (Iwarsson & Ståhl, 2003). The term *perceived housing* addressed a scope of subjective phenomena of experiences related to housing: housing satisfaction, usability, meaning of home, and housing-related control beliefs (Oswald et al., 2007). The findings underscored that participants living in more accessible homes, who perceive their home as meaningful and useful, and who think that external influences are not responsible for their housing situation were more independent in daily activities and had a better sense of well-being. In particular, it was not the number of environmental barriers in the home environment, but the magnitude of accessibility problems that was substantially related to different aspects of healthy aging. Moreover, these results applied consistently to all five national samples. Taken together, the findings of the ENABLE-AGE Project can widen the perspective when striving for barrier-free building standards, to encompass a holistic approach that takes both objective and perceived aspects of housing into account. In practical terms, the insights derived point to the need that home modification and relocation should not simply be prescribed, but need to be negotiated with older persons to take into account their personal preferences as mirrored in terms of perceived aspects of housing.

Conclusions and Future Challenges

Since the 1990s, European research on p-e relations in old age has substantially addressed all the major contents of physical environment and levels of analysis as outlined in Table 1, and there have also been significant contributions to the advancement of methodology in the field of environmental gerontology. Currently, GP as well as OT are playing major roles in the progression of p-e research concerned with aging. A telling example for this is the ENABLE-AGE Project. Furthermore, social scientists and scholars with a background in technology are adding to the development of environmental gerontology in Europe.

Findings of p-e research in Europe are, in many respects, able to underscore that physical environments are critical for maintaining a high quality of life as people age. On the one hand, research demonstrating the importance of objective and perceived housing for a variety of major outcomes such as functional ability and well-being has been important for recent developments. On the other hand, the simultaneous consideration of objective *and* perceived housing aspects reveals substantial and differential relationships with a wider set of healthy aging outcomes. Such a comprehensive perspective probably reflects day-to-day adaptation processes related to housing better than single views, whether concerned with objective or perceived housing. Out-of-home environments also add substantially to the understanding of quality of life in old age. According to recent research, subjective mobility-related aspects such as the importance of going out and satisfaction with the possibilities to pursue leisure time activities, are significant predictors of life satisfaction. The analytic entity of neighborhood or city district is particularly useful in research on out-of-home activities throughout the aging process, because this is the territory beyond the home in which most of the daily life of aging individuals, especially very old persons, unfolds. Finally, findings related to technology and products, particularly regarding assistive technology, revealed on many levels how important it is to concentrate research efforts on the needs of the aging user. As much research has underscored, technology and products such as assistive devices can make a huge difference in the quality of life of older persons, but much depends on adequate fit between the persons' capabilities and needs and the design of the respective product.

Though different levels of analysis have been applied in recent European p-e research, there still is a gap in the literature here, but this also applies to international environmental gerontology research at large (Wahl & Gitlin, 2007). Research strategies involving data collection on the individual level as well as on building regulations and housing policy are a major prerequisite for this approach (Iwarsson et al., 2004). However, the real challenge comes with the conceptual and empirical bridge-building between the micro to meso and the meso to macro levels in all three content areas (home environments, out-of-home environments, technology and products), and convincing research in this regard still seems to be mostly ahead of us.

There has also been substantial progression in terms of cross-country comparisons across Europe in all three content areas. Let us mention here the ENABLE-AGE Project in the context of home environments, MOBILATE and SIZE regarding out-of-home environments, and the Technology Initiative for Disabled and Elderly People (TIDE; see also Mollenkopf et al., 2001) with respect to technology and products. The challenges of comparative research, though a major resource of recent as well as forthcoming European aging research, should not be underestimated (Tesch-Römer & von Kondratowitz, 2006). That is, issues such as different social policy and legislation systems, different languages, and different traditions of what autonomy means all deserve careful consideration in the generation, accomplishment, and interpretation of p-e studies. There is, however, also early evidence that fundamental relationships between objective and perceived housing and major healthy-aging target variables may be rather similar across European countries, even though economic conditions and, thus, objective housing quality for older people remain quite diverse.

References

Baltes, M.M., Maas, I., Wilms, H.-U., Borchelt, M.F., & Little, T. (1999). Everyday competence in old and very old age: Theoretical considerations and empirical findings. In P.B. Baltes & K.-U. Mayer (Eds.), *The Berlin aging study* (pp. 384–402). Cambridge, UK: Cambridge University Press.

Baltes, M.M., & Wahl, H.-W. (1992). The dependency-support script in institutions: Generalization to community settings. *Psychology and Aging, 7,* 409–418.

Bianchetti, A., Benvenuti, P., Ghisla, K.M., Frisoni, G.B., & Trabucchi, M. (1997). An Italian model of dementia special care unit: Results of a pilot study. *Alzheimer Disease and Associated Disorders, 11*(1), 53–56.

Bouma, H., & Graafmans, J.A.M. (Eds.). (1992). *Gerontechnology.* Amsterdam: IOS Press.

Brandt, Å., Iwarsson, S., & Ståhl, A. (2004). Older people's use of powered wheelchairs for activity and participation. *Journal of Rehabilitation Medicine, 36*(2), 70–77.

Burholt, V., & Naylor, D. (2005). The relationship between rural community type and attachment to place for older people living in North Wales, UK. *European Journal of Ageing, 2,* 109–119.

Carp, F.M. (1987). Environment and aging. In D. Stokols & I. Altman (Eds.), *Handbook of environmental psychology* (Vol. 1, pp. 330–360). New York: Wiley.

Cohen, U., & Weisman, G. (1991). *Holding on to home: Designing environments for people with dementia.* Baltimore, MD: Johns Hopkins University Press.

Dahlin-Ivanoff, S., & Sonn, U. (2005). Changes in the use of assistive devices among 90-year-old persons. *Aging Clinical and Experimental Research, 17,* 246–251.

Deeg, D.J.H., & Thomése, F. (2005). Discrepancies between personal income and neighborhood status: Effects on physical and metal health. *European Journal of Ageing, 2,* 98–108.

Elmstahl, S., Annerstedt, L., & Ahlund, O. (1997). How should a group living unit for demented elderly be designed to decrease psychiatric symptoms? *Alzheimer Disease and Associated Disorders, 11*(1), 47–52.

Fänge, A., & Iwarsson, S. (1999). Physical housing environment – development of a self-assessment instrument. *Canadian Journal of Occupational Therapy, 66,* 250–260.

Fänge, A., & Iwarsson, S. (2003). Accessibility and usability in housing – construct validity and implications for research and practice. *Disability and Rehabilitation, 25,* 1316–1325.

Fänge, A., & Iwarsson, S. (2005a). Changes in accessibility and aspects of usability in housing over time – An exploration of the housing adaptation process. *Occupational Therapy International, 12*(1), 44–59.

Fänge, A., & Iwarsson, S. (2005b). Changes in ADL dependence and aspects of usability following housing adaptation – A longitudinal perspective. *American Journal of Occupational Therapy, 59,* 296–304.

Fernandez-Ballesteros, R. (2001). Environmental conditions, health, and satisfaction among the elderly: Some empirical results. *Psicithema, 13*(1), 40–49.

Fernandez-Ballesteros, R., Montorio, M., & Izal, M.I. (1998). Personal and environmental relationship among the elderly living in residential settings. *Archives of Gerontology and Geriatrics, 26,* 185–198.

Haak, M., Dahlin-Ivanoff, S., Fänge, A., Sixsmith, J., & Iwarsson, S. (in press). Home as the base and starting point for participation – Experiences among very old Swedish people. *Occupational Therapy Journal of Research.*

Hedberg-Kristensson, E., Dahlin-Ivanoff, S., & Iwarsson, S. (2006). Participation in the prescription process of mobility devices – Experiences among older patients. *British Journal of Occupational Therapy, 69,* 169–176.

Hedberg-Kristensson, E., Dahlin-Ivanoff, S., & Iwarsson, S. (2007). Experiences among older persons using mobility devices. *Disability and Rehabilitation: Assistive Technology, 2,* 15–22.

Hovbrandt, P., Fridlund, B., & Carlsson, G. (in press). Very old people's experience of occupational performance outside home: Possibilities and limitations. *Scandinavian Journal of Occupational Therapy.*

Iwarsson, S. (1998). Environmental influences on the cumulative structure of instrumental ADL: An example in osteoporosis patients in a Swedish rural district. *Clinical Rehabilitation, 12,* 221–227.

Iwarsson, S. (2004). Assessing the fit between older people and their home environments – An occupational therapy research perspective. In H.-W. Wahl, R. Scheidt, & P. Windley (Eds.), *Focus on aging in context: Socio-physical environments. Annual review of the Gerontological Society of America* (Vol. 23, pp. 85–109). New York: Springer Publishing.

Iwarsson, S. (2005). A long-term perspective on p-e fit and ADL dependence among older Swedish adults. *Gerontologist, 45*(3), 327–36.

Iwarsson, S., Nygren, C., Oswald, F., Wahl, H.-W., & Tomsone, S. (2006). Environmental barriers and housing accessibility problems in three European countries. *Journal of Housing for the Elderly, 20*(3), 23–43.

Iwarsson, S., Nygren, C., & Slaug, B. (2005). Cross-national and multiprofessional interrater reliability of the Housing Enabler. *Scandinavian Journal of Occupational Therapy, 12*(1), 29–39.

Iwarsson, S., & Ståhl, A. (2003). Accessibility, usability, and universal design – Positioning and definition of concepts describing p-e relationships. *Disability and Rehabilitation, 25,* 57–66.

Iwarsson, S., Wahl, H.-W., & Nygren, C. (2004). Challenges of cross-national housing research with older people: Lessons learned from the ENABLE-AGE Project. *European Journal of Ageing, 1,* 79–88.

Iwarsson, S., Wahl, H.-W., Nygren, C., Oswald, F., Sixsmith, A., Sixsmith, J. et al. (2007). Importance of the home environment for healthy aging: Conceptual and methodological background of the European ENABLE-AGE Project. *Gerontologist, 47,* 78–84.

Kielhofner, G. (2002). *Model of human occupation* (3rd ed.). Baltimore: Lippincott, Williams, & Williams.

Lawton, M.P. (1999). Environmental taxonomy: Generalizations from research with older adults. In S.L. Friedman & T.D. Wachs (Eds.), *Measuring environment across the lifespan* (pp. 91–124). Washington, DC: American Psychological Association.

Löfqvist, C., Nygren, C., Széman, Z., & Iwarsson, S. (2005). Assistive devices among very old people in five European countries. *Scandinavian Journal of Occupational Therapy, 12,* 181–192.

Margot-Cattin, I., & Nygård, L. (2006). Access technology and dementia care: Influences on resident's everyday lives in a secure unit. *Scandinavian Journal of Occupational Therapy, 13,* 113–124.

Mollenkopf, H., Kaspar, R., & Wahl, H.-W. (2005). The mobility rich and mobility poor. In H. Mollenkopf, F. Marcellini, I. Ruoppila, Z. Széman & M. Tacken (Eds.), *Enhancing mobility in later life. Personal coping, environmental resources, and technical support. The out-of-*

home mobility of older adults in urban and rural regions of five European countries (pp. 289–294). Amsterdam: IOS Press.

Mollenkopf, H., Marcellini, F., Ruoppila, I., Széman, Z., & Tacken, M. (Eds.). (2005). *Enhancing mobility in later life. Personal coping, environmental resources, and technical support. The out-of-home mobility of older adults in urban and rural regions of five European countries* (Vol. 17). Amsterdam: IOS Press.

Mollenkopf, H., Mix, S., Gäng, K., & Kwon, S. (2001). Alter und Technik [Age and technology]. In Deutsches Zentrum für Altersfragen (Ed.), *Personale, gesundheitliche und Umweltressourcen im Alter* [Person-, health-, and environment-related resources in old age] (Vol. 1, Expertisen zum Dritten Altenbericht der Bundesregierung, pp. 253–438). Opladen, Germany: Leske + Budrich.

Nygren, C., Oswald, F., Iwarsson, S., Fänge, A., Sixsmith, J., Schilling, O. et al. (2007). Relationships between objective and perceived housing in very old age: Results from the EN-ABLE-AGE Project. *Gerontologist, 47*, 85–95.

Oswald, F., Hieber, A., Wahl, H.-W., & Mollenkopf, H. (2005). Ageing and person-environment fit in different urban neighborhoods. *European Journal of Ageing, 2*, 88–97.

Oswald, F., & Wahl, H.-W. (2005). Dimensions of the meaning of home in later life. In G.D. Rowles & H. Chaudhury (Eds.), *Home and identity in later life. International perspectives* (pp. 21–46). New York: Springer Verlag.

Oswald, F., Wahl, H.-W., & Kaspar, R. (2005). Psychological aspects of outdoor mobility in later life. In H. Mollenkopf, F. Marcellini, I. Ruoppila, Z. Széman, & M. Tacken (Eds.), *Enhancing mobility in later life. Personal coping, environmental resources, and technical support. The out-of-home mobility of older adults in urban and rural regions of five European countries* (pp. 173–194). Amsterdam: IOS Press.

Oswald, F., Wahl, H.-W., Martin, M., & Mollenkopf, H. (2003). Toward measuring proactivity in person-environment transactions in late adulthood: The housing-related Control Beliefs Questionnaire. *Journal of Housing for the Elderly, 17*(1/2), 135–152.

Oswald, F., Wahl, H.-W., Mollenkopf, H., & Schilling, O. (2003). Housing and life satisfaction of older adults in two rural regions in Germany. *Research on Aging, 25*, 122–143.

Oswald, F., Wahl, H.-W., Schilling, O., Nygren, C., Fänge, A., Sixsmith, A. et al. (2007). Relationships between housing and healthy aging in very old age. *Gerontologist, 47*, 96–107.

Peace, S.M. (1993). The living environments of older women. In M. Bernard & K. Meade (Eds.), *Women come of age: Perspectives on the lives of older women* (pp. 126–145). London: Edward Arnold.

Peace, S.M. (2005). *Environment and identity in later life.* Berkshire: Open University Press.

Peace, S.M., & Holland, C. (Eds.). (2001). *Inclusive housing in an aging society: Innovative approaches.* Bristol, UK: The Policy Press.

Roelands, M., von Oost, P., Buysse, A., & Depoorter, A.M. (2002). Awareness among community-dwelling elderly of assistive devices for mobility and self-care and attitudes toward their use. *Social Science and Medicine, 54*, 1441–1451.

Rudinger, G. (1996). Alter und Technik [Age and technology]. *Zeitschrift für Gerontologie und Geriatrie, 29*, 246–256.

Saup, W. (2003). *Betreutes Seniorenwohnen im Urteil der Bewohner. Ergebnisse der Augsburger Längsschnittstudie (Bd. 2)* [Assisted living as rated by residents. Findings of the Augsburg Longitudinal Study, Vol. 2]. Augsburg, Germany: Möckl.

Scharf, T., Phillipson, C., & Smith, A.E. (2005). Social exclusion of older people in deprived urban communities of England. *European Journal of Ageing, 2*, 76–87.

Scharf, T., & Wenger, G.C. (2000). Cross-national empirical research in gerontology: The OPERA experience. *Education and Ageing, 15*, 379–397.

Selwyn, N., Gorard, S., Furlong, J., & Madden, L. (2003). Older adults' use of information and communications technology in everyday life. *Ageing and Society, 23*, 561–582.

Sixsmith, A.J., & Sixsmith, J.A. (1991). Transition in home experience in later life. *Journal of Architectural and Planning Research, 8,* 181–191.

Slangen-de Kort, Y. (1999). *A tale of two adaptations. Coping processes of older persons in the domain of independent living.* Eindhoven, the Netherlands: University Press Facilities.

Spillman, B.C. (2004). Changes in elderly disability rates and the implications for health care utilization and cost. *Milbank Quarterly, 82*(1), 157–194.

Ståhl, A., & Iwarsson, S. (2004). "Let's go for a walk" – A project focusing on accessibility, safety, and security for older people in the outdoor environment. Annual Scientific Meeting of the Gerontological Society of America, Washington, USA, Nov. 19–23. *Gerontologist, 44* (Special issue I), 151–151.

Steinfeld, E., & Tauke, B. (2002). Universal designing. In J. Christophersen (Ed.), *Universal design. 17 ways of thinking and teaching* (pp. 165–189). Oslo, Norway: Husbanken.

Tesch-Römer, C., & von Kondratowitz, H.-J. (2006). Comparative aging research: A flourishing field in need of theoretical cultivation. *European Journal of Ageing, 3,* 155–167.

Valdemarsson, M., Jernryd, E., & Iwarsson, S. (2005). Preferences and frequencies of visits to public facilities in old age – A pilot study. *Archives of Gerontology and Geriatrics, 40,* 15–28.

Wahl, H.-W., & Gitlin, L.N. (2007). Environmental gerontology. In J.E. Birren (Ed.), *Encyclopedia of gerontology* (2nd ed., pp. 494–501). Oxford, UK: Elsevier.

Wahl, H.-W., & Mollenkopf, H. (2003). Impact of everyday technology in the home environment on older adults' quality of life. In K.W. Schaie & N. Charness (Eds.), *Impact of technology on successful aging* (pp. 215–241). New York: Springer Verlag.

Wahl, H.-W., Oswald, F., & Zimprich, D. (1999). Everyday competence in visually impaired older adults: A case for person-environment perspectives. *The Gerontologist, 39,* 140–149.

Wahl, H.-W., & Weisman, G. (2003). Environmental gerontology at the beginning of the new millennium: Reflections on its historical, empirical, and theoretical development. *The Gerontologist, 43,* 616–627.

World Health Organization. (2001). *International classification of functioning, disability, and health (ICF).* Geneva, Switzerland: Author.

5. Semantic Memory in Healthy Aging

Herminia Peraita

Introduction

One of the most striking findings in the recent scientific literature on categories and concepts (thus, semantic memory [SM]) is the existence of two theoretical areas. Although these areas have taken different yet parallel paths for more than 25 years and have merged only recently, the fact that there is little literature on SM in healthy aging means that our knowledge thereof has come from our observations on memory disorders. It is this merge that is of interest to us; in particular, memory disorders that occur in pathological aging, such as those resulting from neurodegenerative diseases and other brain pathologies, e.g., cranial-encephalic injury (CEI), cerebro-vascular accidents (CVA), and herpes simplex encephalitis (HSE).

The literature in question is that which, in the 1970s, 1980s, and early 1990s, attempted to analyze in depth the structure, organization, and representation of semantic categories. It did so through an analysis of the different models of representation that intended to overcome the classical model of the representation of concepts and categories, in particular, exemplar models and prototypes, as well as hybrids that emerged from these (Rosch, 1976; Rosch & Mervis, 1975; Smith, Shoben, & Rips, 1974; Smith & Medin, 1981). On the other hand, the neuropsychological literature (mainly the clinical literature) is based on case studies (although groups were later studied) that have had little theoretical basis in categories and concepts and even less in SM. In fact, this literature began to examine certain types of deterioration of this memory system, and found problems in naming, verbal fluency, classification, verification of properties, etc.

Certain types of deterioration found in elderly subjects with specific clinical problems such as those mentioned above were very striking, and one of these meant having a differential knowledge of one of the two main semantic domains that make up what we call natural categories: living (animate) beings and nonliving (inanimate) things. This type of problem is called semantic categorical dissociation and is currently a priority interest in the field (Aronoff, Gonnerman, Almor, Arunachalam, Kempler, & Andersen, 2006; Moss & Tyler, 2000; Sartori & Lombardi, 2004; Zannino & Perri, 2006).

Most neuropsychology studies from the 1980s and 1990s do not refer to the theories, models, experimental findings, and descriptions from the categories and concepts field. Therefore, we believe that the analysis and interpretations have lacked sufficient theoretical support. In fact, this may be one of the reasons for the difficulty in interpreting many of the phenomena found in this field, and for much of the controversy surrounding categorical dissociation (Barbarotto, Capitani, & Laiacona, 2001; Borgo & Schallice, 2003; Bright, Moss, & Tyler, 2004).

This situation began to change at the end of the 1990s and especially from 2000 onward, when a series of authors began to adopt the theories and models of categories and concepts from cognitive psychology as an interpretative framework of the data obtained from subjects with specific semantic problems (Tyler & Moss, 1997).

Currently, after several years of intense debate about the nature, entity, principles of organization, and representation of SM in the brain from the field of cognitive neuropsychology, there is renewed interest in some of the basic principles on which the psychology of natural categories and concepts has been built. Furthermore, there is a need to reconsider the findings, experimental phenomena, and explanatory mechanisms on which a large part of the scientific literature at that time was based, so as to integrate data that is often contradictory (e.g., those stemming from the innumerable empirical studies on categorical dissociations) (Dudas, Clague, Thompson, Graham, & Hodges, 2005).

As Hampton and Moss (2003) say, representation and conceptual processing play the main roles in all cognitive processing, whether it be linguistic processing, reasoning, inferences, decision making, etc. In fact, the themes that are covered in conceptual processing refer to acquisition of meanings and concepts, knowledge about the attributes of objects, the relationship with words and syntax, as well as the interface with sensory-motor systems.

As for the representational format of the conceptual structure, which represents the nucleus of SM, there continues to be controversy as to whether there is a simple static system of amodal conceptual representations, or rather a multimodal distributed network in which the conceptual representations converge. In addition to these two possibilities there exists a third based on categorical domains (Caramazza & Shelton, 1998), although we will not analyze this here, despite its genuine interest.

What is Semantic Memory?

Before approaching the subject of SM in aging itself, it is advisable to examine briefly whether memory in general suffers impairment in old age as is thought, or if, on the contrary, it remains intact. As Maylor (2005) recently indicates in a brief yet illustrative review of the subject, three aspects could affect the impairment of memory in old age: the absence of or decrease in inhibitory control, the decrease in the speed of cognitive processing, and the limited resources in processing, both to encode information and to recover it and bring it to mind at the right time.

Based on these three aspects of cognitive processing, the author offers extensive experimental data as to how each of the memory systems is affected (short-term, long-term: episodic and semantic, implicit, explicit, etc.), concluding that practically all of them, with the exception of implicit memory, are affected in one way or another in old age, more because of the processing problems cited above than to problems of memory itself. At the same time, the author points out the enormous individual differences in this field in old age, as is the case in many other cognitive processes. The author also warns of the excessive generalization to real life of experimental data in memory tasks obtained in the laboratory, as in daily tasks it is perfectly possible to live with mild memory impairments even though constant forgetting can produce high levels of frustration.

Thus, we can affirm that SM is the part of the human memory system that refers to the knowledge the subject has of concepts, the meaning of words, and of the surrounding world (facts, actions, events, persons). It is a declarative, explicit (as opposed to implicit), long-term (as opposed to short-term) memory system, which allows the subject to maintain in memory the meanings of words, concepts and categories, and facts and events of the world (Budson, Bruce, & Price, 2005). It is closely linked to the semantic and pragmatic components of language as well as to the lexical system. According to some authors, SM actually covers all knowledge of the world, with the result that it has become a mixed bag, including geographical, historical, and social knowledge. Therefore, we prefer a stricter conception that makes it equivalent to the system that allows us to know, store, and process the meaning of words and categories of the world (animals, plants, tools, instruments, etc.), as well as their representation and organization in our brain. The connection with the perceptual and linguistic systems is obvious but will not be dealt with here. Therefore, remembering the difficult conditions of the World Wars or the 9/11 attack on the Twin Towers would belong to the episodic memory system, but the fact that we know what a war or terrorist act means belongs to the SM system.

The organization of SM in the brain – the anatomy of memory – is clearly delimited. Semantic memory seems to be situated in the left hemisphere, specifically in the cingulate cortex, in the prefrontal cortex, and in the superior temporal area (Squire & Zola-Morgan, 1991). Not all authors defend this conception, i.e., that semantic memory is akin to declarative knowledge with a basis in some areas of the brain; in fact, some authors support the theory of the temporary activation of a series of neuronal networks that extend over various areas of the brain (Fuster, 2003).

How is the Memory System Affected by Aging? Does it Suffer Deterioration or Dysfunction?

This system, in principle, does not suffer any deterioration in healthy old age or aging. In fact, on the contrary, since the system is very dependent on the knowledge of the world, a greater and deeper knowledge of this and its relationships results in a complex semantic network in which the meanings become intertwined, and the neuronal networks that serve as a support become more diversified. What is affected in healthy old age, but should not be confused with any type of pathology, is the system of lexical access (and of executive function), which is the linguistic system that allows us to select the correct or pertinent word in a specific context. This means that the naming of objects, localization of specific proper nouns, and even fluency in conversation are affected. Therefore, healthy aging is relatively free of semantic problems. Whether we accept the wider definition of SM as an encyclopedic knowledge of the world, or the stricter definition of the knowledge of meanings of things and words, it is clear that both aspects are enriched in old age. Knowledge and concepts tend to be denser and richer in old age than at other points in life, unless the person has had a neurodegenerative condition such as Alzheimer's disease (AD), semantic dementia, etc. As we have already said, what does occur in healthy aging is a diminished ability to access the lexicon, i.e., the words and not their meaning, or a less automatic access, which is what often prevents us from finding a word that a specific situation requires. This should not be confused with any semantic memory disorder, but is in fact a diminished executive function.

However, in aging affected by neurodegenerative disorders, certain areas that support memory systems in the brain and the connections between them may be affected. Semantic memory is affected, with a gradual loss of the knowledge of meanings of words, of concepts, of the use of objects, and the meanings of actions. Despite the controversy of the mid-1980s about this memory system and whether it is affected or not in AD, it seems clear today that this system is greatly damaged (Budson et al., 2005). Even in cases of loss or impairment of SM in neurodegenerative pathologies, such as AD, it is not clear if there is a loss of semantic information or an inability to access it. On the other hand, there are also doubts about the pattern of evolution: Whether category attributes are lost first or if it is the categories themselves. The principal object of investigation in the last 20 years has been the subject of specific deficits of categories, which we refer to below.

Given the difficulty of approaching such a complex system through experimental and measurable tasks, and taking into account all its manifestations of deterioration and loss, research has only focused on some aspects of SM. One of the more controversial aspects has been the interpretation of the differential loss of some types of semantic categories (living beings) in comparison with others (nonliving things), or vice versa. These problems have generated a lively debate for almost 20 years, from the pioneering work of Warrington and Shallice (1984) and Warrington and McCarthy (1987) in the UK until now (Lyons, Kay, Hanley, & Haslam, 2006).

As mentioned above, the interest in studying SM in aging is very recent. It arises from the discovery that certain pathologies and/or cognitive disorders during old age are related to a gradual loss of one of the two large domains in semantic categories. This is generally the category of living beings, while the knowledge of the other large semantic area, that of nonliving things, remains more or less intact for longer. The opposite can also occur, whereby the category of nonliving things is lost first. As a result of these findings, a series of questions arises that researchers in this field have been trying to answer for more than 20 years. This has driven current research to analyze the semantic content of categories and concepts through an analysis of the features, attributes, or properties that configure them (For an extensive review see Capitani, Laiacona, Mahon, & Caramazza, 2003). The questions posed are the following:

– Why do some patients with specific pathologies and/or injuries to the central nervous system (CNS) present a categorical dissociation?
– Why does this categorical dissociation tend to be of a specific type, i.e., the preservation of artifacts and the loss of knowledge of living things, as opposed to the contrary?
– Why are there occasions when the distinction between domains (living/nonliving

and/or animate/inanimate) is not preserved, e.g., with musical instruments and parts of the body considered as living things? Why are there dissociations within a domain?

- Which theory best fits the data obtained over the last 20 years?
- Should conceptual organization based on features and attributes be maintained? Is this now strictly necessary?

Different European groups have tried to give answers to these questions. The main focus of the technical debate is centered on whether the semantic categorical representations are based on features or whether they are based on categorical domains, and, in the first case, what features, attributes, or properties configure the semantic categories both in the domain of living beings and in that of nonliving things.

Recently, the prevailing explanation seems to be the existence of an intrinsic advantage in the processing of categories of nonliving things as opposed to living beings (Perri et al., 2003; Zannino, Perri, Carlesimo, Pasqualetti, & Caltagirone, 2002) that lies in a categorical physiological asymmetry. In other words, healthy elderly people, as with everyone else, process the categories of nonliving things more easily than that of living beings, as seen in explicit tasks (naming and pairing) as well as implicit tasks (semantic priming).

Methodological Criticisms of this Type of Research: The Artifactual Hypothesis

Some authors have argued that most studies on categorical dissociations during the last 20 years lack suitable methodological control of certain variables that may have a decisive effect on the type of task used to evaluate knowledge and semantic deterioration (Funnell & Sheridan, 1992; Stewart, Parkin, & Hunkin, 1992; Gaffan & Heywood, 1993.)

Some of the decisive variables in the duration and preservation of the meaning of words (thus, of concepts) in the mind of the person, in other words, the stability and maintenance of the conceptual and categorical structure, depend on the age of acquisition of the word/concept, the frequency of use, familiarity with it, as well as its structural complexity.

It is not easy to study some of these variables in old people, even though some studies have attempted to do so, through subjective valuation scales (Cuetos, Dobarro, & Martínez, 2005; Moreno-Martínez & Peraita, 2007).

Think of the difficulty that an old person has to remember reliably the age at which he/she acquired the word or concept "zebra," or the subjectivity in the assessment of familiarity with certain concepts. There is also the possibility of an interaction between the familiarity of concepts and categories and the gender of the subjects, which is related to bio-socio-cultural contexts. With regard to the differential processing of semantic categories based on gender, the results are not at all conclusive. Capitani, Barbarotto, and Laiacona (2005), Laiacona, Barbarotto, and Capitani (1998), and Laws (1999) found conclusive results whereas other authors (Fung et al., 2001) did not. How can we explain this? Some authors resort to an explanation based on evolutionary pressure on the brain, which has been influenced by the environment over millions of years.

The complex interaction between the variables cited and the absence of control in many experimental studies has made certain authors doubt the analytical rigor of categorical dissociations and suggest the absolute need to control them.

Methods and Procedures

Measuring the Integrity or Deterioration of Semantic Memory

The procedures and tasks used to evaluate semantic memory are as follows: object-naming or picture-naming task, which is easy to apply yet complex in its interpretation as it can indicate perceptual misidentification as well as impaired lexical access and loss of semantic stores; verbal fluency, in which very different processes are involved, such as lexical retrieval, attentional retrieval, or semantic working memory; and others including categorization tasks, object-word matching, object recognition, object decision, attribute production, and verification.

In summary, the SM that refers to knowledge of natural categories and objects from the surrounding world, as well as knowledge of the meaning of words, actions, and events, presents no problem in aging, except in those cases in which certain types of neurodegenerative problems or conditions appear. In these cases, the whole semantic system suffers, the most widely studied deterioration being that involving a series of specific semantic dissociations of certain categories.

European Groups and Their Contributions to the Field of Semantic Category-Specific Deficits in the Framework of Semantic Memory on Aging

Without doubt, the most active research groups in this field have been those from the UK and Italy, with a minority group formed by authors from the rest of Europe, such as France, Belgium, and Portugal, although these are more "isolated" researchers. Since this chapter has basically focused on a specific problem that emerges when the semantic memory is impaired in aging, and this in turn has led to the creation of models, theories, and hypotheses of the structure, organization, and processing of this memory system in old age, we will use the same idea when citing these groups and their lines of research. It is also important to point out that much of the research is, in fact, indebted to Caramazza and his group (Caramazza, Shelton, Hillis, Rapp, & Romani).

Apart from the pioneering work by Warrington and Shallice (1984), and Warrington and McCarthy (1987) in the UK, Silveri, Daniele, Giustolosi, and Gianotti (1991) were, in Italy, the first researchers to discover categorical dissociations in AD patients and living and nonliving things.

Warrington and others interpreted the cases of their patients within the framework of the *sensory-functional theory* (Warrington & McCarthy, 1987; Warrington & Shallice, 1984), which states that there are two large blocks of attributes or characteristics: sensory characteristics, which are closely linked to visual perception, and functional characteristics, which are closely linked to encyclopedic knowledge of the world. Each of these large blocks characterizes one of the two great domains: the first – sensory/perceptual – the domain of living beings, and the second – functional – that of nonliving things or artifacts. Therefore, SM would be organized on the basis of specific sensory modalities. Furthermore, Moss and Tyler (Tyler, Moss, Durrant-Peatfield, & Levy, 2000; Moss, Tyler, & Devlin, 2002), also from the UK, based their work on the concept of semantic space and on the density of the attributes that are correlated between the exemplars of the categories, i.e., more on this concept of correlation between attributes and distinctiveness thereof than on the analysis of types of attributes and than that of semantic categories (feature *distinctiveness* from the *conceptual structure account*).

For the Caramazza group, however, SM has a genuine categorical structure, and it has been evolutionary adaptation and the subsequent evolutionary pressure that has led to this categorical structure being organized into two large domains.

Therefore, all these concepts (types of features, correlation between them across the different categories, distinctiveness, and relevance) overlap with the two large conceptions of the architecture of SM: that based on sensory modalities and the one based on a unitary amodal system.

Rico Duarte (2004), in France, tackles the methodological difficulties that emerge in the evaluation of SM and analyzes the little existing research on the influence of age on the semantic system. She indicates as an objection to the research the fact that (as mentioned at the beginning of the chapter), in general, SM is evaluated through tasks that have more to do with cultural knowledge and verbal skills (vocabulary, synonyms, geographical knowledge) than with SM as such. She claims that SM in healthy aging is only affected in self-initiated activities and in fast cognitive processing such as verbal fluency, naming, etc. Therefore, it is the exploitation and use of knowledge that would be affected rather than the knowledge itself. She is interested in the processing of living and nonliving concepts in healthy people and not only in pathological aging. In order to explore this question, she subscribes to the accounts considering that this dissociation reflects differences in the internal structure of conceptual domains.

These proposals have the advantage of characterizing the structure of the conceptual domains by advancing several probable factors of organization to explain their dysfunction. Within this framework, we can find the propositions about the feature types from the *sensory-functional theory* (SFT; Warrington & McCarthy, 1987; Warrington & Shallice, 1984), the notion of feature inter-correlation from the *organized unitary content hypothesis* (OUCH; the group of Caramazza, Hillis, Rapp, & Romani), and feature distinctiveness from the *conceptual structure account* (CSA, Tyler et al., 2000; Moss et al., 2002). The last model predicts that the properties characterized by the intercorrelation between perceptual and functional features will be more resistant to the evolution of AD.

In this context, the first aim of Rico Duarte's research is to evaluate this hypothesis with regard to the course of AD. A second and important objective is to test feature processing in normal aging because very few studies have focused on the normal processing of living and nonliving concepts in order to determine the differences or similarities with regard to the pathology. Furthermore, in her approach she gives an important role to the processes mobilized by the tasks in the continuum between automatic and controlled processes (Daum, Riesch, Sartori, & Birbaumer, 1996; Perri et al., 2003). Impairment for a certain class of concepts, in particular those from the living domain, has been observed in tests using controlled processes (e.g., denomination of images, definition of concepts, etc.), whereas no categorical effect has been reported at the time of the realization of the tasks using more automatic processes (e.g., priming, preference task, etc.). In her research, these assumptions were tested not only by tests where the distinctiveness was deduced (the distinctive features were evaluated by a picture-naming task and the shared features by a sorting task), but also by a property-verification task where the indices of distinctiveness and intercorrelation were manipulated and controlled objectively. This made it possible to evaluate the pertinence of defining tasks a priori as relating to a particular kind of distinctiveness without any empirical basis (e.g., distinctive features from picture-naming and shared features from sorting tasks). Moreover, the tasks used represent different levels of complexity (e.g., the picture naming and sorting tasks are based on controlled processes whereas the property-verification task is based on a feeling of familiarity and, therefore, on more automatic processes), which makes it possible to evaluate to what extent the treatment of the conceptual domains of living and nonliving concepts is affected by the cognitive resources mobilized by the tasks (Daum et al., 1996; Perri et al., 2003). The first results show that distinctiveness seems a sensible factor to evaluate SM in normal aging as well as in AD. This factor will be more important than intercorrelation to explain the conceptual evolution of categories of knowledge in AD. In this way, distinctiveness can be a plausible principle of organization of SM. Concerning normal aging, elderly subjects' performance is close to that of young subjects. However, the within-group analysis shows a more important sensitivity in elderly persons to process distinctive rather than shared features, as well as AD. These results underline the modifications in semantic organization with age. Nevertheless, a rupture is observed in comparison with the pathology since the performance of subjects with AD is significantly lower than that of elderly subjects. Currently, researchers are trying to examine the relationships between conceptual domains and metamnemonic processes.

In Portugal, Marques (2005a) has recently developed a naming-from-definition task that can be used for the assessment of SM in the context of both normal aging and dementia. Preliminary data obtained with young adults, normal elderly subjects, and elderly subjects diagnosed with mild AD naming seem to indicate that the task is a potentially interesting and valuable tool for both clinical and research applications (Marques, 2005b).

In Spain, the Costa group (Hernandez, Costa, Juncadella, & Rañé, in preparation) carried out a study whose objective is to investigate the deterioration of SM in patients suffering from AD. Specifically, they aim to assess whether the two basic semantic domains (living entities vs. artifacts) are differentially affected by this disease. Given the hypotheses that (1) living things have more shared properties and less distinctive ones than artifacts and (2) distinctive properties are weaker than shared properties, the following prediction was made. If distinct semantic categories have different internal organization, patients with diffuse lesions such as those suffering from AD would show a dissociation between concepts of living things and artifacts. In concrete, the prediction is that AD patients with SM impairment will have concepts of artifacts affected earlier than concepts of living things.

To test this prediction, they asked AD patients to perform a lexical-decision task in which semantic priming was implemented. In this task, half of the related pairs were animals and the other half were artifacts. Patients were divided into two groups (mild or moderate) depending on the degree of SM impairment, which was assessed by means of the questionnaire developed by the group of Laiacona, Barbarotto, and Capitani (1993). The control group was formed by healthy subjects matched in age and years of education. Results showed that patients with moderate SM impairment had a reduced semantic priming effect for artifacts, while such an effect was around normal levels for living things. No dissociation was found in the control group and, importantly, patients with mild SM impairment performed as well as the control group in the lexical-decision task, thus, excluding the possibility that the dissociation observed in the moderate group of patients is caused by a general cognitive impairment instead of a semantic memory deficit. In conclusion, these results confirm that different semantic categories have a different internal organization.

Our Contribution to the Field of SM in Aging

Our main contribution to the field of SM in old age has been the design of the Alzheimer Dementia Semantic Memory Evaluation (ADSME) battery (in Spanish: Batería EMSDA – Evaluación de la Memoria Semántica en la Demencia tipo Alzheimer; Peraita, González-Labra, Sánchez Bernardos, & Galeote, 2000, 2001). From the theoretical point of view, this battery is based on some of the underlying principles of categories and concepts psychology, this being one of the predominant trends in cognitive psychology in the 1970s, 1980s, and 1990s, and above all, from the investigations of Eleanor Rosch and the school that, to a certain extent, came about as a result of her work (Rosch, 1976; Smith & Medin, 1981).

Consequently, the theoretical frame, predictions, and hypotheses of the ADSME battery assume these same concepts. Stemming from these principles in categories and concepts psychology, a well-balanced selection of items belonging to living and nonliving things was carried out, and eight tests – relevant in terms of semantic processing – were constructed. Furthermore, two levels of generality of items were considered (superordinate and basic), and typicality was controlled on the basis of the only existing norms in Spanish when the battery was designed (Soto, Sebastián, García, & Amo del, 1994). (Currently there is a large series of norms for the production of semantic categories as well as variables that affect the tasks that are designed from them.)

The statistical and psychometric analysis carried out using the ADSME battery showed the construct validity and predictive value of detecting cognitive decline in semantic memory in mild and moderate AD, as well as in patients with possible semantic dementia and other problems of the semantic system (HSE, CEI, etc.).

The ADSME battery consists of eight tests that are structured around the two im-

Table 1. Classification of the tests according to type of processing and sensory modality: visuo-perceptual and auditory verbal

	Visual	Verbal
Production	Naming Classification	Fluency Definition of categories
Comprehension	Matching Analogies	Recognition of attributes Verification

portant cognitive-linguistic processes, production and comprehension, and centered on two sensory modalities of presentation of items: visuo-perceptual and auditory-verbal, as indicated in **Table 1**.

Some of these tests were designed to be complementary, e.g., the definition of categories and recognition of attributes tests, or the verbal fluency and classification. The objective is always to obtain a convergence of indices in the results.

The theoretical framework on which each of the eight tests is based and the objective of processing semantic information are made explicit in each of the tests. The rigorous scoring system adopted is also explained, this being different for each test and going beyond the mere recording of correct answers, errors, and omissions, as is frequent in the majority of tests used in this field.

The total number of categories used during the eight tests is 176: Approximately 50% are presented in a linguistic format and the other 50% in a pictorial format, the latter consisting of black and white drawings designed specifically for this battery, and based on Snodgrass and Vanderwart (1980). Semantic categories of the superordinate and basic generality level are included (see **Table 2**).

Therefore, in its design, the following factors have been combined: two types of categories or semantic domains (living beings and nonliving things), typicality and/or frequency of the items, levels of generality (basic and superordinate), and four types of semantic relationship (functional, part-whole, visual-perceptual, and taxonomic). Even though the number of semantic relationships or attributes is larger than this in the

Table 2. Variables controlled in different tests of the battery

Domains	Subdomains	Typicality values	Levels of generality	Semantic relationships	Difficulties of items
Living beings	Animals	High	Basic	Functional	Low
Nonliving things	Plants	Low	Superordinate	Part-whole	High
	Fruit			Evaluative/perceptual	
	Clothes			Taxonomic	
	Vehicles				
	Furniture				

conceptual model that this work is based on, in the design of some of these tests (matching, verification, analogies) only four have been selected because of the complexity involved in manipulating them.

In conclusion, the four factors cited are categorical factors or variables that affect the selection of the items. However, the design of the battery also takes into account the factors associated with the tests or tasks: modality of presentation (verbal/oral vs. pictorial/visual) and cognitive processes implied in the resolution of such tasks (production vs. comprehension) (see **Table 2**).

Other Studies

In addition to the design and updating of the battery we have just presented, our work in the field of SM during the last six years has been structured around two lines: normative and methodological studies, and experimental studies. In the first line, we obtained norms of production of semantic categories in a sample of healthy elderly subjects, elderly subjects with AD, and young people. These were equally grouped in terms of gender and educational level. The norms of production of attributes of semantic categories and an analysis of their definitions were obtained and we drew up a new controlled set of items in the following relevant variables: familiarity, structural complexity, age of acquisition, and lexical frequency to evaluate the semantic dissociations in AD (Moreno-Martínez & Peraita, 2007).

In the second of these lines, we have concentrated on conceptual processing using property generation tasks, picture-naming tasks, attribute verification paradigms, and psychophysiological measures.

In the line of the production and generation of semantic attributes (and as a continuation of the work carried out in the 1990s on other types of subjects, Peraita, Elosúa, & Linares, 1992), we can highlight our work with F.J. Bueno (Bueno & Peraita, 2006), which tries to find the types of knowledge and/or large blocks of characteristics or attributes that structure and represent semantic categories, in addition to making a comparison with the studies published in English and in an Anglo-Saxon setting.

In the line of the attribute verification paradigm, we will highlight the work carried out with C. Díaz and L. Anllo-Vento (Peraita, Díaz, & Anllo-Vento, submitted). Briefly, we compared the performance of 50 patients with probable AD and that of 30 elderly controls in two semantic tasks: a verbal sentence verification task and a visual test of analogical relationships, both including distinct types of semantic relations. On the sentence verification task, the performance of APs was comparable to that of elderly controls when statements were true, but deteriorated significantly when statements were false. This result was interpreted as a failure of controlled processes to successfully search semantic space when statements were incongruent or false. In addition, all participants found some semantic relations more difficult to process than others, with relative difficulty being consistent across tasks. Taxonomic semantic relationships were the most difficult, while part/whole relationships were the easiest, but also the ones to deteriorate most rapidly. In contrast, functional attributes were comparatively preserved as the disease progressed. These results emphasize the role of attention and semantic context in jointly determining access to relevant attributes and categories. Furthermore, they suggest that semantic memory impairments in AD depend on the type of processing and semantic relationship required by the task.

In this same line of work, using the event-related brain potentials (ERPs) technique, we are currently conducting a study to determine the neural underpinnings and timing of these semantic relationships. In a priming paradigm in which probe and target are joined by one of three possible semantic relationships (functional, taxonomic, or part-whole), we have recorded ERPs to animate and inanimate target words in a group of young subjects. Preliminary data indicate that N400, the ERP component that is most sensitive to the semantic relationship between two words, is modulated by the type of relationship between the probe and target. The amplitude of N400 is greatest when the part-whole relationship is true or false, followed by the taxonomic and, finally, the functional relationship. These results suggest that the part-whole semantic relationship is significantly easier to process than the taxonomic relationship, which, in turn, is significantly easier than the functional one. The N400 results were followed by a sizeable modulation of P6 amplitude by the same three semantic relationships. Thus, it seems that brain activity indexes the type of relationship that exists between two words or concepts in a very short period of time (Anllo-Vento, Hinojosa, Silva, Pozo, & Peraita, 2004).

As for object-naming tasks, we have tried to check if the naming process is helped by the visual cues supplied to the subject, both in people with AD and healthy elderly controls as well as a group of young people (Peraita, Silva, Díaz, Moreno, & Anllo-Vento, 2003). By increasing the wealth of visual cues available to the subject, we investigated whether the naming deficits present in AD would be diminished or prevented. By including stimuli representing animate and inanimate objects, we tested whether naming deficits are disproportionately greater for one of these two categories. We anticipated differences in performance across the groups: young, normal elderly, and AD. Naming performance should improve as the number of visual cues increases, particularly in AD. Also in AD, naming should be better for inanimate than animate objects.

Conclusions and Further Research

Currently, the main challenge is to ascertain whether SM has, or does not have, a categorical structure. That is, if it is organized in the brain-mind system according to more or less extensive and relevant semantic categories present in the environment (category-based models): living beings such as animals, plants, foods, people; and non-living things such as tools, vehicles, furniture, geographic places; or if, on the contrary, organization is based on attributes or characteristics which, in turn, share many of these categories (feature-based models). The wide variety of existing accounts/explanations, especially within the framework of the category-based structure, does not currently make possible a concise explanation of the structure of SM or of its disorders (Garrard, Lambon-Ralph, Hodges, & Patterson, 2001).

In our opinion, it is essential for current cognitive neuropsychology, specifically that dealing with dissociations and categorical dissociations (i.e., category-specific deficits) within the framework of SM impairment, to examine in depth the theoretical and empirical contributions of evolutionary and cognitive psychology in the area of categorization and formation of concepts. By this we mean the area of organization, structure, and representation of the semantic categories in subjects with no pathology (i.e., neither degenerative, nor infectious, nor traumatic), and, basically, in both the ontogenic and phylogenetic evolution of the knowledge of these categories. At the same time, it would be necessary to know some of the contributions, in this case mainly theoretical, of cognitive semantics. If this is not the case, the presentation of an increasingly larger and more specific number of cases of dissociations will not provide us with the necessary interpretive unit and suitable theoretical framework from which we will be able to analyze it.

References

Anllo-Vento, L., Hinojosa, J.A., Silva, A., Pozo, M.A., & Peraita, H. (2004). *Modulation of the N400 by type of semantic relationship connecting word pairs in a semantic priming task.* Paper presented at the CNS, San Francisco & Sevilla 2004 & Lisboa, 2004.

Aronoff, J.M., Gonnerman, L.M., Almor, A., Arunachalam, S., Kempler, D., & Andersen, E.S. (2006). Information content versus relational knowledge: Semantic deficits in patients with Alzheimer's disease. *Neuropsychologia, 44,* 21–35.

Barbarotto, R., Capitani, E., & Laiacona, M. (2001). Living musical instruments and inanimate body parts? *Neuropsychologia, 39,* 406–414.

Borgo, F., & Shallice, T. (2003). Category specificity and feature knowledge: Evidence from new sensory-quality categories. *Cognitive Neuropsychology, 20,* 327–353.

Bright, P., Moss, H., & Tyler, L.K. (2004). Unitary vs. multiple semantics: PET studies of word and picture processing. *Brain and Language, 89,* 417–432.

Budson, A.E, Bruce, H., & Price, M.D. (2005). Memory dysfunction. *The New England Journal of Medicine, 352,* 692–699.

Bueno, J., & Peraita, H. (2006). Análisis de las propiedades de categorías semánticas de seres vivos e inanimados. Un estudio comparativo con el trabajo de Cree & McRae (2003) [Living and nonliving semantic categories property analysis. A comparative study with McRae and Cree (2003)]. Doctoral thesis in preparation.

Capitani, E., Barbarotto, R., & Laiacona, M. (2005). Gender differences and the brain representation of semantic knowledge. *Brain and Language, 95,* 56–57.

Capitani, E., Laiacona, M., Mahon, B., & Caramazza, A. (2003). What are the facts of semantic category-specific deficits? A critical review of the clinical evidence. *Cognitive Neuropsychology, 20,* 213–261.

Caramazza, A., Hillis, A.E., Rapp, B.C., & Romani, C. (1990). The multiple semantics hypothesis: Multiple confusions? *Cognitive Neuropsychology, 7,* 161–189.

Caramazza, A., & Shelton, J.R. (1998). Domain-specific knowledge systems in the brain: The animate-inanimate distinction. *Journal of Cognitive Neuroscience, 10,* 1–34.

Cuetos, F., Dobarro, A., & Martínez, C. (2005). Deterioro de la información conceptual en la EA [Conceptual information problems in Alzheimer's disease]. *Neurología, 20,* 58–64.

Daum, I., Riesch, G., Sartori, G., & Birbaumer, N. (1996). Semantic memory impairment in Alzheimer's disease. *Journal of Clinical and Experimental Neuropsychology, 18,* 648–665.

Dudas, R.B., Clague, F., Thompson, S.A., Graham, K.S., & Hodges, J.R. (2005). Episodic and semantic memory in mild cognitive impairment. *Neuropsychologia, 43,* 1266–1276.

Funnell, E., & Sheridan, J. (1992). Categories of knowledge: Unfamiliar aspects of living and nonliving things. *Cognitive Neuropsychology, 9,* 135–153.

Fung, T.D., Chertkow, H., Murtha, S., Whatmough, C., Peloquin, L., Whitehead, V. et al. (2001). The spectrum of category effects in object and action knowledge in dementia of the Alzheimer's type. *Neuropsychology, 15*, 371–379.

Fuster, J.M. (2003). *Cortex and mind: Unifying cognition.* New York: Oxford University Press.

Garrard, P., Lambon Ralph, M.A., Hodges, J.R., & Patterson, K. (2001). Protypicality, distinctiveness, and intercorrelations: Analyses of the semantic attributes of living and nonliving concepts. *Cognitive Neuropsychology, 18*, 125–174.

Gaffan, D., & Haywood, C.A. (1993). The spurious category specific visual agnosia for living things in normal humans and nonhuman primates. *Journal of Cognitive Neuroscience, 5*, 118–128.

Hampton, J.A., & Moss, H.E. (2003). Concepts and meaning: Introduction to the special issue on conceptual representation. *Language and Cognitive Processes, 18*, 505–515.

Hernandez, M., Costa, A., Juncadella, M., & Rañé, J. (in preparation). *Semantic category-specific deterioration in Alzheimer patients.*

Hillis, A.E., Rapp, B., & Caramazza, A. (1995). Constraining claims about theories of semantic memory: More on unitary versus multiple semantics. *Cognitive Neuropsychology, 12*, 175–186.

Laiacona, M., Barbarotto, R., & Capitani, E. (1993). Perceptual and associative knowledge in category specific impairment of semantic memory: A study of two cases. *Cortex, 29*, 727–740.

Laws. K.R. (1999). Gender affects naming latencies for living and nonliving things: Implications for familiarity. *Cortex, 35*, 729–733.

Laiacona, M., Barbarotto, R., & Capitani, E. (1998). Semantic category disassociations in naming: Is there a gender effect in Alzheimer's disease? *Neuropsychologia, 5*, 407–419.

Lyons, F., Kay, J., Hanley, J.R., & Haslam, C. (2006). Selective preservation of memory for people in the context of semantic memory disorder: Patterns of association and dissociation. *Neuropsychologia, 44*, 2887–2898.

Marques, J.F. (2005a). Naming from definition: The role of feature type and feature distinctiveness. *Quarterly Journal of Experimental Psychology, 58*, 603–611.

Marques, J.F. (2005b). Naming from definition and the assessment of Alzheimer's patients' conceptual knowledge: Some preliminary data. In A. Garriga (Ed.), *Proceedings of the workshop on research on predictors of cognitive impairment and neurodegenerative diseases.* Segovia, Spain: UNED.

Maylor, E.A. (2005). Age-related changes in memory. In M.L. Johnson, V.L. Bengtson, P.G. Coleman, & T.B.L. Kirkwood (Eds.), *The Cambridge handbook of age and aging* (pp. 200–208). Cambridge, UK: Cambridge University Press.

Moreno-Martínez, J., & H. Peraita. (2007). Un nuevo conjunto de ítems para la evaluación de la disociación vivo/artefacto con normas obtenidas de ancianos sanos españoles [A new set of items for the evaluation of living/nonliving dissociations with norms collected from healthy elderly Spanish]. *Psicológica, 28*(1), 1–20.

Moss, H.E., & Tyler, L.K. (2000). A progressive category-specific semantic deficit for nonliving things. *Neuropsychologia, 38*, 60–82.

Moss, H.E., Tyler, L.K., & Devlin, J.T. (2002). The emergence of category-specific deficits in a distributed semantic system. In E.M.E. Forde & G.W. Humphreys (Eds.), *Category-specificity in mind and brain* (pp. 115–148). Hove, UK: Psychology Press.

Peraita, H., Díaz, C., & Anllo-Vento, L. (submitted). Difficulty in processing various types of semantic relations. *Archives of Clinical Neuropsychology.*

Peraita, H., Elosua, R., & Linares, P. (1992). *Representación de categorías naturales en niños ciegos* [Natural categories representation in blind children]. Madrid, Spain: Trotta.

Peraita, H., González-Labra, M.J., Sánchez Bernardos, M.L., & Galeote, M. (2000). Batería de evaluación de la memoria semántica en Alzheimer [Evaluation battery for semantic deterioration in Alzheimer's disease]. *Psicothema, 12*, 192–200.

Peraita, H., González-Labra, M.J., Sánchez Bernardos, M.L., & Galeote, M. (2001). Evaluation battery for semantic memory deterioration in Alzheimer. *Psychology in Spain, 5*, 98–109.

Peraita, H., Silva, A., Díaz, C., Moreno, J., & Anllo-Vento, L. (2003, September). *Object naming efficiency increases with wealth of visual cues in normal elderly and Alzheimer's patients. Symposium: Cognition, aging, and neuroscience.* Paper presented at the XIII Conference of the European Society of Cognitive Psychology. ESCOP-2003. Granada, Spain.

Perri. R., Carlesimo, G.A., Zannino, G.D., Mauri, M., Muolo, B., Pettenati, C. et al. (2003). Intentional and automatic measures of specific-category effect in the semantic impairment of patients with Alzheimer's disease. *Neuropsychologia, 41,* 1509–1522.

Rapp, B., Hillis, A., & Caramazza, A. (1993). The role of representations in cognitive theory: More on multiple semantics and the agnosias. *Cognitive Neuropsychology, 10*(3), 235–249.

Rico-Duarte, L. (2004). L'analyse de la mémoire sémantique dans le vieillissement normal et dans la maladie d'Alzheimer: Mise a l'épreuve du modèle de la structure conceptuelle [Semantic memory analysis in normal aging and Alzheimer's disease: The conceptual structure model]. Doctoral thesis, University Paul Valery, Montpellier, France.

Rosch, E. (1976). Cognitive representations of semantic categories. *Journal of Experimental Psychology: General, 104,* 192–233.

Rosch, E.H., & Mervis, C.B. (1975). Family resemblance studies in the internal structure of categories. *Cognitive Psychology, 7,* 573–605.

Sartori, G., & Lombardi, L. (2004). Semantic relevance and semantic disorders. *Journal of Cognitive Neuroscience, 16,* 439–452.

Silveri, M.C., Daniele, A., Giustolisi, L., & Gianotti, G. (1991). Dissociation between knowledge of living and nonliving things in dementia of the Alzheimer type. *Neurology, 41,* 545–546.

Smith, E.E., & Medin, D.L. (1981). *Categories and concepts.* Cambridge, MA: Harvard University Press.

Smith, E.E., Shoben, E.J., & Rips, L.J. (1974). Structure and process in semantic memory: A featural model of semantic decision. *Psychological Review, 81,* 214–241.

Snodgrass, J., & Vanderwart, M. (1980). A standardized set of 260 pictures: Norms for name agreement, image agreement, familiarity, and visual complexity. *Journal of Experimental Psychology: Learning, Memory, and Cognition, 6,* 174–215.

Soto, P., Sebastián, M.V., García, E., & Amo del, T. (1994). *Las categorías y sus normas en castellano* [Semantic category norms in Castilian]. Madrid, Spain: Visor.

Squire, L.R., & Zola-Morgan, S. (1991). The medial temporal lobe memory system. *Science, 253,* 1380–1386.

Stewart, F., Parkin, A.J., & Hunkin, N.M. (1992). Naming impairments following recovery from herpes simplex encephalitis: Category-specific? *The Quarterly Journal of Experimental Psychology, 11A,* 261–1153.

Tyler, L.K., & Moss, H.E. (1997). Functional properties of concepts: Studies of normal and brain-damaged patients. *Cognitive Neuropsychology, 14,* 511–545.

Tyler, L.K., Moss, H.E., Durrant-Peatfield, M., & Levy, J. (2000). Conceptual structure and the structure of concepts. *Brain and Language, 75,* 195–231.

Warrington, E.K., & Shallice, T. (1984). Category-specific impairment. *Brain, 107,* 829–853.

Warrington, E.K., & McCarthy, R. (1987). Category of knowledge: Further fractionations and an attempted integration. *Brain, 110,* 1273–1296.

Zannino, G.D., Perri, R., Carlesimo, G.A., Palqualetti, P., & Caltagirone, C. (2002). Category-specific impairment in patients with Alzheimer's disease as a function of disease severity: A cross-sectional investigation. *Neuropsychologia, 40,* 2268–2279.

Zannino, G.D., & Perri, R. (2006). Analysis of the semantic representations of living and non-living concepts: A normative study. *Cognitive Neuropsychology, 23,* 515–540.

6. Affect and Emotions

Despina Moraitou and Anastasia Efklides

Introduction

In the last few decades there has been a growing interest in the emotional functioning of older adults. The leading theory in this area is Carstensen's socioemotional selectivity theory (Carstensen, Fung, & Charles, 2003). It posits that older adults are biased toward positive information processing. This is due to their limited time perspective that leads to motivational shifts, which direct attention to emotionally meaningful goals. Moreover, increased attention to emotional goals results in better regulation of emotions and the prioritization of affect optimization in later life.

However, the study of emotions in older age does not focus only on affect regulation. In what follows, we shall focus on emotion changes in aging and we shall argue that emotional functioning is largely spared in old age (see also Carstensen, Mikels, & Mather, in press). Although autonomic reactivity to emotion eliciting stimuli seems to decrease in older age, this proves not to be the case when the stimuli are age-relevant (Kunzmann & Grühn, 2005). Furthermore, the subjective experience of emotions and emotional expressive behavior show less marked age differences, whereas emotion-regulatory skills can improve along with age leading to greater emotional control and a relatively more positive emotional balance (Gross, Carstensen, Tsai, Skorpen, & Hsu, 1997; Isaacowitz & Smith, 2003; Pinquart, 2001). This positive emotional balance is related to relatively stable well-being in old age despite health-related and social losses (Kunzmann, Little, & Smith, 2000). Moreover, positive affectivity facilitates older adults' sociopsychological functioning with growth-related positive involvement in social life (Kunzmann, Stange, & Jordan, 2005). It should be noted, however, that the emphasis of our review is on recent research carried out *in Europe*. We shall refer to studies on emotional development in older age, on emotion regulation, and on the relations of emotion with cognition. Then, we shall relate these findings to older adults' sociopsychological functioning and subjective quality of life.

Emotion Changes in Aging

According to Frijda's (1986) conceptualization, emotions involve four distinct components, namely, physiological arousal, the subjective experience of emotion, face and bodily expression, and behavioral activity. Physiological arousal is related to autonomic reactivity.

Autonomic reactivity, which is linked to the biological substratum of emotion, has been found to decline with age (Carstensen et al., in press; Lawton, 2001). However, based on the evidence of a recent study, it seems that older adults, when exposed to emotion-eliciting stimuli that are particularly meaningful to them, show similar levels of autonomic responding to those of younger adults (Kunzmann & Grühn, 2005). The study investigated old and young participants' physiological reactions to four film clips dealing with a particular class of sadness-evoking events, namely, fundamental and irreversible losses. Results did not show significant differences between the two age groups for four physiological measures. There was even evidence, although limited, for greater autonomic reactivity in older adults as measured with finger pulse amplitude and finger temperature in response to some particular film clips (Kunzmann & Grühn, 2005). This evidence, as compared to previous findings of lower autonomic reactivity in older adults, suggests that what probably changes in older age is not autonomic reactivity per se, but the primary appraisal of the stimuli's relevance to oneself. Thus, for self-relevant stimuli, there is autonomic reactivity comparable to that of younger adults.

As regards the *subjective experience of emotion*, the complexity of the relation between emotion and age becomes even more apparent. Comparisons of older and younger participants' self-assessments of the intensity of emotions, such as pleasure, sadness, and four other negative emotions that they had felt during exposure to four films dealing with irreversible losses (see above), showed greater sadness and anxiety in older adults in response to all films. In addition, the greater affect intensity in older adults generalized to another sample and another film clip of the same type (Kunzmann & Grühn, 2005). Yet, one could argue that older adults' heightened autonomic reactivity and self-assessment of affect is only evident in negative emotions.

Another study, which used meta-analysis to synthesize findings from 125 empirical studies on age differences in positive affect, negative affect, and affect balance in middle-aged and older adults, found that the association of age with affect differed between particular positive and negative emotions. The meta-analysis showed an age-associated decrease of self-assessed affect intensity and frequency mainly with regard to high-arousal positive and negative emotions (e.g., feeling excited or angry), whereas low-arousal emotions (e.g., feeling calm or bored) showed an age-associated increase (Pinquart, 2001). Furthermore, there was a tendency for decline of positive affect and increase of negative affect in older samples. More concretely, positive affect was not related to age in the youngest samples ($M = 55$ years), but was negatively related to age in the oldest samples ($M = 75$ years). Negative affect decreased in the youngest samples, but increased in the oldest samples. Affect balance decreased in the youngest samples whereas no significant age effects were found in the oldest samples.

Looking also at changes of specific emotions, Gross et al. (1997) used a self-report questionnaire to examine how frequently Norwegian younger and older participants experienced each of five emotions (happiness, sadness, fear, anger, disgust). In this study, the single age-related effect for frequency of emotional experiences was for anger. Specifically, older women reported a lower frequency of anger experience than younger women. This finding is in line with the Pinquart (2001) finding that older adults do not report emotions of high arousal, such as anger. On the other hand, the self-report data of this study seem to contradict Pinquart's (2001) and Kunzmann and Grühn (2005) findings of increased negative affect or decreased positive affect in older adults, since there were no age differences in other positive or negative emotions.

As regards positive affect, Kunzmann et al. (2005) focused on two broader and highly distinct dimensions of positive affectivity, labeled pleasant affect and positive involvement. *Pleasant affect* is indicated by positive affective states with a relatively low arousal component (e.g., happiness), and is characterized by self-centered feelings. On the contrary, *positive involvement* encompasses positive affective states with high arousal (e.g., interest), and is characterized by process-oriented and environment-centered feelings. In the Kunzmann et al. (2005) study, young, middle-aged, and older participants were asked to indicate how frequently they had experienced each of five pleasant-affect feelings, five positive-involvement feelings, and ten negative affective states during the previous year. In this case the results showed that younger adults were more likely to experience pleasant feelings, whereas older adults were more likely to experience feelings of positive involvement.

Therefore, the age-associated decline of high-arousal positive emotions (Pinquart, 2001) may reflect a difference in the source of positive emotions in older adults. The source of happiness or pleasant affect is not so much their own self but the environment, such as family, grandchildren, etc. (Efklides, Kalaitzidou, & Chankin, 2003). Of course, we should bear in mind that self-reports rely on memory and are prone to biases of various types due to beliefs, attitudes, social desirability effects, etc. Thus, the physiological reactivity data show that older adults are capable of high intensity emotions to self-relevant stimuli, while the self-report data suggest lower frequency of them, possibly because older adults avoid recalling them, giving priority to other emotions that are deemed more "appropriate" to their age, such as positive involvement feelings.

In general, as regards age-associated changes in self-reported affect frequency and valence, a steady stream of research (see Carstensen et al., in press; Mroczek, 2001; Pinquart, 2001; Teachman, 2006) has come to the conclusion that the relationship between age and frequency of positive and negative emotions appears to be curvilinear, with the least optimal emotional experiences in young adulthood and the most optimal ones in early old age. In other words, according to the findings of these studies, older adults tend to report experiencing the same or more positive emotions and, mainly, less negative emotions than younger adults. However, positive affect diminishes and negative affect increases again in very old age, resulting in the decrease of the quality of emotional experience in the oldest old. Health and functional constraints may account for this decrease of positive affect and increase of negative affect in very old age. Kunzmann et al. (2000) investigated samples of old and very old adults from the Berlin Aging Study (age range 70–100+ years), using a self-report positive and negative affect questionnaire that referred to specific emotions with a high-arousal component. Participants were asked to indicate how frequently they had experienced each emotion during the previous year. They were also tested for functional health constraints in vision, hearing, and mobility. In initial cross-sectional and longitudinal analyses, age was negatively related to positive affect but unrelated to negative affect. On the contrary, when cross-sectional data were controlled for functional health constraints, age was associated with high positive affect and low negative affect.

On the other hand, the longitudinal evidence showed that negative affect in the samples remained stable over 4 years suggesting that the valence of affect may not change with age and the cross-sectional age differences may be the result of cohort effects. In any case, the findings of this study generally corroborated the notion that age, per se, is not a risk factor for the emotional well-being of older adults as indicated by the balance of positive and negative affect. More recently, analysis of cross-sectional data from the Berlin Aging Study of very old individuals aged 70 to 100+ years (Isaacowitz & Smith, 2003) examined whether the unique effects of age on positive and negative affect remained after the statistical control for demographic, personality, and health and cognitive functioning variables. The results showed no unique age effects on either positive or negative affect in the sample, while personality and general intelligence emerged as the strongest predictors of affect. Therefore, the increase of negative affect in very old adults (see also Pinquart, 2001) is associated with the constraints imposed by ill health and limited functionality rather than with age per se.

However, the person's emotional response to health constraints seems to be mediated by personality and intelligence factors, and this may explain the contradictory findings in the various studies. Pinquart (2001) also found that the association between age and affect varied as a function of study characteristics; there were differences between cross-sectional and longitudinal studies, between past and more recent studies, published and unpublished, as well as differences based on the type of measure used. A noticeable finding was that the representativeness of the samples (probability samples versus convenience samples such as visitors of *senior centers*) was positively associated with positive affect and affect balance, and negatively associated with negative affect. This may indicate that nonrepresentative samples are often biased toward healthy and active older adults.

What was also interesting was the finding that there were national differences in the association of age with affect valence and balance (Pinquart, 2001). Older adults from the former communist Eastern European countries showed the strongest age-associated decline of positive affect and the strongest age-associated increase of negative affect. Thus, besides health and functionality constraints, major cultural or financial changes in one's life, or loss of meaning of life that occur at a late stage of one's life – when coping is difficult – are critical for the quality of affect experienced. This is probably due to the fact that optimization of emotional well-being is hard to achieve in such situations.

Overall, the evidence on autonomic reactivity as well as on the frequency, intensity, and valence of emotional experiences suggests that there is increase of positive affect and decrease or stability of negative affect in aging. However, as regards the very old age (75+) it seems that this type of affect balance is reversed. The increase of negative affect and the decrease of positive affect are mainly related to health problems and other constraints rather than to age itself. The findings from all the aforementioned studies are summarized in a simplified form, in terms of gain, stability, or loss, in **Table 1**.

Table 1. Summary of findings from European studies of the nature of emotion in old age

	Emotional components														
	Autonomic reactivity			Intensity			Frequency			Valence					
										Positive			Negative		
Type of measure	Gain	Stability	Loss	Gain	Stability	Loss	Gain	Stability	Loss	Increase	Stability	Decrease	Increase	Stability	Decrease
Sad films	✓	✓													
Meta-analysis	✓[1]			✓[1]		✓[2]	✓[1]		✓[2]	✓[3]		✓[4]	✓[4]		✓[3]
Self-reports								✓						✓	
Self-reports									✓[5]	✓[6]					
Self-reports										✓				✓	✓
Self-reports											✓			✓	

Note. The evidence summarized in this table comes from Kunzmann & Grühn, 2005; Pinquart, 2001; Gross et al, 1997; Kunzmann et al., 2005; Kunzmann et al, 2000; Isaacowitz & Smith, 2003, respectively. The superscripts indicate: 1 = low-arousal emotions; 2 = high-arousal emotions; 3 = representative samples of older adults; 4 = very old age; 5 = the specific emotion of anger; 6 = positive involvement.

Emotion Decoding

Another component of emotion that has been differentially associated with aging is the ability to *decode and interpret emotional cues*, which is referred to as *emotional understanding* (Phillips, Smith, & Gilhooly, 2002). Socio-cognitive approaches propose that with age there should be an increased ability to understand emotions mainly because of the accumulated life experiences of analyzing emotional cues in interpersonal communication (Carstensen et al., 2003). However, neuropsychological evidence suggests that there might be impairments in the interpretation of emotional cues in older adults, due to the rapid decline in normal aging of brain areas known to be involved in decoding emotional identity (Phillips & Della Sala, 1998).

Phillips et al. (2002a) tested young and older adults on a range of emotional ability measures, in order to investigate the pattern of age effects on the understanding of emotions inherent in verbal and nonverbal material. The results showed that there were no age effects on the ability to decode emotions from verbal material. Likewise, there was no overall age effect on decoding emotions from faces. However, older adults were less able to identify facial expressions of anger and sadness. They were also less able to interpret mental states from pictures of eyes as well as to recognize and share others' feelings (i.e., empathy). According to Phillips et al. (2002a), these findings may indicate that empathy involves determining another person's thoughts or feelings on a moment-to-moment basis. However, age effects found on empathy were explained in terms of age-related differences due to years of education and intelligence. Fluid intelligence can influence empathy, mainly in terms of facilitating emotional understanding that requires analysis of complex information (Phillips et al., 2002a), whereas crystallized intelligence and education can facilitate empathy through acquired knowledge and learned skills. Thus, based on the above findings there is no evidence of an age-associated improvement in emotion understanding, nor of a general decline in the decoding of emotional cues. The results indicated only specific age-related deficits in understanding sadness and anger from facial cues.

In the same vein, MacPherson, Phillips, and Della Sala (2002) examined young, middle-aged, and older adults in the labeling of emotions from color photographs of faces. Consistent with the above findings, they found that older adults were impaired in decoding only one type of emotion out of seven studied, namely, sadness. These findings suggest that whereas older adults may experience heightened negative emotions, they have difficulty in perceiving them in others' faces. This may be due to differential processing of cues related to negative affect in older age. Fischer, Sandblom, Gavazzeni, Fransson, Wright, and Baeckman (2005) examined age-related differences in the neural circuitry involved in the perception of negative facial affect, using functional magnetic resonance imaging (fMRI). Younger and older adults were presented with blocks of angry and neutral faces. The fMRI data analysis of the angry versus neutral faces contrast indicated that aging is associated with lower subcortical activation and higher cortical activation during perception of angry faces. These finding suggests that learned self-regulatory processes of affect may intervene in older adults' decoding of anger in others' faces.

In another study, Phillips and Allen (2004) tested young and older participants on the perceived intensity of four different emotions (happiness, sadness, fear, anger) presented in pictures of faces and in text. The results indicated a lowering of perceived intensity of facial expressions of sadness and happiness in old age. With regard to the written text tasks, younger adults displayed higher perceived intensity of fear than did the older ones. However, all these age differences were explained in terms of the higher levels of anxiety and depression in young adults, and the decreases in fluid and increases in crystallized intelligence seen in normal aging. On the other hand, there was an age difference in perceived intensity of anger in neutral faces, which was not explained by mood or cognitive ability variables; on the basis of this finding, it was suggested that young adults may be more likely than older adults to perceive anger in facial expressions, when no such emotion is intended to be communicated.

Overall, then, the above studies indicate that advancing age may result in poorer ability to decode emotions from faces, but this deficit tends to be restricted to some negative emotions, such as sadness and anger, as well as to understanding complex emotional states from eyes. From a neuropsychological viewpoint, these age-related changes may reflect less efficient processing of emotional facial expressions in old age. However, another possibility is that young and older adults are processing differentially negative affective information from faces and stories, as a result of differences in the regulation of negative emotions. This differential processing, in turn, may cause differences in brain activation (see Fischer et al., 2005; Phillips & Della Sala, 1998).

Another possibility could be that older adults have difficulty in the categorization of emotional stimuli rather than in decoding them. Kiffel, Campanella, and Bruyer (2005) focused on a specific aspect of perception of faces and facial expressions, which is referred to as *categorical perception*. A common requirement in perception is to assign stimuli to discrete categories, in order to simplify their interpretation. To do so, people enhance the differences of stimuli belonging to two different categories while the differences of within-category stimuli are reduced. This phenomenon is known as the *categorical perception effect* (see Kiffel et al., 2005). Specifically, this study investigated the effect of aging on categorical perception of emotional facial expressions; young, middle-aged, and older adults were tested in a discrimination task with facial stimuli displaying happiness, sadness, and disgust. The results showed that, independently of age, participants discriminated more easily (with better accuracy and faster correct response latencies) faces representing two different emotions than faces representing the same one. Thus, the categorical perception effect was verified in emotion perception. From the perspective of aging, these findings indicate that the representations of emotions are stable in the life span, and older adults display similar perceptual sensitivity to this of young adults when they have to determine emotional category membership. The same conclusion was reached by D'Argembeau and Van der Linden (2004), who examined age-related differences in memory for identity and emotional expression of unfamiliar faces. Therefore, older adults have no difficulty with the categorization of emotional cues in faces. Consequently, the differential processing by older adults of facial stimuli that denote sadness and anger cannot be attributed to changes in the categorization process in aging, but either to changes in brain activity or to changes in the regulation of emotions. **Table 2** sums up the findings from the aforementioned studies on emotional understanding in older age.

Table 2. Summary of findings on emotion decoding and categorization from European studies comparing older, middle-aged, and young adults as a function of type of stimuli

Studies/Similarity of processing	Verbal material		Facial expressions		Mental states from eyes	
	Similar	Different	Similar	Different	Similar	Different
Phillips et al., 2002	✓		✓	✓*		✓
MacPherson et al., 2002			✓	✓*		
Fischer et al., 2005				✓*		
Phillips & Allen, 2004	✓			✓*		
Kiffel et al., 2005			✓			
D'Argembeau & Van der Linden, 2004			✓			

Note. *indicates the specific negative emotion of anger or sadness or both of them. Similar/different = similar/different processing across age groups.

Emotion Regulation

Explicitly differentiating between emotion and emotion regulation is a very difficult –if not an arbitrary– attempt (see Diamond & Aspinwall, 2003). Generally speaking, *emotion regulation* refers to the processes through which individuals consciously or unconsciously modify either their own emotional experience and behavior or the emotion-eliciting stimulus, so that they attain a relatively pleasant, not-too-distracting state that allows them to turn their full attention onto the task at hand (see Carstensen et al., 2003). Seen in this light, phenomena such as the decreasing intensity and frequency of high arousal emotions during the life span, the decreasing ability to perceive sadness or anger in others' faces, and the stability or optimization of affect balance could be interpreted as regulatory and/or compensational moves appropriate to the time of life when biological and social resources are diminishing.

However, there are other aspects of emotion regulation as well. In general, older adults use coping strategies for the regulation of their emotional states (response-focused emotion regulation) as well as strategies for proactively avoiding negative emotions (antecedent emotion regulation) (see Carstensen et al., 2003). In this vein, Winkeler, Filipp, and Boll (2000) examined whether older adults tend to perceive and construe close social relationships in a generalized positively biased manner or if this is a specific tendency that applies only to the parent-child relationship. Scenarios describing two family members (i.e., aged parent and adult child versus two adult siblings) discussing a controversial issue were presented to middle-aged and older participants. Each scenario was followed by participants' appraisals of the protagonists' behavior and the quality of their relationship. Results showed that older adults perceived both inter- and intra-generational relationships more positively, that is, as being less conflictual and more affectionate, than the middle-aged adults. Thus, a "positivity bias" was verified in the older adults' perceptions of social relationships, indicating an attempt to regulate their own emotional experience and to preserve harmony with their surroundings.

As regards the specific strategies the participants proposed in order to handle a conflictual situation, older adults clearly favored avoidance of the controversial topic altogether, in contrast to middle-aged participants who were far more inclined to recommend communicating constructively or turning to confrontation. So, consistent with previous research findings (Carstensen et al., 2003), these results indicated that older adults seem to prefer the use of emotion-focused strategies – such as the strategy of distancing themselves from negative emotions – than the use of problem-focused ones, when confronted with emotionally charged problems.

Another study (Garnefski & Kraaij, 2006) examined how the use of cognitive emotion-regulation strategies unfolds during the life span. Five specific samples (ranging from adolescents to older adults) were compared as to their reported use of nine conceptually different cognitive strategies for emotion regulation. Measures of depressive symptomatology were also collected. The results showed that older adults differed from all the other age groups in their higher preference of the following three cognitive strategies: "putting into perspective," i.e., referring to the relativity of an event when compared to other, more serious events; "positive refocusing," i.e., thinking about pleasant situations instead of thinking about the actual threatening or stressful event; "acceptance," i.e., accepting the negative experience and/or adopting a passive form of resignation. In older adults acceptance was associated mainly with depressive symptomatology. This kind of coping may represent a passive, negative life-adjustment style for older adults (Garnefski & Kraaij, 2006).

Thomsen, Mehlsen, Viidik, Sommerlund, and Zachariae (2005), in a similar empirical work, focused on two specific cognitive strategies of emotion regulation: "rumination," that is, recurrent thoughts and/or images of past negative events, and "defensiveness," that is, self-deception as an attempt to downregulate negative affect. Specifically, they investigated whether age and gender differences in negative affect could be explained by emotion-regulation processes such as defensiveness and rumination, while controlling the effects of life events. Young and older participants completed self-report questionnaires concerning negative affect such as anger, anxiety and sadness, depressive symptoms, stress (as experience of stressful events within the last year), rumination (as rehearsal of negative thoughts), and defensiveness (as self-assessed social desirability). With regard to age differences in negative affect, the results generally confirmed previous findings, showing that older adults generally scored lower on self-reported negative affect and affective-cognitive depressive symptoms (but not on depressive somatic symptoms). On the other hand, the results revealed that age differences in negative affect were in part due to the young women's higher preference for rumination. Defensiveness and experience of stressful events also appeared to mediate the age effects; particularly in the case of sadness, older adults reported higher sadness than younger participants when controlling for defensiveness and stressful events. Moreover, the mediation effects of defensiveness and rumination remained even after controlling for life stressors.

Thus, as regards emotion regulation and aging, on the basis of the aforementioned

Table 3. Coping strategies for emotion regulation preferred by older adults according to the findings from European studies

Type of measure	Coping strategy
	General
Scenarios of social relationships	"Positivity bias:" Perception and construal of social relationships in a generalized positively biased manner.
Self-reports	"Greater internal control of emotion:" Greater ability to control internal emotional experiences.
	Specific
Scenarios of social relationships	"Avoidance:" Distancing the self from negative emotions.
Self-reports	"Putting into perspective:" Referring to the relativity of an event when compared to other events.
Self-reports	"Positive refocusing:" Thinking about pleasant situations instead of thinking about the actual stressful event.
Self-reports	"Acceptance:" Accept the negative experience and/or adopt a passive form of resignation.
Self-reports	"Defensiveness:" Self-deception as an attempt to downregulate negative affect.
Self-reports	"Greater internal control of anger"

Note. Findings in this table come from Garnefski & Kraaij, 2006; Gross et al., 1997; Thomsen et al., 2005; Winkeler et al., 2000.

findings it can be concluded that, although defensiveness has traditionally been viewed as a nonadaptive strategy, it may hold advantages in older age when uncontrollable stressors, such as irreversible losses, emerge. Besides the specific strategies, Gross et al. (1997) investigated age differences in emotional control, using a self-report questionnaire. Young and older participants indicated their ability to control their inner experience and the outer expression of five emotions (happiness, sadness, fear, anger, and disgust). Results indicated greater internal control with aging, whereas external control of emotion did not show any age-related changes. In addition, older women reported a greater ability to control their internal experience of anger compared to younger women. This finding is in line with the evidence already presented regarding less reported anger in older age, albeit in this case it refers to women only. In general, emotion regulation in old age is characterized by increased inner control of emotions, more flexible handling of emotionally charged problems through the use of a wide range of emotion-focused strategies, and a stronger tendency to perceive social life positively. However, at this point it must be noted that questions remain as concerns potential changes in the adaptive value of specific emotion regulation strategies during the life span. The findings from the aforementioned studies are summarized in **Table 3**.

Emotion-Cognition Interactions

Another source of evidence regarding emotions in older age comes from research on the memory of emotions and emotion-cognition interactions. Although there is evidence showing an age difference in the ratio of positive to negative material in information processing, with older adults disproportionately preferring the processing of positive information as compared to younger ones (see Carstensen et al., in press, for a review) there is also evidence for the opposite. There are studies that demonstrated an enhancing cognitive processing of negative information in later life (e.g., Denburg, Buchanan, Tranel, & Adolphs, 2003). In either case it seems that emotional variables influence older adults' cognitive performance mainly in tasks requiring attention and memory (Carstensen et al., in press).

D'Argembeau and Van der Linden (2004) examined age-related differences in face recognition and memory of emotional expression of unfamiliar faces. More specifically, younger and older adults were shown happy and angry faces, and, later on, were asked to recognize the same faces displaying a neutral expression. They were also asked to remember what the initial emotional expression of each face was. Results showed that emotional information from faces was retrieved similarly well by older and younger participants in contrast to identity information, i.e., face recognition. On the basis of this finding it was suggested that episodic memory regarding emotional characteristics of faces is preserved in old age.

Likewise, Comblain, D'Argembeau, Van der Linden, and Aldenhoff (2004) investigated age-related differences in recognition memory for emotional and neutral pictures. Younger and older participants were asked to rate pictures according to their emotional valence, arousal, and visual complexity. Two weeks later they were tested on recognition of these pictures. States of awareness that accompanied recognition memory were also assessed with the "remember/know/guess procedure:" briefly, this is an experiential and qualitative approach to estimate the contribution of familiarity and recollection processes in recognition memory tasks. In the case of this study, if participants recollected something they had consciously experienced at the time the picture was first presented, they made a "remember" response. If participants simply "knew" that the picture had been presented earlier and felt familiar, but they were unable to recollect any details about its first exposure, they made a "know" response. Finally, they made a "guess" response if they were not sure whether the picture had been presented previously and they had guessed. Results indicated that, although recognition accuracy (i.e., the ability to discriminate between previously presented pictures and new pictures) was better for younger than for older adults, there was an enhancing effect of emotion on accuracy in both age groups. However, this effect seemed to be weaker in older adults, as regards their ability to consciously retrieve the picture-stimulus together with the associated specific emotional, cognitive, or perceptual information in detail. When asked to state reasons for the "remembering" of a picture, older participants reported more often than younger ones recollection of their emotional reactions toward the picture (Comblain et al., 2004).

Thus, on the basis of these findings it seems that older adults tend to place greater emphasis on subjective and interpretative aspects of information rather than on factual details, as compared to younger adults. This tendency may be at least partially responsible for age-related source-memory failures or for the undermining of possible benefits in memory retrieval derived from the emotional character of the information.

Another study (Hill, van Boxtel, Ponds, Houx, & Jolles, 2005) investigated the relationship of positive affect with episodic memory in a sample of middle-aged and older adults from the Maastricht Aging Study. The role of positive affect – defined as self-reported positive emotional state – was examined as predictor of performance on a serial list learning task that included a recognition-recall and a free recall component. Results showed that positive affect predicted only free recall in the older age group. This finding supported the hypothesis that positive affect facilitates episodic memory in later life only when nonsupporting task conditions are present, which place heavy demands on cognitive processing resources (Hill et al., 2005).

According to Hill et al. (2005), an explanation for this function of positive affect may lie in that it offers enhanced information processing resources, when one is facing a strenuous engagement with a cognitively demanding task. If this is true, then older adults' reporting of lower frequency of negative emotions can be explained as the outcome of self-regulatory processes based on their awareness of the debilitating effect of negative emotions on information processing.

Grühn, Smith, and Baltes (2005) examined the contribution of selective processing of positively toned material (i.e., positivity effect) to memory in older adults. They examined young and older participants' memory for emotionally toned words using a multitrial task which compared memory performance on mixed valence (e.g., including positive, negative, and neutral words) and single valence word lists. The lists were matched for word frequency, word length, and imagery. The findings indicated no age differences in recall of emotionally toned words, and this was the case for both mixed and single valence conditions. However, a differential pattern of retrieval of positive and negative material across the two conditions emerged. Specifically, there was a processing prioritization in memory for negatively toned material (negativity effect), and this was greater for young adults than for older ones. This finding suggests that there is no memory bias for positive information in older adults, but there is reduced memory bias for negative information. Consequently, the question is if the proposed positivity effect in older adults is actually a reduced negativity effect, due either to better emotion regulation in later life or to age-related limitations in cognitive processing of negative information (Grühn et al., 2005).

In the same vein, another study (Comblain, D'Argembeau, & Van der Linden, 2005) explored age-related differences in qualitative characteristics of autobiographical memories for positive, negative, and neutral events. Young and older participants were asked to recall two specific personal experiences of each type and then to rate these memories on 16 sensorial and contextual dimensions. In corroboration of the suggestions of Grühn et al. (2005), this study showed that emotional memories, independently of their valence, contained more qualitative details than neutral ones in both age groups, and positive and negative memories did not differ on most dimensions. In addition, memories for positive events were not qualitatively different between younger and older adults. However, negative memories were associated with a higher intensity of positive feelings and a reduced complexity of storyline in older as compared to younger participants. This finding suggests that older adults tend to reappraise negative events in a more positive light.

Executive Functions

Besides memory, affect valence may have effects on executive functions as well. Phillips et al. (2002b) focused their attention on executive functioning, deficits in which have been found as a result of aging and positive and negative mood states. More specifically, Phillips et al. (2002b) used a film and music for mood induction, a self-report questionnaire on mood states, and a commonly used executive function task, namely, Tower of London. Their aim was to investigate whether executive functioning (in this case planning) in older adults can be impaired by the induced mood. The results indicated that age and mood state interacted in their effect on planning. Older adults needed similar number of moves to carry out the task in the neutral condition, but more moves under both positive and negative mood states as compared to younger adults. This finding suggests impaired executive functioning of older adults in both positive and negative mood states, possibly because mood interfered with their working memory capacity. Moreover, whereas under positive mood state planning time was decreased in younger adults, this did not happen in older adults. Older adults spent about the same time (and less than the time spent in the neutral condition) in both positive and negative mood states. Finally, mood interfered in the estimation of moves needed to carry out the task. Older adults, as compared to younger ones, underestimated the number of moves needed to carry out the task, mainly under the negative mood state. Overoptimism for younger adults was evident only under positive mood state.

These findings suggest that the best condition for older adults to exercise their executive functions, i.e., effortful, analytic processing, is the affectively neutral condition. In younger adults it is the negative mood state that enhances analytic processing (Kuhl, 2001). However, as working memory capacity is impaired in older age (Light, 1991; Philips & Della Sala, 1998; Phillips et al., 2002b), any interference caused by a heightened mood state further impairs older adults' ability to apply their full working memory resources onto the task. Moreover, it impairs their ability to correctly estimate task demands.

This facilitating effect of the neutral affect condition, as regards executive functions, fits with the evidence suggesting that older adults have similar autonomic reactivity as younger adults to self-relevant stimuli (Kunzmann & Grühn, 2005), but they report lower incidence of high arousal emotions, both positive and negative (Pinquart, 2001). It seems that older adults are aware of the debilitating effects of strong emotional states on their executive functioning and for this reason they downregulate them. However, downregulation of negative affect makes them less aware of the actual processing demands of the task and, thus, more optimistic. This may have a motivational side effect, that is, makes them willing to get involved in effortful processing.

In sum, research concerning emotion-cognition interactions in aging suggests that emotion regulation in later life emerges as one of the most important protective factors against cognitive impairment. **Table 4** sums up the findings from the above mentioned studies on emotion – cognition interactions in old age, in terms of gain, stability, or loss in specific aspects of cognitive functioning that are affected by emotion.

Table 4. Summary of findings from European studies on emotion-cognition interactions in old age

| Measures | Cognitive processes affected by emotional information | | |
	Gain	Stability	Loss
Face recognition and memory of expression of faces	Memory retrieval		
Emotional and neutral picture recognition	Recognition accuracy		Source memory
Self-reported positive affect and serial list learning task	Free recall		
Multitrial task of memory performance on mixed valence and single valence word lists			Processing prioritization in memory for negative information (negativity bias)
Recalling of personal positive and negative versus neutral events	Autobiographical memory		
Recalling of personal positive and negative versus neutral events	Positivity bias in memory for negative information .		Source memory
Self-reported affect, mood induction, and a planning task			Executive functioning
Tasks of executive functioning and working memory, and tasks of emotional processing and social decision making		Abilities mediated by the ventromedial prefrontal area (emotional and social behavior)	

Note. Findings in this table come from D' Argembeau & Van der Linden, 2004; Comblain et al., 2004; Hill et al., 2005; Grühn et al., 2005; Comblain et al., 2005; Phillips et al., 2002; MacPherson et al., 2002.

Implications of Emotion Regulation for Well-Being

The evidence on emotions and emotion regulation in aging suggests that older adults downregulate negative emotions and affect in order to compensate for the diminishing cognitive resources but also for maintaining or enhancing social relations. This perspective may explain Efklides and colleagues' (2003) finding that adaptation to old age involves adapting one's goals to one's capability, exercising emotional control and maintaining self-efficacy, as well as strategies, such as perception of health problems relative to others and downward social comparison. These aspects of adaptation to aging reflect an awareness of one's limitations as well as emotion regulation and adoption of emotion-focused strategies in order to handle health and social problems (see also Carstensen et al., 2003).

On the other hand, subjective quality of life involves happiness and enthusiasm for life, as well as life satisfaction (Efklides et al., 2003). Therefore, maintaining positive affect is critical for subjective quality of life. Yet, Efklides et al. (2003) found that both positive and negative emotional states are critical for the reported happiness. Since happiness reflects the extent to which positive affect prevails over negative (Diener, 2000), older adults' efforts to maintain emotional balance between increased negative affect and decreasing positive affect is of great importance. Downregulating negative affect and increasing positive affect through positive involvement (Kunzmann et al., 2005) helps maintain the balance on the positive side. Moreover, positive affect is contributing to life satisfaction and to morale (Efklides et al., 2003). In addition, the effects of most demographic and health factors on subjective quality of life in older adults were partially explained by affect (Efklides et al., 2003). The only demographic factor that appeared to have a direct effect on all aspects of subjective quality of life, except subjective well-being, was the existence of children in the family. Having children supports the sense of family belonging, gives perspective to older adults' life and, possibly, opportunities for positive involvement.

The importance of positive involvement was shown in the study of Kunzmann et al. (2005), who investigated whether two distinct facets of positive affectivity, namely positive involvement and pleasant affect (for details see above), differentially predicted two lifestyles (growth-related and hedonic). Self-reported value orientations, everyday activities, and activity aspirations were measured. In terms of age, the results indicated that older adults may be less likely to pursue everyday activities related to a pleasurable life, intimacy, and social approval (hedonic life style), which are related to pleasant affect (i.e., self-focused). On the contrary, they are more likely to pursue activities related to personal growth, well-being of friends and family, and societal engagement (growth-related life style) because they experience feelings of positive involvement more frequently than younger adults. For the same reason they may be more inclined to hold growth-related values. These findings are in line with evidence provided by the Efklides et al. (2003) study showing that generativity (i.e., offering to younger generation) holds a distinct position in older adults' adaptation to old age. Moreover, older adults may thrive in domains that require integration of world knowledge, expertise, and positive affect as in wisdom (Moraitou & Efklides, 2005). In the same vein, Kunzmann and Baltes (2003) examined the connection between wisdom, as expert knowledge about the conduct and meaning of life, and positive and negative affectivity. Results showed that wisdom-related knowledge was positively associated with positive involvement and negatively associated with pleasant affect.

Caprara, Caprara, and Steca (2003) examined affective self-regulatory efficacy as an agentic personality mechanism. Affective self-regulatory efficacy refers to the perceived capacity to manage negative affect and to express positive affect (Caprara et al., 2003). Consistent with what was found in the case of emotional stability, these findings indicated that males appear to enter adulthood with a robust sense of efficacy in dealing with negative affect, but this sense weakens in old age. On the other hand, females' perceived capability of regulating their negative affects seems to improve along with advancing age. Yet, both males' and females' sense of personal efficacy in expressing positive affect declines with age.

In another study, Kunzmann et al. (2002) focused their attention on the role of control beliefs in emotion regulation in old and very old age (sample from the Berlin Aging Study; age range: 70–103 years). They examined longitudinal changes in perceived personal/internal control over desirable outcomes, perceived personal responsibility for undesirable outcomes, and perceived others'/external control, and their relation to emotional well-being (positive and negative affect). Whereas beliefs about internal control over positive and negative aspects of life were stable over time, the belief that others determine the events in one's life increased with age. Perceived internal control over desirable outcomes was associated with high emotional well-being, while perceived external control was shown to be associated with low emotional well-being in the later years of life.

Finally, Moraitou, Kolovou, Papasozomenou, and Paschoula (2006) found that dispositional hope is another psychological dimension that can be involved in emotion regulation in old age. Hope as perceived ability to generate and sustain alternative cognitive strategies toward valued goals (i.e., pathways thought, see Snyder et al., 1991) appears to facilitate positive involvement tendencies of older adults in terms of generativity. Likewise, it seems to enhance mainly emotional control in old age as well as the use of emotion regulation strategies, such as "downward social comparison" and "putting into perspective." On the other hand, hope as goal-pursuit beliefs based on past successes (i.e., agency thinking), seems to facilitate primarily intra-individual processes of adaptation to old age, such as inner emotional control and the sense of self-efficacy (Moraitou et al., 2006).

In general, on the basis of the above findings, it can be concluded that affect-related functioning in old age may be resilient against decline at least as regards positive affect and emotion regulation. The role of individual difference factors as well as of social and cultural context factors (Diener, 2000) should be investigated in order to fully understand the subjective quality of life, positive life-span development, and emotion regulation in old age.

Concluding Remarks

In this chapter, we presented recent research carried out in Europe on affect and emotions in old age. The literature overview focused on (1) emotion changes and emotion regulation in old age, (2) emotion-cognition interactions, and (3) implications of emotional functioning for older adults' well-being. European research on emotions and affect extends current theories of aging such as the socioemotional selectivity theory (Carstensen et al., 2003), which posits that older adults' awareness of limited time perspective leads to motivational shifts that direct their attention to emotionally meaningful goals.

Shifts in older adults' motives, however, cannot explain the mechanism underlying emotion-regulation in old age. European research on emotions aims at doing this. Thus, there is evidence showing that older adults show similar or greater levels of autonomic reactivity to emotional stimuli than those of younger adults, when emotion-eliciting stimuli are highly age-relevant. This finding suggests selectivity in the processing of information and explains why older adults are often seen as emotionally less involved as compared to younger adults. Moreover, affect intensity, frequency, valence, and balance undergo changes – the most of them of a compensational character, such as the decreasing intensity and frequency of high arousal positive and, particularly, negative emotions (especially of anger) and increasing frequency of low arousal emotions. Furthermore, there is stability or increase of affect balance until very old age, indicating an optimization of the affect process. From this point of view, Baltes' (Baltes, 1997) "metatheory," which stresses the role of the processes of selection, optimization, and compensation in successful adaptation to old age, nicely captures the emotional functioning of older adults. Heckhausen and Schultz's (Schulz & Heckhausen, 1998) theory of control, which stresses the compensational nature of control on self-regulation of emotion in older age, is also relevant.

The empirical studies on emotional understanding reveal that advancing age is associated with deficits in decoding negative emotions, such as sadness and anger, from faces, as well as in understanding complex emotional states from eyes. Considering that older adults are capable of high autonomic reactivity to stimuli eliciting negative emotions, it is interesting to understand why they show deficits in decoding negative emotions in faces. There are two possible explanations: (1) The emotion loop is distinct from the cognition loop, that is, the cognitive processes underlying the representation and understanding of emotions, as suggested by Labouvie-Vief and Medler (2002). (2) There is downregulation of negative affect triggered by facial cues of anger as a self-regulatory process of the increased autonomic reactivity to negative emotional stimuli.

Specifically, Labouvie-Vief and Medler's (2002) developmental model of self-regulation in adulthood distinguishes between two affect regulation strategies: affect optimization and cognitive-affective complexity. The former has to do with the emotional experience. The latter refers to the conceptual representation and understanding of the emotional experience, which reflects the role of cognition in affect regulation. Based on findings of cognitive and emotional aging, Labouvie-Vief argues that these two strategies of emotion regulation display different aging trajectories, with the ability to optimize affect remarkably improving but conceptual understanding of emotion slightly declining as adults move from middle to old age.

However, the evidence on categorization of facial expressions of emotions suggests that older adults do not differ from younger ones (Kiffel et al., 2005). Therefore, it might not be a cognitive deficit that explains older adults' lower perception of negative emotions in pictures of faces, but a downregulation of negative affect that prevents older adults from experiencing high arousal negative emotions, which interfere with cognitive processing. This explanation is supported by the evidence regarding cognition-emotion interactions. As stated above, there seems to be reduced processing prioritization for negative information in memory and negative affect has adversive effects on executive functioning in older adults as compared to younger ones. This tendency to reduce negativity bias appears to be connected with less sophisticated or analytic processing of information.

On the other hand, the emotional nature, either positive or negative, of the to-be-processed information appears to enhance cognitive performance in memory and social decision making, and positive affect seems to facilitate memory in later life when task-conditions – such as lack of contextual support – place heavy demands on cognitive processing resources. Thus, downregulation of negative affect facilitates cognitive processing without burdening cognitive resources. On the basis of these findings, "affect optimization" seems to be a defensive strategy which, according to several theories of affect (see Labouvie-Vief & Medler, 2002) may foster highly stereotyped thinking and heuristic information processing.

According to Kuhl (2001) downregulation of negative affect activates extension memory (i.e., extended networks of possible goals, meanings, or objects) and representations of the integrated self, namely personal needs, values, attitudes, etc. Furthermore, it facilitates the pathway between extension memory and the recognition of previously encountered objects. Thus, downregulation of negative affect facilitates openness and, presumably, personal involvement in an environment-focused lifestyle rather than a self-focused one that is mediated by intension memory.

Consistent with socio-cognitive theories and, especially, with the socioemotional selectivity theory (Carstensen et al., 2003), European research findings concerning emotion regulation indicate that advancing age is associated with increasing inner control of emotion, and more flexible handling of emotionally charged problems. Older adults prefer to apply a wide range of emotion-focused strategies along with problem-focused ones, as compared to younger adults' preference to handle these problems using primarily the latter. Although some of the emotion-focused coping strategies are nonadaptive for younger adults, it seems that they help older adults to maintain affective resilience as well as their social network and subjective well-being.

In conclusion, the above review of European studies on emotion and aging suggests that emotion represents one of the few psychological dimensions in which functioning remains relatively intact or even improves during the life span and until very old age. Thus, with regard to everyday life, emotions can help both the older adults to successfully cope with the increasing challenges of old age and younger individuals to learn from older adults how to effectively handle emotional problems in social relationships.

Future Perspectives

The European research on emotions and affect we reviewed was overwhelmingly cross-sectional, self-report studies, and to a lesser extent experimental. The findings help us understand the changes that occur in emotional functioning and emotion regulation in old age and the possible mechanism that underlies them. However, emotional development is a lifelong process and more longitudinal studies are needed in order to understand general patterns as well as individual variation in it. Moreover, there is great need for observational research of emotional behaviors in the social and cultural context in which they occur. Specific emphasis must also be given to the study of discrete emotions and the possible situational effects on them, particularly situations and conditions that foster positive affective functioning despite negative life events. The role of personality, intelligence, and individual difference factors in emotion regulation and coping strategies of older adults is also important when seen in a situational and cultural perspective. Such an approach can also elucidate the process involved in subjective quality of life and positive life span development.

References

Baltes, P.B. (1997). On the incomplete architecture of human ontogeny. *American Psychologist, 52*, 366–380.

Caprara, G.V., Caprara, M., & Steca, P. (2003). Personality's correlates of adult development and aging. *European Psychologist, 8*, 131–147.

Carstensen, L., Fung, H., & Charles, S. (2003). Socioemotional selectivity theory and the regulation of emotion in the second half of life. *Motivation and Emotion, 27*, 103–123.

Carstensen, L., Mikels, J., & Mather, M. (in press). Aging and the intersection of cognition, motivation and emotion. In J. Birren & K.W. Schaie (Eds.), *Handbook of the psychology of aging* (6th ed.). San Diego, CA: Academic Press.

Comblain, C., D'Argembeau, A., Van der Linden, M., & Aldenhoff, L. (2004). The effect of aging on the recollection of emotional and neutral pictures. *Memory, 12*, 673–684.

Comblain, C., D'Argembeau, A., & Van der Linden, M. (2005). Phenomenal characteristics of autobiographical memories for emotional and neutral events in older and younger adults. *Experimental Aging Research, 31*, 173–189.

D'Argembeau, A., & Van der Linden, M. (2004). Identity but not expression memory for unfamiliar faces is affected by aging. *Memory, 12*, 644–654.

Denburg, N., Buchanan, T., Tranel, D., & Adolphs, R. (2003). Evidence for preserved emotional memory in normal older persons. *Emotion, 3*, 239–253.

Diamond, L., & Aspinwall, L. (2003). Emotion regulation across the life span: An integrative perspective emphasizing self-regulation, positive affect, and dyadic processes. *Motivation and Emotion, 27*, 125–156.

Diener, E. (2000). The science of happiness and a proposal for a national index. *American Psychologist, 55*, 34–43.

Efklides, A., Kalaitzidou, M., & Chankin, G. (2003). Subjective quality of life in old age in Greece: The effect of demographic factors, emotional state, and adaptation to aging. *European Psychologist, 8*, 178–191.

Fischer, H., Sandblom, J., Gavazzeni, J., Fransson, P., Wright, C., & Bäckman, L. (2005). Age-differential patterns of brain activation during perception of angry faces. *Neuroscience Letters, 386*, 99–104.

Frijda, N.H. (1986). *The emotions.* Cambridge, UK: Cambridge University Press.

Garnefski, N., & Kraaij, V. (2006). Relationships between cognitive emotion regulation strategies and depressive symptoms: A comparative study of five specific samples. *Personality and Individual Differences, 40*, 1659–1669.

Gross, J., Carstensen, L., Pasupathi, M., Tsai, J., Skorpen, C., & Hsu, A. (1997). Emotion and aging: Experience, expression, and control. *Psychology and Aging, 12*, 590–599.

Grühn, D., Smith, J., & Baltes, P. (2005). No aging bias favoring memory for positive material: Evidence from a heterogeneity–homogeneity list paradigm using emotionally toned words. *Psychology and Aging, 20*, 579–588.

Hill, R., van Boxtel, M., Ponds, R., Houx, P., & Jolles, J. (2005). Positive affect and its relationship to free recall memory performance in a sample of older Dutch adults from the Maastricht Aging Study. *International Journal of Geriatric Psychiatry, 20*, 429–435.

Isaacowitz, D., & Smith, J. (2003). Positive and negative affect in very old age. *The Journals of Gerontology Series B: Psychological Sciences and Social Sciences, 58*, 143–152.

Kiffel, C., Campanella, S., & Bruyer, R. (2005). Categorical perception of faces and facial expressions: The age factor. *Experimental Aging Research, 31*, 119–147.

Kuhl, J. (2001). A functional approach to motivation: The role of goal-enactment and self-regulation in current research on approach and avoidance. In A. Efklides, J. Kuhl, & R.M. Sorrentino (Eds.), *Trends and prospects in motivation research* (pp. 239–268). Dordrecht, The Netherlands: Kluwer.

Kunzmann, U., & Baltes, P. (2003). Wisdom-related knowledge: Affective, motivational, and interpersonal correlates. *Personality and Social Psychology Bulletin, 29*, 1104–1119.

Kunzmann, U., & Grühn, D. (2005). Age differences in emotional reactivity: The sample case of sadness. *Psychology and Aging, 20*, 47–59.

Kunzmann, U., Little, T., & Smith, J. (2000). Is age-related stability of subjective well-being a paradox? Cross-sectional and longitudinal evidence from the Berlin Aging Study. *Psychology and Aging, 15*, 511–526.

Kunzmann, U., Little, T., & Smith, J. (2002). Perceiving control: A double-edged sword in old age. *The Journals of Gerontology Series B: Psychological Sciences and Social Sciences, 57*, 484–491.

Kunzmann, U., Stange, A., & Jordan, J. (2005). Positive affectivity and lifestyle in adulthood: Do you do what you feel? *Personality and Social Psychology Bulletin, 31*, 574–588.

Labouvie-Vief, G., & Medler, M. (2002). Affect optimization and affect complexity: Modes and styles of regulation in adulthood. *Psychology and Aging, 17*, 571–588.

Lawton, M.P. (2001). Emotion in later life. *Current Directions in Psychological Science, 10*, 120–125.

Light, L.L. (1991). Memory and aging: Four hypotheses in search of data. *Annual Review of Psychology, 42*, 333–376.

MacPherson, S., Phillips, L., & Della Sala, S. (2002). Age, executive function, and social decision making: A dorsolateral prefrontal theory of cognitive aging. *Psychology and Aging, 17*, 598–609.

Moraitou, D., & Efklides, A. (2005). Developmental patterns as regards the formation of laymen's implicit theories of wisdom. Comparison with cleverness, creativity, and humanity [in Greek]. In F. Vlachos, F. Bonoti, P. Metallidou, I. Dermitzaki, & A. Efklides (Eds.), *Scientific annals of the Psychological Society of Northern Greece: Vol. 3. Human behavior and learning* (pp. 271–361). Athens, Greece: Ellinika Grammata.

Moraitou, D., Kolovou, C., Papasozomenou, C., & Paschoula, D. (2006). Hope and adaptation to old age: Their relationship with individual-demographic factors. *Social Indicators Research, 76*, 71–93.

Mroczek, D. (2001). Age and emotion in adulthood. *Current Directions in Psychological Science, 10*(3), 87–90.

Phillips, L., & Allen, R. (2004). Adult aging and the perceived intensity of emotions in faces and stories. *Aging Clinical and Experimental Research, 16*(3), 1–10.

Phillips, L., & Della Sala, S. (1998). Aging, intelligence, and anatomical segregation in the frontal lobes. *Learning and Individual Differences, 10*, 217–243.

Phillips, L., MacLean, R., & Allen, R. (2002a). Age and the understanding of emotions: Neuropsychological and sociocognitive perspectives. *The Journals of Gerontology Series B: Psychological Sciences and Social Sciences, 57*, 526–530.

Phillips, L., Smith, L., & Gilhooly, K. (2002b). The effects of adult aging and induced positive and negative mood on planning. *Emotion, 2*, 263–272.

Pinquart, M. (2001). Age differences in perceived positive affect, negative affect, and affect balance in middle and old age. *Journal of Happiness Studies, 2*, 375–405.

Schulz, R., & Heckhausen, J. (1998). Emotion and control: A life span perspective. In K.W. Schaie & M.P. Lawton (Eds.), *Annual review of gerontology and geriatrics: Vol. 17. Emphasis on emotion and adult development* (pp. 185–205). New York: Springer-Verlag.

Snyder, C.R., Harris, C., Anderson, J.R., Holleran, S.A., Irving, L.M., Sigmon, S.T. et al. (1991).

The will and the ways: Development and validation of an individual-differences measure of hope. *Journal of Personality and Social Psychology, 60,* 570–585.

Teachman, B.A. (2006). Aging and negative affect: The rise and fall and rise of anxiety and depression symptoms. *Psychology and Aging, 21,* 201–207.

Thomsen, D.K., Mehlsen, M.Y., Viidik, A., Sommerlund, B., & Zachariae, R. (2005). Age and gender differences in negative affect – Is there a role for emotion regulation? *Personality and Individual Differences, 38,* 1935–1946.

Winkeler, M., Filipp, S-H., & Boll, T. (2000). Positivity in the aged's perceptions of intergenerational relationships: A "stake" or "leniency" effect? *International Journal of Behavioral Development, 24,* 173–182.

7. Personality and Self-Beliefs

Mariagiovanna Caprara, Patrizia Steca, and Gian Vittorio Caprara

Introduction

The world is in the midst of an unprecedented demographic change. Longevity is increasing at an extraordinary rate and incontrovertible statistics tell us that despite tremendous disparities in the conditions of life across continents and countries, we will have many older people in the coming decades. For the first time in human history, most people live to see old age. Infant mortality and disease that formerly took the lives of young people, now affect only a very small proportion of the population and this is true in most parts of the world. No other demographic group is growing as quickly as older people, and the percentage of the population made up of older adults is growing faster than any other. The average age of the global population moved from 23.5 years in 1950 to 26 years in 1998 and is expected to reach 38 years before 2050. Overall, the "oldest" area of the world will continue to be Europe with over 14% of older adults in Italy (see Chapter 1).

In order to face these changes, new psychological knowledge is needed to grant full expression to human potentials over the life span to the largest portion of the population, to extend healthy aging and to enable communities to deal effectively with the unavoidable declines associated with extended aging. Until the last few decades very little information was available about old age, which people generally thought was characterized by illness, loss of autonomy, and dependence upon others. Today, people between the age of retirement and their early eighties, represent a significant part of the population in most developed countries whose habits and attitudes toward life are quite different from prior generations. Although many stereotypes about older people still persist, today, elderly people often stay in business, contribute actively to governance, manage their families, and enjoy a wide variety of personal interests. Recent changes largely follow from significant changes in conditions of work and life as well the tremendous progress of medicine.

In reality, psychological research plays a key role in fostering the needed changes in mentalities and habits, by leading to the acknowledgment of the extraordinary resources of old age, by promoting their fulfilment, by contrasting stereotypes, and ultimately, by enabling communities to benefit both economically and socially from old age. Personality psychology, in particular, plays a key role in addressing the personal and social processes that can contribute to the full expression of individuals' capacities, pointing to the agentic role people may exert over the course of their life and focusing on their strength no less than on their vulnerabilities.

Although very old age usually carries loss and pain, many of the elderly experience the demands and setbacks of aging without any loss of psychological well-being. Thus, the capacities that enable old people to overcome adversities and contribute to keeping intact their trust in life deserve utmost attention. Even in old age, people have a large degree of freedom in selecting activities, environments and interpersonal relations that are most congenial given their age.

Personality research should help the elderly to better appreciate their strengths and potentials and implement the changes in attitudes and behaviors needed to achieve optimal adaptation. Along this line of reasoning, cross-sectional findings are presented which indicate that elderly people, while being perceptive of age-related developmental losses, are quite effective in maintaining a sense of control and a positive view of self- and personal development.

Social policy makers may benefit from knowing and regularly monitoring what people report about their habits, beliefs, and aims, so that they may make people better equipped to face the challenges and changes of various seasons of life in accordance with the spirit of the times.

Looking at Personality Over the Life Course

Decades of research attest to the fact that both change and stability mark personality over the course of life, albeit differently, depending on the features of personality one considers and on the extent to which situations constrain or promote their expression (Baltes, 1997; Roberts & Del Vecchio, 2000). Personality may be defined as the complexity of structures, processes and patterns of cognition, affect, and behavior functioning; a self-regulatory system in the service of adaptation. It can be viewed as both a construction and an agentic system, resulting from psychological processes and structures that emerge in the course of development and gradually evolve into coherent psychological systems. As a construction, personality is the whole architecture which results from the transactions between the individual and the environment over the entire course of life and which conveys the sense of unity, continuity and coherence which distinguishes any individual from others. As an agency, personality is the complex of capacities to make things happen by one's own action from which one derives the sense of one's own identity as a unique agent being. A variety of self-referent processes operating in concert enable people to guide behavior purposefully, to transform the environments they encounter, and to actively shape their own personality and the course of their life.

As the term "personality" encompasses a great variety of phenomena, it is not surprising that different ideas and conceptualizations appear in the traditional and common use of the word. Nor it is surprising that different assumptions and research strategies have marked the study of personality since the beginning of the discipline (Caprara & Cervone, 2000). A number of "key areas" have been identified in the study of personality, reflecting different conceptualizations and theoretical positions.

In the present chapter, we will address various aspects of personality: (1) traits, (2) values, (3) motives, (4) self-esteem, (5) self-efficacy beliefs, and (6) subjective and psychological well-being. Each of these aspects corresponds to the concerted action of mental structures and processes that contribute to personality functioning as a self-regulatory system; each serves to capture the uniqueness that distinguishes one person from another; each may highlight important changes in individual functioning with aging in response to the different demands and tasks of the life course.

It is likely that both stability and change in habits, attitudes, goals, interaction and adaptation strategies are necessary along the various stages of life. Stability is critical for preserving one's own identity, as well as for establishing and keeping stable relations with others. Change is needed in order to face a continuously changing environment. Yet, it is not fully clear which changes take place in the above dimensions over the course of adulthood, nor is it clear which change in direction is most desirable after the entrance into old age.

To address these issues, we will report recent findings from ongoing Italian cross-sectional studies aimed at investigating personality in the elderly. First, we will examine the extent to which old people locate themselves at different levels along the various dimensions. Then we will look at sociodemographic variables such as gender, education, and marital status. Ultimately, we will examine the extent to which old people show different patterns of correlations between traits, motives, values, self-esteem, self-efficacy beliefs, psychological well-being, life satisfaction, and health and happiness.

Traits

Throughout much of its history, personality psychology has been concerned with individual differences in observable variations in styles of behavior, affect, and cognition traceable to a limited number of dispositional constructs. As people exhibit stable patterns of experience and action that distinguishes them from one another, traits have been posited to account for the tendencies to exhibit one versus another type of response across different settings and across time. Traditionally, dispositional theorists conceived personality as a hierarchical organization and focused on high level traits (e.g., extraversion) which organize lower level tendencies (e.g., sociability), which in turn supervise lower level behavioral habits (e.g., talkative) (Eysenck, 1970).

After alternative taxonomies have been confronted with each other over the decades, the five-factor model of personality, or the "Big Five," is currently the most common and most largely accepted classification of personality traits. This model proposes that at the broadest level of description and classification of the individual personality, five basic dimensions (factors) can be distinguished: Extraversion (or Energy), Agreeableness (or Friendliness), Conscientiousness, Neuroticism (vs. Emotional stability), and Openness to experience (or Culture) (Caprara & Cervone, 2000; Digman, 1990).

Most research dealing with personality stability and change over the course of life has focused on traits, leading to the conclusion that linear changes are no more important than nonlinear changes and that intra-individual variability is no more important than inter-individual variability (Helson, Kwan, John, & Jones, 2002; Nesselroade,

1987). Age-related changes and age differences in personality traits have been assessed in many studies (Heatherton & Weinberger, 1994; Helson, Jones, & Kwan, 2002; Helson, & Wink, 1992; McCrae & Costa, 1990; Costa & McCrae, 1997). In their effort to summarize all of the available longitudinal evidence on personality development across the life-span, Costa and McCrae (e.g., 1992, 1994) showed that stability coefficients declined but are still relevant with increasing time intervals between measurements, from a mean value of .78 (6 or 3 years) to a mean value of .61 (30 years). Studies across age groups have reported higher stability in Neuroticism than other factors over prolonged periods of time, and negative age trends for Extraversion/Energy and Openness (Costa & McCrae, 1994; Smith & Baltes, 1999). In general, findings attest to both stability and change, and similar changes across countries, but figures may vary between countries and within countries for different distances of time.

Earlier studies on Italian adults have investigated differences in the Big Five across ages (Caprara, Gentilomo, Barbaranelli, & Giorgi, 1993; McCrae et al., 1999). The first study reported lower scores in extraversion and friendliness and higher scores in conscientiousness in older people (55+ years) compared to young people (18–28 years). The second study reported lower scores in openness and extraversion and higher scores in conscientiousness in older people (50+ years) compared to young people (18–29 years). These findings are consistent with other cross-cultural findings (Fernández-Ballesteros et al., 2004; McCrae et al., 1999).

On the other hand the studies are inconsistent with other European findings that report higher friendliness in the elderly than in young people (e.g., Smith & Baltes, 1999).

Recent findings from a study involving a large population of Italian adults, ranging in age from 20 to 80 years old, confirmed a decline in energy, conscientiousness, and

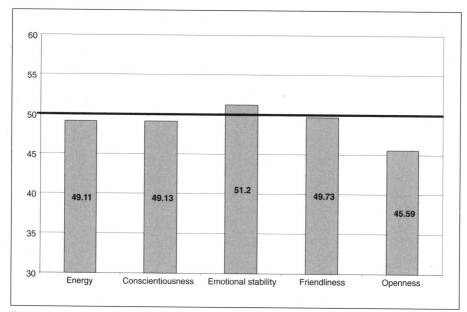

Figure 1. Mean standardized *t*-scores of Big Five personality traits in older adults

mostly in openness, in the elderly (Caprara, Caprara, & Steca, 2003). **Figure 1** reports mean values of the Big Five personality dimensions for 293 adults (140 males and 153 females) over 65 years of age (mean age = 74.81, SD = 5.85). The Big Five were measured using the Big Five Questionnaire (BFQ; Caprara, Barbaranelli, & Borgogni, 1993) that contains five-domain scales: "energy/extraversion," "friendliness," "conscientiousness," "emotional stability," and "openness."

As for all the figures reported below, means are expressed in standardized t-scores (M = 50, SD = 10), based on a large population of Italian adults of different ages (N = 1433, M = 49.3, SD = 18, range 20–92 years). Scores higher than 50 indicate that the dimension in the elderly people is higher than the one observed in the total population while scores lower than 50 indicate that the dimension in the target group is lower than the one for the total population. Findings are in accordance with previous research showing a decline in extraversion/energy and openness, and an increase in emotional stability in the elderly respect to the general population (Roberts, Walton, & Viechtbauer, 2006; Srivastava, John, Gosling, & Potter, 2003; McCrae & Costa, 1999). Nevertheless, only openness displayed a significant decrease with respect to the normal population.

Values

Values are cognitive representations of desirable, abstract, transituational goals that serve as guiding principles in peoples lives (Schwartz, 1992). Whereas values are related to both traits and motives, they help to uncover aspects of personality functioning mostly related to the ideals that guide people's lives and to the standards that serve as criteria for their judgments about behavior, events, others, and the self.

The theory of values' content and structure proposed by Schwartz (1992) is a comprehensive theory enabling the explication of the relations among different sets of values that largely differ in terms of the motivational goals they express. The identified sets of values represent, in the form of conscious goals, three universal requirements of human existence: biological needs, requisites of coordinated social interaction, and demands of group survival and functioning.

The theory distinguishes ten basic values, found in cross-cultural research in 44 countries: universalism, benevolence, conformity, tradition, security, power, achievement, hedonism, stimulation, and self-direction (Schwartz, 1992; Schwartz & Sagiv, 1995). These ten value types are organized into four higher-level types: self-transcendence, emphasizing acceptance of others as equals and concern for their welfare; self-enhancement, emphasizing pursuit of one's own relative success and dominance over others; openness to change, emphasizing independent thought and action and favoring change; and conservatism, emphasizing submissive self-restriction to preserve one's status quo.

Studies on value development across the life span are certainly fewer than those focused on personality traits. As supposed by Schwartz (e.g., 2003), with age, security values should be more important because a safe, suitable environment is more critical as the capacities to cope with change decrease. A similar increasing importance has

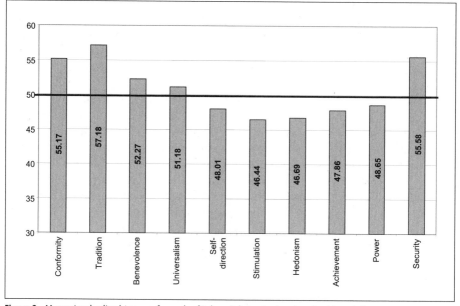

Figure 2. Mean standardized *t*-scores for each of Schwartz's ten basic values in older adults

been hypothesized for conformity and tradition values, because habits and accepted ways of doing things are less demanding and threatening. On the contrary, stimulation values should be less important because novelty and risk are too challenging and threatening for older people who tend to become more embedded in social networks, more committed to habitual patterns, and less exposed to arousing and exciting changes and challenges (Tyler & Shuller, 1991). Hedonism values also should be less important because dulling of the senses reduces the capacity to enjoy sensual pleasure. Achievement and, perhaps, power values should also be less important for older people who are less able to perform demanding tasks successfully and to obtain social approval.

Findings from our studies corroborated the expected significant positive correlations between age and security, tradition, and conformity, as well as significant negative correlations between age and self-direction, stimulation, hedonism, and achievement. A decrease in old age of openness to change and self-enhancement values, and an increase of conservatism values was also found (Caprara et al., 2003).

Figure 2 reports mean *t*-scores for the elderly on Schwartz's ten basic values, measured by the Portrait Values Questionnaire (PVQ) (Schwartz, Melech, Lehmann, Burgess, & Harris, 2001), a self-report questionnaire that includes 40 short verbal portraits, each describing a person's goal, aspiration, or wish pointing implicitly to the importance of specific values.

As found in previous studies old adults reported above mean scores on conformity, tradition and security; benevolence and universalism were also slightly above the population's mean. On the contrary, both self-enhancement and openness to change values for elderly were below the mean; as hypothesized the lowest scores were reported in stimulation and hedonism values.

Motives

Motives refer to dispositions within the person to strive to reach certain kinds of positive incentives, rewards or goals, or to avoid certain kinds of threats. Motives have been often used as synonymous with needs; as enduring dispositions to strive for particular kinds of aims, namely, particular kinds of goals accompanied by feelings of satisfaction.

The priority assigned to the pursuit of certain aims like achievement, affiliation or power, across situations, is associated to preferences for certain kind of activities which lead to distinguish individuals one from another on the basis of their motivational orientation: as people may seek satisfaction by accomplishing a challenging task or by having positive affective relationships with other persons, or by exerting control over other people.

David McClelland (1987) has proposed of a taxonomy of basic motives that includes power, affiliation, and achievement, each being characterized by major desires and concerns. The power motive is characterized by a desire to control others, to persuade and prevail, and often by a subtle concern to be controlled. The affiliation motive is characterized by a desire to belong and by the concern about being abandoned. The achievement motive is characterized by the desire to meet challenges and to master complex tasks and situations, and by a major concern for failure.

As motives are conducive to pursue satisfaction through actions that can result more or less congenial to different ages, one may expect that successful adaptation may imply significant changes over the life course. In reality, this is what resulted from our findings. **Figure 3** reports mean *t*-scores for the elderly on McClelland's three major

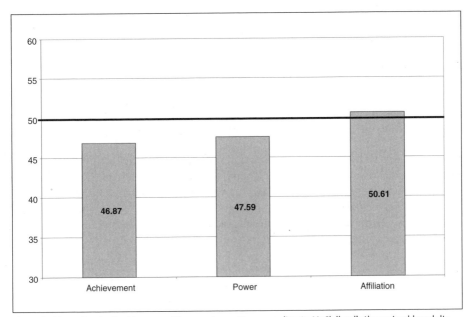

Figure 3. Mean standardized *t*-scores of three major motives according to McClelland's theory in older adults

motives, assessed through the Motivational Orientations Test (Borgogni, Petitta, & Barbaranelli, 2004). In accordance with a life condition in which people retire from work and increasingly depend upon others' assistance, older people showed lower mean scores in both achievement and power motives. While the elderly demonstrated higher values in affiliation, the differences were not statistically significant.

Self-Esteem

Self-esteem corresponds to the global regard and acceptance that one has for oneself as a person (Harter, 1993). This overall judgment reflects the manifold person/situation transactions that mark one's course of life, as people draw recognition from what they have accomplished with others over the course of time and across diverse life contingencies.

Although one should not underestimate the costly pursuit of self-esteem under severe contingencies (Crocker & Park, 2004), or the risky consequences of an exaggerated opinion of oneself (Baumeister, Campbell, Krueger, & Vohs, 2003), one cannot doubt the beneficial effects of self-esteem along the entire lifespan and in various life domains (DuBois & Tevendale, 1999; Emler, 2001). People with high levels of self-esteem are at lower risk for anxiety and depressive symptoms and have better health outcomes (Baumeister, 1993; Greenberg et al., 1992; O'Connor & Vallerand, 1998). They also adopt more efficacious strategies in pursuing their goals, are less prone to give up in the face of obstacles and adversities (Kernis, 1995), feel more control over life events (Tedeschi & Norman, 1985), and have more self-confidence, especially following an initial failure (e.g., McFarlin & Blascovich, 1981).

A number of longitudinal studies have documented the beneficial effects that self-esteem exerts over the course of life (DeLongis, Folkamn, & Lazarus, 1988; Egan & Perry, 1998; Murrel, Meeks, & Walker, 1991), acting as a protective factor and fostering personal and interpersonal resources. The positive effect of self-esteem is particularly lasting, even if the personal amount of self-esteem may vary across time as a consequence of changes in personal capacities and attitudes toward the self, and the variation in the surrounding social environment that the individual uses to compare his or her own characteristics, capacities, and attainments (i.e., Damon & Hart, 1988; Harter, 1998).

A recent review by Robins, Trzesniewski, Tracy, Gosling, and Potter (2002) showed that self-esteem levels are high in childhood, drop during adolescence, rise gradually throughout adulthood, and decline sharply in old age. This trajectory generally held across gender, socioeconomic status, ethnicity, and nationality (U.S. citizens vs. non-U.S. citizens). However, differences in self-esteem, as assessed by the Rosenberg scale (1965), between older people and the rest of the population did not reach statistical significance ($M = 49.4$).

Self-Efficacy Beliefs

Various self-referent processes operate in concert allowing people to function as self-regulating agents who actively negotiate with the social world and exert control over personal experiences. Among knowledge structures that mostly contribute to self-regulation and adaptation, self-efficacy beliefs, namely individuals' beliefs in their capacity to exert control over the events that affect their lives, play a central role in personality functioning (Bandura, 1997; Caprara & Cervone, 2000).

Whatever other factors may operate as guides and motivators in people's efforts to reach desired results, they are rooted in the core belief that one has the power to produce effects by one's own actions. Unless people believe they can be successful in obtaining desired outcomes, they have little incentive to undertake activities or to persevere in the case of difficulties or failures.

Findings from diverse lines of research have documented that self-efficacy beliefs regarding distinct life contexts and specific tasks contribute to distinct outcomes in various life domains of functioning such as learning, work, sports, health, social adjustment, and well-being (for a review, see Bandura, 1997, 2001). However, self-efficacy beliefs do not operate in isolation from one another. As people reflect on their experiences across specific settings, they construct beliefs about their capabilities that pertain to domains of life that include a cluster of interrelated circumstances.

Although much previous research has centered on the effects of self-efficacy beliefs on cognitive processes, motivation, and performance, recent research has broadened and extended analyses of the functional properties of perceived self-efficacy to the regulation of one's affective life and interpersonal relations, and their impact on psychosocial functioning and well-being (Bandura, Caprara, Barbaranelli, Gerbino, & Pastorelli, 2003; Caprara & Steca, 2005a, 2005b, 2006; Caprara, Steca, Gerbino, Paciello, & Vecchio, 2006).

Efficacious measures have been developed to assess emotional and interpersonal self-regulatory efficacy beliefs related to peoples capacity to manage negative emotions, to express positive emotions, to deal effectively with others (social efficacy) and to be sensitive to others needs and request for help (empathetic efficacy) (Caprara & Gerbino, 2001; Caprara, Gerbino, & Delle Fratte, 2001).

While previous findings report a decrease across ages of the perceived capacity to express and manage positive affects, as well as of the perceived capacity to manage interpersonal relationships (social self-efficacy beliefs) and of empathic self-efficacy beliefs (Caprara et al., 2003), only social self-efficacy differences reached statistical significance.

However, recent findings only in part replicate the above differences as shown in **Figure 4**. Whereas older adults scored moderately below the mean in both empathic and social self-efficacy as in previous studies, they scored slightly above the mean in emotional self-efficacy. It is likely that older people benefit more from effective management of negative and positive emotions rather than from being socially assertive and from being too empathetic with other's request of comfort and support.

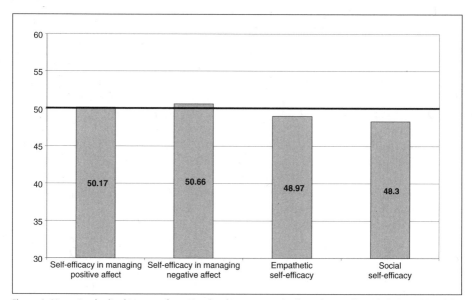

Figure 4 Mean standardized t-scores of emotional and interpersonal self-regulatory efficacy beliefs in older adults

Subjective Well-Being: Life Satisfaction and Happiness

In the study of the positive, much attention has been given to the concept of subjective well-being (SWB). In the last two decades, Ed Diener has been the researcher who has probably dedicated the most effort to the conceptualization and empirical study of the components of SWB. According to his theoretical perspective, SWB corresponds to one's individual experience of the quality and emotional states of individual life conditions, as they are perceived, evaluated and reported by the person (Diener, 1984, 1994, 2000; Diener, Lucas, & Oishi, 2002; Diener, Suh, Lucas, & Smith, 1999).

Two components are usually distinguished in the subjective experience of well-being: a cognitive component and an affective component. The cognitive component corresponds to the individual's evaluation of life satisfaction, according to subjectively determined standards, and may be formulated at a general level when it refers to life as a whole, or at more specific levels when it refers to particular life domains (e.g., family, job environment, leisure, friendship, etc.). The affective component corresponds to the degree of happiness resulting from individual's hedonic balance, namely by the predominance of pleasant (or positive) affective experiences over unpleasant (or negative) affective experiences (Diener, 1984, 1994, 2000; Diener et al., 1999).

Researchers on SWB's change across ages have spoken of a "paradox of well-being," because despite the difficulties of aging (e.g., physical deterioration, loss of friends and relatives), older people do not report concomitant decreases in most aspects of well-being. Numerous studies using cross-sectional data have found negligible age differences in life satisfaction and other forms of subjective well-being (for a review, see Diener & Suh, 1998), whereas some other studies have found an increase in feelings of well-being among older adults, in that they report less anxiety (Lawton, Kleban, &

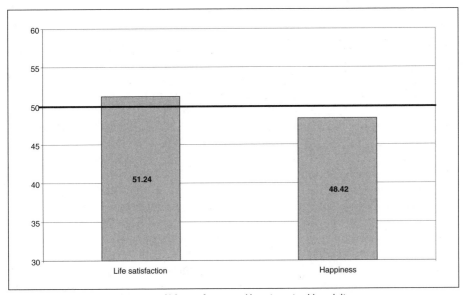

Figure 5 Mean standardized *t*-scores of life satisfaction and happiness in older adults

Dean, 1993), better emotional regulation (Gross, Cartensen, Tsai, Skorpen, & Hsu, 1997; Lawton et al., 1993; Lawton, Klebam, Rejagopal, & Dean, 1992) and have a better balance of positive to negative affect (Ryff, 1989b).

In particular, older people may continue to experience and report high levels of life satisfaction and happiness when they benefit from the advantages of high socioeconomic status, enjoy a vast network of friendly relationships and can fully express their autonomy (Diener & Suh, 1997; Field & Minkler, 1988; Carstensen, 1992; Carstensen, Pasupathi, Mayr, & Nesselroade, 2000; Mroczek & Kolarz; 1998; Ryff, 1989b; Zamarrón & Fernandez-Ballesteros, 2000). Thus, it is not surprising that quality of life, well-being, life satisfaction, and successful aging are all major issues in Europe, as attested by several research programs such as EXCELSA (2003), SHARE (2006), and ESAW (2004).

Figure 5 reports the mean scores of life satisfaction and happiness (hedonic balance) for older adults, measured by the Satisfaction with Life Scale (Diener, Emmons, Larsen, & Griffin, 1985) and the Positive and Negative Affect Scale (Watson, Clark, & Tellegen, 1988), respectively.

As older adults scored slightly above the mean in life satisfaction and slightly below the mean in happiness, one may guess that life satisfaction is more stable than is happiness. Whereas the former reflects an overall evaluation of life, the latter, resulting from positive minus negative affect, is more sensitive to contingent mood fluctuations due the current conditions of life. Thus, older people may capitalize on previous experiences to keep a positive evaluation of their life, but cannot avoid acknowledging the loss, adversities and pains associated with aging.

Psychological Well-Being

Several psychological and philosophical theories have investigated and described what makes life worth living. From a thorough review of the literature, Carol Ryff has derived a multidimensional formulation of psychological well-being that is articulated in six fundamental dimensions. According to the author, to be psychologically well, a person needs to have positive feelings about oneself and one's past life and to accept personal incapacities and limitations *(Self-acceptance)*, as well as to have high quality, supporting, and gratifying connections with others *(Positive relationships with others)*. He/she also needs to be able to effectively manage everyday demands and tasks *(Environmental mastery)* and to have the capacity to follow one's own ideas and convictions even if they go against convention and others' opinions *(Autonomy)*. Finally, central features of psychological well-being include the need to find meaning in one's life, which comprises having goals that give direction to life *(Purpose in life)* and experiencing a sense of ongoing development and realization of personal talents and potentials *(Personal growth)* (Ryff, 1989a, 1995, 1998; Ryff, Kwan, & Singer, 2001).

Findings derived from large cross-sectional samples have showed large age differences in the six dimensions. Environmental mastery and autonomy demonstrated incremental patterns with age, whereas personal growth and purpose in life showed decreasing patterns, especially from midlife to old age (Ryff, 1989b, 1991; Ryff & Singer, 1998; Ryff, Lee, Essex, & Schmutte, 1994; Seeman, Singer, McEwen, Horwitz, & Rowe, 1997). Other aspects of psychological well-being, namely, self-acceptance and positive relationships with others are characterized by little variation across the periods of young adulthood, midlife, and old age.

Previous findings from Italian studies on large samples of subjects from young to middle and old adulthood showed a significant decrease in personal growth and posi-

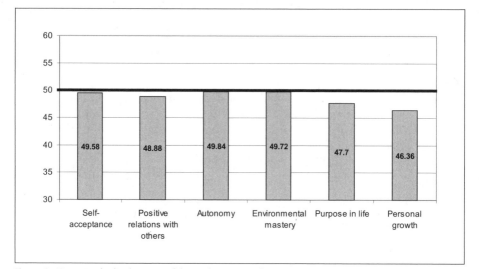

Figure 6. Mean standardized *t*-scores of the six dimensions of psychological well-being according to Ryff's model in older adults

tive relationships with others, but no significant variations due to age in other dimensions of psychological well-being (Caprara et al., 2003).

Recent findings, reported in **Figure 6**, corroborate these findings, although suggesting a general decline as people advance in old age.

The Role of Gender, Education, Marital Status, and Health

The following figures show the differential effect that gender, education, marital status and health status may exert on the above variables in old age. Nonstandardized mean values are reported for each variable only in the case of significant differences. **Figure 7** does report nonstandardized mean scores of the considered constructs separately for old men and women.

As found in previous studies, men reported higher energy and openness than did females (Caprara et al., 2003). With respect to values, previous studies reported scarce differences between men and women; women tend to give higher priority to self-transcendence values and lower priority to self-enhancement values than do men (Capanna, Vecchione, & Schwartz, 2005; Caprara et al., 2003; Schwartz, 2003). Our results confirmed the lower priority that older women give to both self-enhancement and openness to change values; they also showed that older females give higher importance to tradition values than their male counterparts. Similar results were found for motives: men reported higher scores on power and achievement motives than did women.

Men reported higher scores than women in social self-efficacy beliefs, confirming previous findings (Caprara et al., 2003; Caprara & Steca, 2005). On the contrary, and

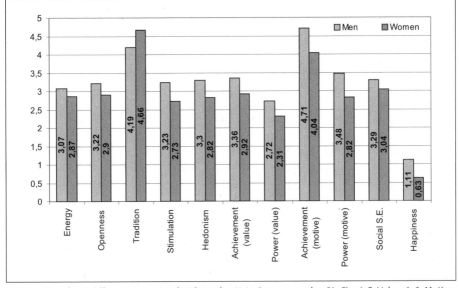

Figure 7. Significant differences associated with gender. *Note:* Response scales: Big Five 1–5; Values 1–6; Motives 1–7; Self-efficacy beliefs 1–5; Happiness 1–5; *p* < .01 with Bonferroni correction

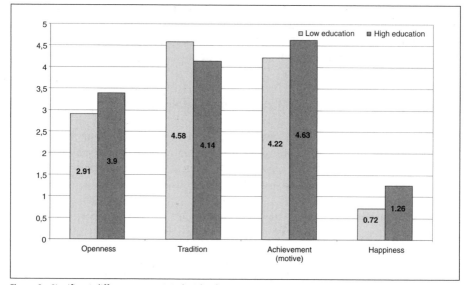

Figure 8. Significant differences associated with education. *Note:* Response scale: Big Five 1–5; Values 1–6; Motives 1–7; Happiness 1–5; *p* < .01 with Bonferroni correction

differently from previous findings, no gender differences were found in self-efficacy beliefs in managing affect and empathic self-efficacy (i.e., Caprara et al., 2003; Caprara & Steca, 2005), nor in self-esteem (i.e., Brody, 1997; Daley, 1991; Kling, Hide, Showers, & Buswell, 1999; Larsen, 1992). Also, no differences were found between older males and females with respect to the six dimensions of psychological well-being. These findings disconfirmed previous results showing that women of all ages consistently rate themselves higher on positive relations with others (Ryff, 1991, Ryff et al., 1994; Ryff & Keyes, 1995) while men score higher on autonomy, environmental mastery, personal growth, purpose in life and self-acceptance (Caprara et al., 2003; Steca et al., 2002). **Figure 8** reports nonstandardized mean scores of the considered constructs, separately for older adults with low (elementary and junior high school) and high education (high school). Also in this case, only significant differences due to the level of education are reported.

Older adults with high education reported higher scores on openness, achievement motive, and hedonic balance; they also reported lower scores on tradition values than did their counterparts with low education. These results, only in part, confirm previous differences due to education on the Big Five, as well as on values and well-being. In addition, these results are partly consistent with findings from a study that examined age differences on the Big Five in both an Italian and Spanish sample (Caprara & Steca, 2004). In this study, educational level was associated with both heightened openness to experience and emotional stability in both Italian and Spanish participants. Educational level appears to be a factor that encourages adaptation and well-being in the elderly.

As reported by Capanna et al. (2005) and Schwartz (2003), higher levels of education correlated positively with self-direction and stimulation and negatively with secu-

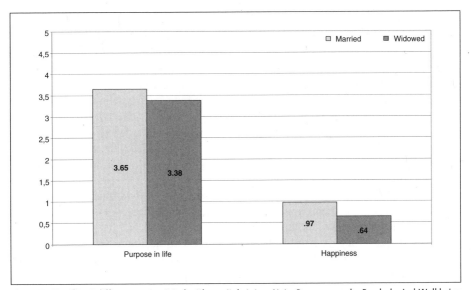

Figure 9. Significant differences associated with marital status. *Note:* Response scale: Psychological Well-being 1–5; Happiness 1–5

rity, tradition, and conformity. As suggested by Schwartz (2003), the further one goes through education, the more likely one is to experience freedom from close supervision, complex problem-solving, rewards for independent thought, encouragement of intellectual flexibility, and openness to novelty. Education also provides knowledge and skills that enhance people's confidence and efficacy in coping with challenges and uncertainties and helps them find more financially secure jobs.

Furthermore, Franks, Herzog, Holmber, and Markus (1999) investigated how aging selves are defined and represented as a function of educational attainment. They showed that those with more education have more complex and detailed selves, and suggested that self-definition and process (e.g., self-esteem, sense of personal control and capacities, etc.) may be implicated in understanding variability in later life health and well-being. Ryff, Magee, Kling, and Wing (1999) summarized findings from several studies showing that those with higher levels of income and education tend to have higher levels of psychological well-being in terms of self-acceptance, purpose in life, and personal growth. **Figure 9** reports nonstandardized mean scores of the considered constructs, separately for married and widowed individuals. As in the case of previous figures, the figure only reports variables that showed significant differences due to marital status.

Married older adults reported higher purpose in life and hedonic balance. As reported by previous studies, marriage appears to guarantee reciprocal support and occasions to share pleasant activities that are particularly valuable in the late phases of life (Gove & Umberson, 1985; Hendrick & Hendrick, 1997).

Covariation Patterns for Traits, Motives, Values, and Self-beliefs, Psychological Well-Being, and Life Satisfaction with Health and Happiness

Figure 10 show correlations for traits, motives, values, self-beliefs, psychological well-being and life satisfaction with health and happiness (hedonic balance) in three age groups: young adults, adults, and people over 65 years, namely, the turning point for retirement in most countries. Correlations do not represent causation however, their changes over the course of life can be informative to a certain degree of the effect that stable characteristics of personality may exert on health and happiness as well as of the effect that a decline in health associated to aging may exert on habits, goals and attitudes toward self and others.

Most correlation patterns with health are similar in adult and older persons. However, health is related to emotional stability, perceived efficacy in managing negative emotions, self-acceptance, environmental mastery, purpose in life, personal growth, and life satisfaction less in the elderly than in the rest of the population. Thus, one may say that these dimensions are more independent from health in the elderly than in the rest of the population. On the one hand, one may guess that other factors, likely social factors, covary with health, more than psychological factors. On the other hand, one may guess that the unavoidable decline in health as a result of aging carries no significant changes in emotional stability, concern for others, effort to master the environment, investment in the future, self-acceptance, positive relations with others, purpose in life and ultimately, lower satisfaction.

Also, most correlations with happiness are similar in older people as in the rest of the adult population. Yet, one may guess that happiness more than health, is affected in aging by stable personality characteristics like traits, motives, values, and self-beliefs as well as by views about the self and life that derive from previous experiences and influence one's current mood.

It is likely that energy, openness, stimulation, self-direction, autonomy, self-esteem, self-acceptance, and life satisfaction contribute less to happiness in old age than in the rest of the population. On the contrary, friendliness, the capacity to express positive emotions and to be empathic with others may significantly contribute to happiness as modesty and closeness to others helps to compensate for loss in agency by cultivating communion.

Conclusions

The above findings demonstrate that the image that older people report of themselves does not differ much from the one reported by younger people as far as traits, motives, values, self-beliefs, psychological well-being, and life satisfaction are concerned. Yet, both health and happiness covary differently with the above variables at different ages. There is no doubt that a number of life changes that tend to occur in old age might have a negative impact on well-being. However, findings suggest that aging may also entail improved coping and emotional regulation abilities that may represent a protective

	Health			Happiness		
	20–40	41–65	>65	20–40	41–65	>65
BIG FIVE						
Energy	.006	.096*	.048	.414***	.423***	.330***
Friendliness	−.038	.009	−.057	.126**	.236***	.284***
Conscientiousness	.089	.073	.071	.353***	.328***	.347***
Emotional stability	.340***	.294***	.189**	.553***	.553***	.542***
Openness	−.001	.091*	.052	.325***	.427***	.378***
VALUES						
Conformity	−.032	−.058	.086	.050	−.002	.021
Tradition	−.064	−.077	−.002	−.002	−.079	−.167**
Benevolence	−.090	.010	−.010	.118**	.199***	.169**
Universalism	−.052	.028	.136*	.115	.158***	.166**
Self-direction	.049	.138**	.080	.388***	.388***	.280***
Stimulation	−.070	.111**	.035	.256***	.228***	.303***
Hedonism	−.020	.097*	.076	.180***	.208***	.129*
Achievement	−.051	.026	.002	.185***	.202***	.144*
Power	−.037	.045	.095	.188***	.147***	.077
Security	.028	−.010	.050	.123**	.022	−.032
MOTIVES						
Achievement	.083	.138***	.096	.390***	.404***	.417***
Power	−.023	.053	.013	.222***	.206***	.194**
Affiliation	−.104*	−.030	−.040	−.123**	.056	.069
SELF-ESTEEM	.342***	.266***	.242***	.605***	.543***	.458***
SELF-EFFICACY BELIEFS						
Managing positive emotions	−.018	.022	.043	.305***	.272***	.314***
Managing negative emotions	.214***	.226***	.167**	.479***	.439***	.428***
Empathic	−.074	−.001	.113*	.221***	.223***	.402***
Social	.021	.140***	.071	.428***	.471***	.435***
PSYCHOLOGICAL WELL-BEING						
Self-acceptance	.333***	.303***	.223***	.614***	.555***	.472***
Positive relationships with others	.104*	.170***	.067	.333***	.383***	.351***
Autonomy	.195***	.169***	.123*	.410***	.422***	.368***
Environmental mastery	.290***	.286***	.204***	.564***	.547***	.550***
Purpose in life	.244***	.264***	.155**	.527***	.537***	.506***
Personal growth	.196***	.172***	.092	.404***	.468***	.477***
LIFE SATISFACTION	.213***	.254***	.158**	.413***	.381***	.355***

*$p < .05$, **$p < .01$, ***$p < .001$

Figure 10. Correlation coefficients for traits, values, motives, self-beliefs, psychological well-being, and life satisfaction with health and happiness in three age groups

factor against declining feelings of well-being (Baltes & Baltes, 1990). It is likely that the gain in personality functioning of older people mostly derives from their capacity to capitalize upon experiences and to compensate for the unavoidable loss associated with aging.

Throughout this chapter, we have looked at personality over the course of life using cross-sectional findings related to traits, motives, values, self-esteem, self-efficacy beliefs, psychological well-being, and health and happiness. Traits showed a decline in extraversion, energy, openness to experience, and an increase in emotional stability in old age. Motives demonstrated a decline in achievement and power, but an increase in affiliation. Our findings indicate that aging people tend to assign more value to security and tradition and less to stimulation and change.

With respect to self-esteem, it has been repeatedly shown that the beneficial effects of high self-esteem are maintained over the course of a lifetime. Despite the many changes associated to aging, older people do not show less self-esteem than younger adults. Our findings also suggest a decline in empathic and social self-efficacy beliefs, but a slight increase in emotional self-efficacy. It is likely that older people can manage negative emotions and benefit from expressing positive ones better than younger adults due to the wisdom associated with experience, self-knowledge, and better understanding of one's own emotions.

Psychological well-being during old age goes hand in hand with having positive relations with others and having a sense of environmental mastery, a resource gained through experience.

Our findings further attest to the beneficial effects associated with high educational level. Older people with higher levels of education tend to report higher levels of self-direction, self-acceptance, purpose in life, and personal growth. Marital status is also an important factor that grants support and companionship, both resources that are particularly valuable in old age. Traditional role expectations persist in old age. While women tend to value self-transcendence values, interpersonal relations, and communion more than men, men show more autonomy and environmental mastery than women. Men are more concerned with personal growth, and purpose in life, while reporting higher self-acceptance than women.

Health is fundamental for older people. It may be a source of worries, but at the same time, it contributes greatly to life satisfaction and general well-being. Despite the inevitable decline in health status as time passes, older people maintain a certain level of emotional stability and self-esteem. This fact favors the resilience or resistance to adversity theory, in the sense that an adaptation capability is developed in this age group. In the elderly, health is related less to emotional stability, perceived efficacy in managing negative emotions, self-esteem, self-acceptance, environmental mastery, purpose in life, personal growth, and life satisfaction than it is in younger individuals. It has been said, and we generally expect, that the natural decline in health may bring lower mastery of the environment, lower investment in the future, and higher recognition of one's own vulnerability and, therefore, lower the scores in life satisfaction. However, studies have contradicted these hypotheses, emphasizing the powerful role that accommodative strategies can play in old age when control over the environment becomes less available. People compensate for their evident losses by approaching their friends, developing the capacity to express positive emotions, and being empathetic with others. Communion and closeness to others compensates for the evident losses and contributes to happiness.

We believe that our samples can be taken as representative of a large part of the Italian population. Yet, we cannot underestimate the role played by the different changes occurring in our times, for instance, the prolonged education and delayed occupation of youth, the massive feminization of work, and the later retirement of older people. The extended life expectancy associated with significant changes in family life and work organization carry important changes for the relations among generations and expectations of people at various ages.

The majority of the differences between the elderly and the rest of the adult population appear to reflect, in a large part, functional and congenial changes in current life conditions. Thus, the elderly appear to revise their behavior and habits to better adapt to the circumstances of the present time rather than attempt to change others or the environment. For instance, less energy and openness to experience is consistent with a life phase in which there is less energy to spend and few opportunities for new experiences. Similarly, less need for power and success and more attention to interpersonal relationships is in harmony with a time in life wherein the majority of people are retired and life satisfaction is mostly derived from affective rather than professional successes. Obviously, much still depends on the resources and life conditions available to best help preserve one's own capacities and best enhance one's experiences.

The importance of interpersonal relationships is not only maintained, but increases with age. Being able to count on the help of close friends and family is undoubtedly a significant protective factor against feelings of isolation and loneliness. Numerous studies in social epidemiology have documented that those who are more socially integrated show lower profiles of morbidity and delayed mortality (Berkman, 1995; Seeman et al., 1997). The importance of affiliation as a resource in a life phase that requires more than anything else, the help of others, is evident.

Although we cannot yet impede diseases encoded within our DNA or those caused by pathogenic factors, we can keep our mind in shape and strengthen our interpersonal relationships. Thus, we can focus on changing our environment (selectively) and make an effort to change our dysfunctional ways of thinking and behaving. When primary control is unavailable (modification of the environment), we can focus on areas under secondary control (changing ourselves, our ways of seeing things, our objectives) (Heckhausen & Schulz, 1993).

Acknowledging the role of personal agency over the life span expands one's view of human nature. People do not consist merely of a set of tendencies that progress in determined sequence towards inevitable end states. In many cases, people must actively take steps to expose themselves to environmental settings that can contribute to the development of their potential. As developmental potentials are not unlimited, it is critical to make available strategies through which people may maximize their potentials across the life course. In this regard, the metaphor of the clock can prove particularly useful to investigate the constraints and opportunities that biologically, socially and psychologically may condition optimal adaptation in old age. The bio-

logical clock refers to the constraints of nature; the social clock refers to the obliga-
tions of society; the psychological clock refers to individual's plans and expectations.
As the three clocks do not operate separately from one another, optimal adaptation
reflects the ability to set goals and develop strategies that allows the full realization
of individual potentials in all three domains of functioning. In this regard, we are
indebted to Paul and Margareth Baltes for their extraordinary contribution to better
value old age, and their attention to the resources and strategies that permit people to
efficaciously confront aging. Successful aging can be achieved through a balancing
of three factors: selection, optimization and compensation.

Our findings call attention to the importance that self-beliefs, habitual behaviors,
motivational orientation and values may exert as determinants and indicators of successful aging. In fact, it seems unlikely that one can enable people to make the best use
of their capacities and potentials without taking into serious consideration their habitual
behaviors, the activities and goals they believe are within their reach, and the principles
guiding their lives. In this regard, our preliminary findings further recommend extending our knowledge of personality and aging to make possible the full expression of
individual potentials at all ages of life.

References

Baltes, P.B. (1997). On the incomplete architecture of human ontogeny: Selection, optimization,
    and compensation ad foundation of developmental theory. *American Psychologist, 52,*
    366–380.

Bandura, A. (1997). *Self-efficacy: The exercise of control.* New York: Freeman.

Bandura, A. (2001). Social cognitive theory: An agentic perspective. *Annual Review of Psychol-
    ogy, 52,* 1–26.

Baumeister, R.F. (1993). *Self-esteem: The puzzle of low self-regard.* New York: Plenum.

Baumeister, R.F., Campbell, J.D., Krueger, J.I., & Vohs, K.D. (2003). Does high self-esteem
    cause better performance, interpersonal success, happiness, or healthier lifestyle? *Psycholog-
    ical Science in the Public Interest, 4,* 1–44.

Berkman, L.F. (1995). The role of social relations in health promotion. *Psychosomatic Medicine,
    57* (Special issue: Superhighways for disease, May/June), 245–254.

Borgogni, L., Petitta, L., & Barbaranelli, C. (2004). *Test di orientamento motivazionale* [Moti-
    vational Orientation Test]. Florence, Italy: Organizzazioni Speciali.

Brody, J.E. (1997). Personal health: Girls and puberty: The crisis years. *The New York Times,*
    November 4, p. F9.

Capanna, C., Vecchione, M., & Schwartz, S. (2005). Un contributo alla validazione del Portrait
    Values Questionnaire su un campione italiano [The validation of the Portrait Values Question-
    naire in an Italian sample]. *Bollettino di Psicologia Applicata, 246,* 29–41.

Caprara, G.V., Barbaranelli, C., & Borgogni, L. (1993). *BFQ Big Five questionnaire.* Florence,
    Italy: Organizzazioni Speciali.

Caprara, G.V., Barbaranelli, C., Bermudez, J., Maslach, C., & Ruch, W. (2000). Multivariate
    methods for the comparison of factor structures in cross-cultural research: An illustration with
    the Big Five questionnaire. *Journal of Cross-Cultural Psychology, 31,* 437–464.

Caprara, G.V., Caprara, M.G., & Steca, P. (2003). Personality's correlates of adult development and aging. *European Psychologist, 8,* 131–147.

Caprara, G.V., & Cervone, D. (2000). *Personality: Determinants, dynamics, and potentials.* Cambridge: Cambridge University Press.

Caprara, G.V., Gentilomo, A., Barbaranelli, C., & Giorgi, P. (1993). Profili di personalità nell'arco vitale [Personality profile across the life span]. *Archivio di Psicologia, Neurologia e Psichiatria, 54,* 25–39.

Caprara, G.V., Gerbino, M., & Delle Fratte, A. (2001). Autoefficacia Interpersonale [Interpersonal self-effiacy]. In G.V. Caprara (Ed.), *La valutazione dell'autoefficacia* [Self-effiacy assessment] (pp. 87–104). Trento, Italy: Edizioni Erickson.

Caprara, G.V., & Gerbino, M. (2001). Autoefficacia emotiva percepita: La capacità di regolare l'affettività negativa e di esprimere quella positiva [Emotional self-effiacy: The capacity to regulate negative affect and to express positive affect]. In G.V. Caprara (Ed.), *La valutazione dell'autoefficacia* [Self-effiacy assessment] (pp. 35–50). Trento, Italy: Edizioni Erickson.

Caprara, G.V., & Steca, P. (2005a). Affective and social self-regulatory efficacy beliefs as determinants of positive thinking and happiness. *European Psychologist, 4,* 275–286.

Caprara, G.V., & Steca, P. (2005b). Self-efficacy beliefs as determinants of prosocial behavior conducive to life satisfaction across ages. *Journal of Social and Clinical Psychology, 24,* 191–217.

Caprara, G.V., & Steca, P. (2006). Affective and interpersonal self-regulatory efficacy beliefs as determinants of subjective well-being. In A. Delle Fave (Ed.), *Dimensions of well-being: Research and intervention.* Milan: Franco Angeli.

Caprara, G.V., Steca, P., Gerbino, M., Paciello, M. & Vecchio, G.M. (2006). Looking for adolescents' well-being: Self-efficacy beliefs as determinants of positive thinking and happiness. *Epidemiologia e Psichiatria Sociale, 15,* 30–43.

Caprara, M., & Steca, P. (2004). Personalidad y envejecimiento [Personality and aging]. *Intervención Psicosocial, 13*(1), 85–98.

Carstensen, L.L. (1992). Social and emotional patterns in adulthood: Support for socioemotional selectivity theory. *Psychology and Aging, 7,* 331–338.

Carstensen, L.L., Pasupathi, M., Mayr, U., & Nesselroade, J.R. (2000). Emotional experience in everyday life across the adult lifespan. *Journal of Personality and Social Psychology, 79,* 644–655.

Costa, P.T., & McCrae, R.R. (1992). *Revised NEO Personality Inventory (NEO-PI-R) and NEO Five-Factor Inventory (NEO-FFI) professional manual.* Odessa, FL: Psychological Assessment Resources.

Costa, P.T., & McCrae, R.R. (1994). Stability and change in personality from adolescence through adulthood. In C.F. Halverson, G.A. Kohnstamm, & R.P. Martin (Eds.), *The developing structure of temperament and personality from infancy to adulthood* (pp. 139–150). Hillsdale, NJ: Erlbaum.

Costa, P.T., & McCrae, R.R. (1997). Longitudinal stability of adult personality. In R. Hogan, J. Johnson, & S. Briggs (Eds.), *Handbook of personality psychology* (pp. 269–290). San Diego: Academic Press.

Crocker, J., & Park, L.E. (2004). The costly pursuit of self-esteem. *Psychological Bulletin, 130,* 392–414.

Daley, S. (1991). Little girls lose their self-esteem on way to adolescence, study finds. *The New York Times,* January 9, p. B6.

Damon, W., & Hart, D. (1988). *Self-understanding in childhood and adolescence.* New York: Cambridge.

DeLongis, A., Folkamn, S., & Lazarus, R.S. (1988). The impact of daily stress on health and mood: Psychological and social resources as mediators. *Journal of Personality and Social Psychology, 54,* 486–495.

Diener, E. (1984). Subjective well-being. *Psychological Bulletin, 95,* 542–575.

Diener, E. (1994). Assessing subjective well-being: Progress and opportunities. *Social Indicators Research, 31,* 103–157.

Diener, E. (2000). Subjective well-being: The science of happiness, and a proposal for a national index. *American Psychologist, 55,* 34–43.

Diener, E., & Suh, E.M. (1997). Measuring quality of life: Economic, social, and subjective indicators. *Social Indicators Research, 40,* 189–216.

Diener, E., & Suh, E.M. (1998). Subjective well-being and age: An international analysis. In K.W. Schaie & M.P. Lawton (Eds.), *Annual review of gerontology and geriatrics* (Vol. 17). New York: Springer Verlag.

Diener, E., Emmons, R.A., Larsen, R.J., & Griffin, S. (1985). The Satisfaction with Life Scale. *Journal of Personality Assessment, 49,* 71–75.

Diener, E., Lucas, R.E., & Oishi, S. (2002). Subjective well-being: The science of happiness and life satisfaction. In C.R. Snyder & S.J. Lopez (Eds.), *The handbook of positive psychology* (pp. 63–73). Oxford: Oxford University Press.

Diener, E., Suh, E.M., Lucas, R.E., & Smith, H. (1999). Subjective well-being: Three decades of progress. *Psychological Bulletin, 125,* 276–303.

Digman, J.M. (1990). Personality structure: Emergence of the five factor model. *Annual Review of Psychology, 41,* 417–440.

DuBois, D.L., & Tevendale, H.D. (1999). Self-esteem in childhood and adolescence: Vaccine or epiphenomenon? *Applied and Preventive Psychology, 8,* 103–117.

Egan, S.K., & Perry, D.G. (1998). Does low self-regard invite victimization? *Developmental Psychology, 34,* 299–309.

Emler, N. (2001). *Self-esteem: The costs and consequences of low self-worth.* York, UK: York Publishing Services.

Eysenck, H.J. (1970). *The structure of human personality* (3rd ed.). London: Methuen.

Fernández-Ballesteros, R., Zamaron, M.D., Rudinger, G., Schroots, J.J.F. et al. (2004). Assessing competence: The European survey on aging protocol (ESAP). *Gerontology, 50,* 330–347.

Field, D., & Minkler, M. (1988). Continuity and change in social support between young-old and old old or very-old age. *Journal of Gerontology: Psychological Sciences, 43,* 100–106.

Franks, M.M., Herzog, A. R, Holmberg, D., & Markus, H.R. (1999). Educational attainment and self-making in later life. In C.D. Ryff & V.W. Marshall (Eds.), *The self and society in aging processes* (pp. 223–246). New York: Springer-Verlag.

Gove, W.R., & Umberson, D. (1985, August). *Marriage and the well-being of men and women.* Paper presented at the annual meeting of the American Sociological Association, Washington, DC.

Greenberg, J., Solomon, S., Pyszczynski, T., Rosenblatt, A., Burling, J., Lyon, D. et al. (1992). Why do people need self-esteem? Converging evidence that self-esteem serves an anxiety-buffering function. *Journal of Personality and Social Psychology, 63,* 913–922.

Gross, J.J., Carstensen, L.L., Tsai, J., Skorpen, C.G., & Hsu, A.Y.C. (1997). Emotion and aging: Experience, expression, and control. *Psychology and Aging, 12,* 590–599.

Harter, S. (1993). Causes and consequences of low self-esteem in children and adolescents. In R.F. Baumeister (Ed.), *Self-esteem: The puzzle of low self-regard* (pp. 87–116). New York: Plenum.

Harter, S. (1998). The development of self-representations. In W. Damon & N. Eisenberg (Eds.), *Handbook of child development, Vol. 3: Emotional and personality development* (5th ed., pp. 553–617). New York: Wiley.

Heatherton. T.F., & Weinberger, J.L. (Eds.). (1994). *Can personality change?* Washington, DC: American Psychological Association.

Heckhausen, J., & Schulz, R. (1995). A life-span theory of control. *Psychological Review, 102,* 284–304.

Helson, R., Jones, C.J., & Kwan, V.S.Y. (2002). Personality change over 40 years of adulthood: HLM analyses of two longitudinal samples. *Journal of Personality and Social Psychology, 82,* 752–766.

Helson, R., & Wink, P. (1992). Personality change in women from the early 40s to the early 50s. *Journal of Personality and Social Psychology, 7,* 46–55.

Helson, R., Kwan, V.S.Y., John, O.P., & Jones, C. (2002). The growing evidence for personality change in adulthood: Findings from research with personality inventories. *Journal of Research in Personality, 36,* 287–306.

Hendrick, S.S., & Hendrick, C. (1997). Love and satisfaction. In R.J. Sternberg & M. Hojjat (Eds.), *Satisfaction in close relationships* (pp. 56–78). New York: Guilford.

Kernis, M. (1995). *Efficacy, agency, and self-esteem.* New York: Plenum.

Kling, K.C., Hide, J.S., Showers, C.J., & Buswell, B.N. (1999). Gender differences in self-esteem: A meta-analysis. *Psychological Bulletin, 12,* 470–500.

Lawton, M.P., Kleban, M.H., & Dean, J. (1993). Affect and age: Cross-sectional comparisons of structure and prevalence. *Psychology and Aging, 8,* 165–175.

Lawton, M.P., Kleban, M.H., Rejagopal, D., & Dean, J. (1992). Dimensions of affective experience in three age groups. *Psychology and Aging, 7,* 171–184.

McClelland, D.C. (1987). *Human motivation.* Cambridge, UK: Cambridge University Press.

McCrae, R.R., & Costa, P.T. (1990). *Personality in adulthood.* New York: Guilford.

McCrae, R.R., & Costa, P.T., Jr. (1999). A five-factor theory of personality. In L.A. Pervin & O.P. John (Eds.), *Handbook of personality: Theory and research* (2nd ed., pp. 139–153). New York: Guilford.

McCrae, R.R., Costa, P.T., De Lima, M.P., Simoes, A., Ostendorf, F., Angleitner, A. et al. (1999). Age differences in personality across the adult life span: Parallels in five cultures. *Developmental Psychology, 35,* 466–477.

McFarlin, D.B., & Blascovich, J. (1981). Effects of self-esteem and performance feedback on future affective preference and cognitive expectations. *Journal of Personality and Social Psychology, 80,* 472–488.

Mroczek, D.K., & Kolarz, C.M. (1998). The effect of age on positive and negative affect: A developmental perspective on happiness. *Journal of Personality and Social Psychology, 75,* 1333–1349.

Murrel, S.A., Meeks, S., & Walker, J. (1991). Protective functions of health and self-esteem against depression in older adults facing illness or bereavement. *Psychology and Aging, 6,* 352–360.

Nesselroade, J.R. (1987). Some implications of the trait-state distinction for the study of development over the life span: The case of personality. In P.B. Baltes, D.L. Featherman, & R.M. Lerner (Eds.), *Life-span development and behavior* (Vol. 8, pp. 163–189). Hillsdale, NJ: Erlbaum.

O'Connor, B.P., & Vallerand, R.J. (1998). Psychosocial adjustment variables as predictors of morality among nursing home residents. *Psychology and Aging, 13,* 368–374.

Rosenberg, M. (1965). *Society and the adolescent self-image.* Princeton, NJ: Princeton University Press.

Roberts, B.W., & Del Vecchio, W. (2000). The rank-order consistency of personality traits from childhood to old age: A quantitative review of longitudinal studies. *Psychological Bulletin, 126,* 3–25.

Roberts, B.W., Walton, K.E., & Viechtbauer, W. (2006). Patterns of mean-level change in personality traits across the life course: A meta-analysis of longitudinal studies. *Psychological Bulletin, 132*, 1–25.

Robins, R.W., Trzesniewski, K.H., Tracy, J.L., Gosling, S.D., & Potter, J. (2002). Global self-esteem across the life span. *Psychology and Aging, 17*, 423–434.

Ryff, C.D. (1991). Possible selves in adulthood and old age: A tale shifting horizons. *Psychology and Aging, 6*, 286–295.

Ryff, C.D. (1995). Psychological well-being in adult life. *Current Directions in Psychological Science, 4*, 99–104.

Ryff, C.D. (1989a). Happiness is everything, or is it? Explorations on the meaning of psychological well-being. *Journal of Personality and Social Psychology, 57*, 1069–1081.

Ryff, C.D. (1989b). In the eye of the beholder: Views of psychological well-being among middle-aged and older adults. *Psychology and Aging, 6*, 286–295.

Ryff, C.D. (1998). Life course profiles of positive mental health in women. In E. Blechman & K. Brownell (Eds.), *Behavioral medicine for women: A comprehensive handbook*. New York: Guilford.

Ryff, C.D., & Keyes, C.L.M. (1995). The structure of psychological well-being revised. *Journal of Personality and Social Psychology, 69*, 719–727.

Ryff, C.D., Kwan, C.M.L., & Singer, B. (2001). Personality and aging: Flourishing agendas and future challenges. In J.E. Birren & K.W. Schaie (Eds.), *Handbook of the psychology of aging* (5th ed., pp. 477–499). San Diego, CA: Academic Press.

Ryff, C.D., Lee, H., Essex, M., & Schmutte, P. (1994). My children and me: Midlife evaluations of grown children and of self. *Psychology and Aging, 9*, 195–205.

Ryff, C.D., Magee, W.J., Kling, K.C., & Wing, E.H. (1999). Forging macro-micro linkages in the study of psychological well-being. In C.D. Ryff & V.W. Marshall (Eds.), *The self and society in aging processes* (pp. 247–278). New York: Springer-Verlag.

Ryff C.D., & Singer B. (1998). Middle age and well-being. In H.S. Friedman (Ed.), *Encyclopedia of mental health* (pp. 707–719). San Diego, CA: Academic Press.

Schwartz, S. (1992). Universals in the content and structure of values: Theoretical advances and empirical tests in 20 countries. In M.P. Zanna (Ed.), *Advances in experimental social psychology* (Vol. 25, pp. 1–65). New York: Academic Press.

Schwartz, S.H. (2003). Basic human values: Their content and structure across cultures. In A. Tamayo & J. Porto (Eds.), *Valores e trabalho* [Values and work]. Brasilia, Brazil: Editora Universidade de Brasilia.

Schwartz, S.H., Melech, G., Lehmann, A., Burgess, S., & Harris, M. (2001). Extending the cross-cultural validity of the theory of basic human values with a different method of measurement. *Journal of Cross Cultural Psychology, 32*, 519–542.

Schwartz, S.H., & Sagiv, L. (1995). Identifying culture specifics in the content and structure of values. *Journal of Cross-Cultural Psychology, 26*, 92–116.

Seeman T.E., Singer, B.H., McEwen, B.S., Horwitz, R.J., & Rowe, J.W. (1997). The price of adaptation and its health consequences: McArthur studies of successful aging. *Archives for Internal Medicine, 157*, 2259–2268.

Smith, J., & Baltes, P.B. (1999). Trends and profiles of psychological functioning in very old age. In P. Baltes & K. Mayer (Eds.), *The Berlin aging study: Aging from 70 to 100* (pp. 197–226). Cambridge, UK: Cambridge University Press.

Srivastava, S., John, O.P., Gosling, S.D., & Potter, J. (2003). Development of personality in early and middle adulthood: Set like plaster or persistent change? *Journal of Personality and Social Psychology, 84*, 1041–1053.

Steca, P., Ryff, C., D'Alessandro, S., & Delle Fratte, A. (2002). Il benessere psicologico: differenze di genere e di età nel contesto italiano [Psychological well-being: Gender and age differences in the Italian context]. *Psicologia della Salute, 2,* 121–143.

Tedeschi, J.T., & Norman, N. (1985). Social power, self-presentation, and the self. In B.R. Schlenker (Ed.), *The self and social life* (pp. 293–322). New York: McGraw-Hill.

Tyler, T.R., & Schuller, R.A. (1991). Aging and attitude change. *Journal of Personality and Social Psychology, 61,* 689–697.

Watson, D., Clark, L.A., & Tellegen, A. (1988). Development and validation of brief measures of positive and negative affect: The PANAS Scales. *Journal of Personality and Social Psychology, 54,* 1063–1070.

Zamarrón, M.D., & Fernández-Ballesteros, R. (2000): Satisfacción con la vida en personas mayores que viven en sus domicilios y en residencias. Factores determinantes [Life satisfaction in the elderly living at home or in residential homes for the aged. Determining factors]. *Revista de Geriatría y Gerontología, 35* (S2), 17–29.

8. Old-Old People

Major Recent Findings and the European Contribution to the State of the Art

Constança Paúl

Introduction

In developed regions, people aged 80 years and over constitute 3% of the population and are the fastest growing segment of the aged population (WHO, 2002). This age boundary is said to mark the transition from the third to the fourth age that takes place when 50% of the people who reached age 50 or 60 have died, which is between 80 and 85 years (Baltes & Smith, 2003).

It is expected that in 2050 people 80 years old and more will be 3.4% of the total population of the world, 8% of the population of the more developed regions, 10.6% of the Southern Europe population, and 10.1% of the Western Europe population (United Nations, 1996a,b). To live a long life constitutes a challenge to the self and to the all community. Although the trend in population health, associated with improvements in life expectancy, seems to be positive, the patterns will vary widely from country to country (Hayward & Zhang, 2001). The disability-free life expectancy and life free of functional limitation (measured in DALYs – disability adjusted life years) is crucial when looking at very old people, and a major component of quality of life.

What is the profile of the old-old people, or, as some authors call this age group, "oldest old" or the "very old"? Is the aging process continuous until very old age or is there a discontinuity of the aging process beyond the 8th decade of life (Poon, Jang, Reynolds, & McCarthy, 2005). Are the old-old people survivors, and do they have distinctive characteristics as a group for that reason alone, or is living to a very old age just prolonging the same trajectory, even though very few succeed in extending their life span beyond a certain age? With the expanded life expectancy what should we expect in terms of autonomy for this very old population?

The profile of the old-old throughout the world show that they are mostly females, probably living alone, with lower levels of education and higher poverty rates compared to the younger-old (Poon et al., 2005). According to these authors, at least in the United States, it is estimated that approximately one third of the oldest-old are healthy enough to live independently in the community, one third are functionally impaired, and one third are extremely impaired and disabled. These figures are similar to the ones presented by Deep and Jeste (2006), based in a meta-analysis, which show that around one third of old people have aged successfully. However, the predictors include younger age in first place, plus not smoking, no disabilities, musculoskeletal diseases, or diabetes, and to a lesser extent, continuing physical activity, more social contacts, better self-perception of health, less depression, and less cognitive decline or medical conditions. According to this data it seems that the probability of finding a "successful" old individual diminishes with advancing age and diminishing health. However, according to Poon et al. (2005) there is still "one third of success" within the very old population. The claimed heterogeneity of old people is even larger for centenarians compared with younger cohorts. Maybe the success of these old-old is explained by factors different from the ones of younger cohorts, namely efficient coping strategies, developed throughout the lifetime, which helped them face stresses and led to positive evaluations of themselves. This constitutes, in our view, one of the major issues for this area of research in the near future.

We completed a literature review in PsycINFO searching for *old-old*, *very old*, and *centenarians*. We also searched the European longitudinal studies on aging (e.g., BASE, ELSA, Lundt 80+, Octo-twin) to find results on people aged 80 years and over. There is a great variability in what constitutes the concept of old-old, particularly the age boundary of age groups. Although most of the studies classify people aged 80+ years as old-old or very old, others put those aged 75+ in this same category, and a few consider the old-old as those aged 85+. Our main interest is on the protective factors associated with successful and active aging, and on the adaptation process to the challenges of this last stage of life.

To adapt to the challenges of getting older, people have to cope with illness and aging-related losses. The range of possible outcomes of the aging process is sufficiently large to include completely different trajectories above and below a disability threshold. The concept of wisdom (Baltes & Staudinger, 2000) is defined as an expertise in the conduct, meaning, and interpretation of life. It is hypothesized that old people regulate the subjective impact of health-related losses by internally adapting and reconstructing reality, and so report positive well-being even when objective life circumstances are negative. The proposed SOC model (selection, optimization, compensation) explains how elderly people can cope successfully with age-related losses, mainly by using the compensation mechanism later in life. More recently, Baltes (1997) updated his own theory focusing attention on the dilemmas of the so-called *fourth age*. These very old populations are characterized, according to the author, by a reduced potential to compensate for losses because of cognitive decline and increased frailty. Evidence from the BASE study (Baltes & Mayer, 2001) shows an accumulation of chronic problems in the fourth age (80% of old-old people experience losses in 3–6 areas: vision, hearing, strength, functional capacity, instrumental activities of daily living [IADL]-activities of daily living [ADL], illness, cognition), increased systemic breakdown in psychological adaptability, and increased losses in positive aspects of life (happiness, social contacts). The profile of functioning 2 years prior to death appears increasingly negative with losses in cognitive functions and in identity, greater loneliness, and psychological dependence. Even though the news is not very good, the heterogeneity of the aging process can shed light on the future and teach us how to prevent or postpone decline and intervene to raise the quality of life of this very old population.

Baltes and Smith (2003) summarize their current view on the dilemmas of the fourth age in a core article that appeared in *Gerontology*. The main idea is that recent findings about the oldest-old point toward a biocultural incompleteness, vulnerability, and unpredictability of the fourth age. They stress the losses in cognitive potential and ability to learn, increase in chronic stress syndrome, sizeable prevalence of dementia, high prevalence of frailty, dysfunctionality, and multimorbidity, all endangering human dignity in dying at older ages. The meta-theoretical proposition about the biocultural architectures of the fourth age argues that the efficacy of culture to compensate for biological decline decreases in very old age. The authors consider that the fourth age is not a simple continuation of the third age and that healthy and successful aging has its age limits. They consider that resources should be allocated to children, youth, and young adults to guarantee age fairness, and that societal resources continue to be available to support old age.

We begin by reviewing the more recent findings on cognition and personality, and finally physical and mental health. Next we focus on adaptation, quality of life, and life satisfaction within an integrative view of very old age. Looking at the positive aspects of a successful long life we will arrive at preventive interventions, avoiding, or at least postponing, disability, to as close to death as possible, and questioning the recent pessimistic view of Baltes, described above. The shortage of research with old-old people in Europe make it difficult to restrict the literature reviewed to European research, although there are major contributions coming from European teams.

Cognition in Very Old Age

Based in a systematic review of cognitive decline in the general elderly population, Park, O'Connell, and Thomson (2003) showed that some degree of cognitive impairment was almost universal and could be expected in the majority of the oldest-old. The prevalence of cognitive impairment and the rate of decline increased with age. Studies excluding people with dementia at baseline showed smaller rates of decline. The intra- and interindividual variation was great. The Cambridge Project for Later Life (Brayne, Huppert, Paykel, & Gill, 1992) was cited to illustrate the proportion of participants whose cognition was unchanged (15%), with a further 28% improving over the 28-month follow-up. In the Baltimore Epidemiologic Catchment Area Study, 32% of the participants did not change their cognitive function over a period of 11.6 years follow-up (Lyketsos, Chen, & Anthony, 1999). If the cognitive decline seems normative, its extension and temporal limits are not, as we could see from a vast number of reviewed papers.

Howieson et al. (2003) examined the occurrence and outcome of cognitive decline in healthy, community-dwelling, old-old people who at entry had no cognitive impairment and were followed for up to 13 years. Three outcomes of aging were determined: intact cognition, persistent cognitive decline without progression to dementia, and dementia. Whereas 49% remained cognitively intact, 51% developed cognitive decline. Those who remained cognitively intact had better memory at entry and were less likely to have the gene APOE4 that has been linked to late onset of Alzheimer's disease, than those who developed cognitive decline. Of the 48 participants with cognitive decline, 27 (56%) developed dementia about 2.8 years later. The old are at high risk for developing cognitive decline but many will not progress to dementia during the next 2 to 3 years or even beyond. Hong, Zarit, and Johansson (2003) examined participants from the larger Origins of Variance in the Old-Old: Octogenarian Twins (OCTO-Twin) study. Mild cognitive impairment was rated at baseline, however, neither set of criteria predicted subsequent dementia. The failure to confirm subsequent dementia suggests that there may be many sources of mild cognitive impairment in very late life besides incipient dementia, and once again the progress is not unidirectional.

Higher age was related to lower performance in all cognitive measures, except synonyms. For digit span forward, symbol digit, and general cognitive ability tasks, there was an interaction between sex and age with greater deficits in the performance of women compared with those of men at higher ages. They did not found sex-specific genetic influences, and the magnitude of genetic effect was similar for men and women (Read, Vogler, Pederson, & Johansson, 2006).

McGinnis and Zelinski (2003) find that there is a subgroup of older adults who experience verbal processing and comprehension deficits and a subgroup that does not. The size of the verbal deficit subgroup increases with age. One of the hypotheses to explain the cognitive performance of older adults is the abstraction deficit. According to this, there is a tendency for over-abstracted processing, characterizing inferential processes, that increases with age, which means that the old-old individuals are more likely to focus on thematic interpretations instead of processing at more optimal levels of abstraction.

The extent to which the characteristics and behaviors of an individual change or remain stable over the life span is an important issue for the study of cognitive aging. It seems that performance variability, which refers to change that is relatively rapid and transient, is related to changes in cognition and may be considered a marker of cognitive aging (MacDonald et al., 2003).

Cognitive performance seems not to benefit from training in very old age. Singer, Lindenberger, and Baltes (2003) trained old-old people from the BASE study in mnemonic skills but did not obtain any gains, particularly in the crystallized-ability domain. These differences in plasticity could be predicted by six years prior to loss in perceptual speed. More precisely, perceptual speed, memory, and fluency declined with age whereas knowledge remained stable up to age 90, declining thereafter. It seems that rates of decline vary by distance to death, age, and intellectual ability (Singer, Verhaeghen, Ghisletta, Lindenberger, & Baltes, 2003).

In the Lund 80+ study, Svensson et al. (1993) report cognitive decline with advancing age regardless of the health status of the individuals. The authors present a comparison of their own data on reasoning and spatial ability with those from the Gothenburg Health Study and found significant decline comparing baseline measures at 70 years with those 9 years after, and no differences between people aged 79 from Gothenburg and people aged 80 from Lund.

Data from the second wave of ELSA (English Longitudinal Study of Ageing) directed by Michael Marmot (Banks, Breeze, Lessof, & Nazroo, 2006), showed that one third of the sample reported that their memory had worsened over the previous years. Older groups have a double disadvantage in relation to their memory performance, that is: they remember fewer words immediately and they forget more. Around two thirds of participants aged 75+ have a striking impairment in prospective memory – remembering to carry out an action without being reminded. The most sensitive measure of cognitive decline, particularly for the older group, was speed of information processing. Literacy was strongly age related and the impairment was greater in people aged 80+ years. The trend for literacy impairment to increase with age was evident even when controlling for level of education. The higher the level of wealth, the better the cognitive performance, on all measures except speed of processing (Huppert et al., 2006).

The proximity to death seems to accelerate decline in memory, reasoning, speed, and verbal abilities (Johansson et al., 2004). According to Small et al. (2003), mortality is related to deficits observed in old people in cross-sectional studies, and mortality is also related to longitudinal changes in cognitive performance among a group of very old individuals. These associations were independent of cause of death.

Both physical and cognitive activities were related to better cognitive performance. Cognitive activity was a stronger predictor than physical activity of the complex but not the simple tasks, suggesting that physical and cognitive stimulation are useful in protecting against cognitive decline with age (Newson & Kemps, 2006b). Actually, fitness was a strong predictor of cognition and accounted for more variance in processing resources than in higher-order functions. Newson and Kemps (2006a) found that cardiorespiratory fitness may have a selective protective effect against age-associated cognitive decline. Ghisletta et al. (2006), based on data from SWILSO-O (Longitudinal Study on the Oldest-Old; Lalive d'Espinay et al., 2001) suggest that increased leisure activity engagement may lessen decline in perceptual speed but not in verbal fluency or performance, whereas cognitive performance does not affect change in activity engagement.

Cognitive decline is concurrent with sensory decline in old age. It seems that there is a common factor explaining a small proportion of variability of both (memory and visual aging) but that there are also independent factors influencing cognitive and sensory decline in agreement with neuroimaging studies showing different rates of changes in different regions within an individual (Anstey, Hofer, & Luszcz, 2003)

There are two main hypotheses to explain cognitive aging: (1) The source of age-related declines on a wide variety of cognitive tasks is based on changes in a single mechanism underlying many functions, on random changes caused by life experiences, or (2) there are process specific changes. The first hypothesis is consistent with the idea of dedifferentiation of specialized abilities (Baltes, Cornelius, Spiro, Nesselroade, & Willis, 1980), and the common aging factor could be, for example, the general slowing observed in old people (Salthouse, 1998). The second hypothesis is consistent with the research of Zelinski and Lewis (2003) as they concluded that there may be multiple processes in aging, some associated with stability and others associated with change but that the process-specific models of change better explain cognitive aging.

In summary, some degree of cognitive impairment is almost universal and can be expected in the majority of the old-old, however, its extension and temporal limits vary widely. Cognitive decline is concurrent with sensory decline in old age and the proximity to death seems to accelerate decline.

Personality Along the Life Span

Although many studies have examined the issue of personality stability in early and middle adulthood, few have explored the limits of personality stability in the very old, who are often confronted with major changes in their health and life circumstances, which can severely impact adaptive behavior. Maiden, Peterson, Caya, and Hayslip (2003) conducted a longitudinal study of women with a mean age of 80 years. They were assessed on the personality traits of neuroticism, extroversion, and openness. Although multiple regression analyses revealed moderate stability on all three traits, their stability was found to be influenced by negative changes in life circumstances. For example, decreased social support and increased unmet needs were associated with more neuroticism. Less extroversion was associated with poorer health and greater psychosocial needs. The trait of openness was very stable and was the least affected by life events. These contradictory findings are reconciled by considering personality development within an interaction framework. Other findings report small changes, for instance, the cross-sectional study of Weiss, Costa, Karuza, Duberstein, Friedman, and McCrae (2005), which found no age differences in personality as measured with the NEO, although the old-old people aged 80–100 years, particularly the men, were higher in agreeableness.

Svensson et al. (1993) showed that persons from the Lund 80+ study who experienced a negative change in health showed more neuroticism and experienced lower life satisfaction depending on the coping mechanism used (e.g., avoidance coping leads to less neuroticism).

It seems that personality stability extends to very old age. Read et al. (2006) studied the stability and change in genetic and environmental components of personality in pairs of twins 80 years and over and found high mean level stability in extroversion and neuroticism. Mortality was related to lower scores in extroversion and higher scores in neuroticism. The genetic effects were moderate for extroversion and neuroticism. Nonshared environmental effects were less stable over time. No new genetic effects were found over time, thus, showing more stability. New environmental effects emerged but this does not show cumulative long-lasting effects.

As a synopsis, it seems that personality stability extends to very old age, although negative changes in life circumstances was found to influence some variation.

Physical Health in the Old-Old People

Health is a major factor of quality of life particularly in very old age. During the 20th century, mortality among the old declined about 1% per year (Crimmins, 2004). Although according to Olshanansky, Carnes, and Desesquelles (2001) the future increase in life expectancy will be minimal and implies deep knowledge, and intervention, in the basic mechanisms of aging. Trends in the health of the elderly can be summarized in two opposite hypotheses from the 1980s – one by Fries (1980) assuming the "compression of mortality" with disease and disability postponed to later ages, and the other by Kramer (1980), considering the "expansion of morbidity" that assumes that people will simply live longer with greater burdens of disease and disability. The actual general trend shows that older people are healthier then they were two decades ago, with improvements in most dimensions of health. People live longer and have fewer disabilities, have less functioning loss and report themselves to be in better health. Because people live longer a greater percentage of people have some specific common diseases and on average live with more diseases, on the other hand having a disease appears to be less disabling. There is a strong cohort effect in the improvement of health that seems to favor those in their 60s. The key for continuing improved health seems to be to delay the onset of risk factors, disease, and disability in older-age people (Crimmins, 2004).

Results from ELSA (Banks et al., 2006) shows from the first wave of data (cross-sectional) that there is considerable variation in the level of physical impairment between age groups. Of the respondents in their 80s and older, 58% report no difficulties with basic activities of daily living and 17% report no difficulty with mobility functions; walking speed slows dramatically with age; and chronological age is the strongest determinant of scores on the objective cognitive tests, whereas scores on the subjective measure (self-reported memory) are more strongly influenced by education and occupational class than by age). Breeze, Cheshire, and Zaninotto (2006) reported that in the second wave of ELSA, only 1 in 10 of those aged 80 years and over were without a diagnosis of any chronic condition. Older age was also associated with greater likelihood of multiple falls. The association between wealth and health indicators largely disappeared in those older than 75 years.

The conclusions of the Rotterdam Study (Hofman, Jong, van Duijn, & Breteler, 2006) show that the neurological diseases (dementia, stroke, Parkinson's disease, and macular degeneration) are extremely common and increase with age. The rise of incidence seems to continue in very old people. The authors stressed the fact that longitudinal studies, like that one, made clear that silent and nonsilent strokes predict dementia and that stroke is often a precursor of dementia. They also found a strong predictive value of diabetes mellitus for Alzheimer's disease and cognitive function. Their point was the possibility of prevention or at least postponement of the diseases by looking carefully to the vascular factors, to the oxidative stress, and the inflammatory factors earlier in life.

Data from five annual interviews of people 80–84 years old, living in the community, of The Swiss Interdisciplinary Longitudinal Study on the Oldest-Old (SWILSO-O; Lalive d'Espinay et al., 2001) shows that 17% of people were dependent at base line and that 5 years later this number rose to 37%. However, the most common individual health trajectory was stability (be it in good or bad health), which means that decline was not the rule. Moreover, in the first wave, 58% were helping others (children) and 45% were still helping others in the second wave. At the same time, the number of those receiving help rose from 21% to 42%.

In the Lund 80+ study two thirds of the subjects were not dependent on any kind of regular formal or informal support. Regarding medical examination, only 13% had symptoms requiring additional treatment, 51% had diagnoses and were being treated, and 24% were found to be healthy (Svensson et al., 1993).

Pain is an important factor influencing quality of life in very old age and we should be more attentive and proactive about it. Among old-old subjects living in the community, daily pain is highly prevalent and this condition is associated with impaired muscle strength and lower physical performance (Onder, Cesari, Russo, Zamboni, Bernabei, & Landi, 2006). Sleep is another area of discomfort and complaint for the old-old. Research on this subject is difficult, mainly because of the medication taken by most old people and their sleep behavior during the day. McCrae et al. (2003) report that the old-old slept longer each night, but took longer to fall asleep, napped more, and were more likely to complain of insomnia than the young-old; otherwise, the young-old/old-old distinction did not explain sleep differences among different types of sleepers. Data from the Lund 80+ study (Svensson et al., 1993) show that sleep was judged very good or fairly good for 76% of the sample although 31% of people took hypnotics.

Nutrition is a very important issue during old age. The old-old people believed they were doing well nutritionally despite reduced independence and physical limitations. They were positive about their lives and creative in problem solving to remain independent. Social relationships were the major factor for maintaining independence into old age. The leading barrier to maintaining nutritional health was health problems. Those with more barriers were more likely to be depressed. Knowledge of aids and barriers to nutritional health, from a personal perspective, gives an understanding of the issues and concerns of old-old people (Callen & Wells, 2003). Besides these problems, the old-old people were less likely than the old and young-old ones to do health check-ups. Model testing found that age, chronic illnesses, degree of physical and mental health, and cognitive status directly or indirectly influenced older adults participation in primary and secondary health behaviors (Resnick, 2003). The health status effects on health behavior change differ by age group and health status. Food consumption, food preparation, and medical care show negative change for old-old persons (Zanjani, Shaie, & Willis, 2006). Health interventions need to focus on the old-old individuals with physical disability, and on smoking and seat-belt use, to limit future onset of disability and morbidity and prevent premature death.

It is well established from the health psychology literature that subjective health is more influential on quality of life than objective health. Benyamini, Blumstein, Lusky, and Modan (2003) investigated gender differences in the association between self-rated health (SRH) and mortality. The study was based on an Israeli nationally representative sample (aged 75–94 years), who were interviewed about their SRH, as well as sociodemographic information and other measures of health, physical functioning, cognitive status, and depression. For both genders, SRH was associated only with shorter term mortality and not with longer-term mortality. This association was strongest among the old (ages 75–84) women, compared with the old men and with the old old (85–94) women and men. The SRH-mortality association may differ among age and gender groups.

Svensson et al. (1993) found that 25% of the 80+ individuals rated their health as very good and an additional 49% rated health as fairly good. The correlation between the individuals' and physicians' ratings was highly significant, which is very interesting considering the predictive value of these measures in terms of mortality and morbidity. In ELSA three fifths of people at age 80 or over described their health as good, very good, or excellent (Marmot, 2006).

According to Ben-Ezra and Shmotkin (2006), the more significant predictors of mortality in the old-old in Israel (CALAS study) are age, sex, disability, and self-rated health, although their predictive effect seems to diminish in very old age.

Personality also seems to be associated with perceived health and functioning status in older people (Duberstein et al., 2003) and lifetime trauma (e.g., sexual and physical abuse, witnessing crime, premature loss of a parent) appears associated with worse health in later life, although the risk is greater for the young-old than for the old-old individuals (Krause, Shaw, & Cairney, 2004).

In summary, we can assert that the actual general trend in health shows improvements in most dimensions of health of old-old people when compared to twenty years ago.

Mental Health in the Old-Old People

The association between physical health problems and depression is well documented even though the direction of the association is not clear. Late-life depression is common, disabling, and frequently comorbid with physical illness. Physical health and depression are closely related in the elderly (Beekman, Deeg, van Tilburg, Smit, Hooijer, & van Tilburg, 1995) as reported in cross-sectional and longitudinal studies. The relation between four aspects of physical health and depressive symptom levels were studied in a community-based sample of older inhabitants of a small town in the Netherlands. Results indicate that depression is sufficiently different from physical health to be distinguished from it, and that it is sufficiently related to physical health to be relevant for further study. The more subjective measures of physical health used in this study (pain and subjective health) appear to have a much stronger relation with depression than the more objective health-measures (chronic diseases and functional limitations). Physical health and aspects of the social environment such as marital status appear to have independent effects on mood. In this study these effects were moderated by age and sex. In women and the young-old none of the associations between physical health and depression were significant. In men and the old-old all associations were highly significant.

Most longitudinal studies report increases in depression contrarily to cross-sectional studies that are more likely to report stability or even decrease of depression. Rothermund and Brandtstädter (2003) concluded that there are two phases: One to about 70 years characterized by stability and a subsequent phase with an increase of depressive tendencies may be because of the expectation of impending death.

We found in a representative sample of UK old and very old people living in the community that when adjusting for other variables (e.g., health problems, disability), age is not a predictor of depression. There were positive associations between depression and loneliness, number of health problems, and limitations caused by illness and a negative association with knowing neighbors and self-rated good quality of life (Paúl, Ayes, & Ebrahim, 2006).

According to Zhang, Ho, and Woo (2005) physical health is not the only aspect associated with depression. Income was significantly associated with cognitive functioning and geriatric depression in elderly persons in Hong Kong. Mental health, ADL deficiency, major chronic conditions, and resource utilization are interrelated. The fact that aging is associated with increasing cognitive impairment and geriatric depression presents new challenges for the health care system.

Depression is a serious problem for the oldest-old but a number of correlates are consistently identified in this age group as well as in the elderly population in general. Financial strain, poor self-rated health, loneliness, and heart disease were significantly and positively related to depression in the oldest-old, after gender, marital status, education, living arrangement, functional disability, sensory impairment, cognitive ability, and the presence of eight medical conditions were controlled. Interestingly, financial strain, self-rated health, and loneliness were found to be significant correlates of depression in the young-old and in the old-old groups. Therefore, they should be carefully considered for prevention and treatment of depression (Chou & Chi, 2005).

Mental well-being seems to benefit from physical and leisure activity in older adults, as was found by Lampinen, Heikkinen, Kauppinen, and Heikkinen (2006) in an 8-year follow-up study. Therefore, activity, health, and mobility should be targeted for preventive intervention in old age.

In general, we learn that late-life depression is common, disabling, and increasing with advancing age.

Quality of Life and Resilience in Very Old Age

Adapting to the challenges of aging is a major task for very old people. It is generally accepted that there are resource deficits, namely, in physical and functional health, social networks, and cognitive capacity in old-old people (e.g., Jopp & Smith, 2006), which enforce constant adaptation and a continuous redefinition of quality of life. Regardless of this, very old people reported happiness and a positive outlook on life, both good predictors of well-being during very old age. Most centenarians of the Heidelberg Centenarian Study felt happy, although they were experiencing decline in certain domains of functioning (Jopp & Rott, 2006). We found in a community sample of English people aged 80 years and over that 66% had long standing illness, disability, or infirmity; 53% had limitations in social participation, and 86% had limitations in activities of daily living. However, more then 70% rated their health and quality of life as good. Despite this apparent paradox between health and quality of life, deeper analyses showed that those in better health were more optimistic, and those with more health problems and more limitation of activity expressed lower self-perceived health status, lower quality of life, and less optimism. This observation points, on one hand, to the importance of health for quality of life and, on the other hand, to the "low expectancies" people have for their health in later years, easily surpassed in our time (Paúl, Ayis, & Ebrahim, in press). Similar results were obtained by Samuelsson et al. (1997) in the Swedish Centenarian Study. The authors show that centenarians who reported high quality of life were healthier than those with lower levels.

Freund and Baltes (1998) reported a negative age correlation for the use of optimization and SOC strategies in a sample of old and very old people. The protective effect of SOC in determining successful aging was dependent of the resource level of the old-old individuals. The old-old people who profited more from SOC were those with low resources showing that SOC strategies serve as protective buffers when resources are limited (Jopp & Smith, 2006).

Autonomous living is the main objective of old people. People want to live on their own, taking care of themselves, engaged in the community, and being able to cope with the challenges of getting older and with the declines associated with age. To succeed in doing so people need to stay competent even in very old age. Competence comes out as a key aspect of old age and particularly of very old age.

Mastery of daily living is essential and a major component of competence during old age. Usually this mastery is measured by one's ability to perform the ADL strictly related to survival and IADL, also essential to independent living. In a chapter devoted to everyday competence in old and very old age, Baltes and colleagues (2001) reviewed the concept of competence and showed evidence of its progression in old people. Their perspective of competence includes skills, mastery and the context, and is differentiated into two components: a basic level of competence (BaCo) and an expanded level of competence (ExCo). The BaCo reflects the basic personal maintenance of daily life (ADL), and the ExCo reflects the optional leisure and social activities, as well as the IADL, including relating the self to the world, and influencing quality of life. In any case, we are looking at not only capacities but behaviors. The reported findings show that older people differ from younger ones in resting time, which lasts longer in the oldest group, and in instrumental and leisure activities, that take up less time in the very old age group. Participants aged 85 and above report more difficulty in almost all the activities (except eating and grooming). In fact, the older people are less engaged in all activities. One conclusion of this study is that age and basic competence are important independent predictors of expanded competence. At the same time it becomes clear that there is a great variability between people, reinforcing the concept of differential aging. The authors propose balance/gait, intelligence, and personality as moderating factors between age and competence. That means that it is not age but health and psychosocial factors that are affecting competence.

Wilms, Riedel-Heller, and Angermeyer (in press) showed in a representative sample of the Leipzig population 75+ years old that 61.8% had relevant deficits in their capacity of independent living (ADL and IADLs). Most of the limitations were the result of variance shared by dementia and mobility-related declines suggesting caution when interpreting results from scales of ADL and IADL.

In brief, in spite of some physical and functional health problems, most of the very old people reported happiness and a positive outlook on life. Evidence shows great variability of aging between people and that not age but health and psychosocial factors are affecting competence and many of those are modifiable.

Adapting to Very Old Age

Depending on the type of study (cross-sectional or longitudinal) data about people aged 80+ vary widely. In general, we can say that cross-sectional studies show more age-related decline then longitudinal ones. However, most of the studies show health and cognitive decline particularly close to death. Regarding personality and the emotions, although some papers found minor changes over time, it seems that it is quite stable or even that old people can better adapt to aging challenges.

Future research to study this very old group is urgent and should adopt a longitudinal approach. Cross-sectional studies will continue to have a role as exploratory pilot studies or as a first stage of prospective longitudinal studies (Shaie, 2000).

Takkinen and Suutama (2004), based on a study of lifelines of 83–87-year-old Finnish people, reported that the interindividual variance was greater during childhood and old age comparing with middle adulthood. Most of the lowest points in life were located in childhood and the highest points in the present old age. The densest period of major events and their affective meaning was in youth and young adulthood. The content is human relationships and school oriented in women and work and war oriented in men. These results seem to corroborate those of Field (1997). He found that when people were asked the period of life that brought them the most satisfaction "right now" was the most frequent answer.

Some psychological characteristics of the individuals can predict the long-term likelihood or severity of disability in older adults. According to Caplan and Schooler (2003) fatalism measured 20 years earlier predicted greater difficulty in everyday cognitive tasks as well as illness; on the contrary self-confidence was associated with lesser degrees of cognitive and fine-motor difficulty and intellectual resources (flexibility and education) predicted less cognitive and gross motor difficulty as well as lesser degrees of illness 20 years after. Most of these associations were stronger for the oldest group, and even though they were more fatalistic, they considered themselves as competent as the youngest to deal with unavoidable events in their lives. The way these characteristics influence illness and disability is not clear. It may be that people with more intellectual resources, less fatalism, and more self-confidence engage in more preventive behaviors. On the other hand, it may be that people higher in fatalism or lower in self-confidence might experience more stress and so became more vulnerable to disease and disability.

According to the findings of the Cross-Sectional and Longitudinal Study (CALAS) from Israel (Walter-Ginzburg, Shmotkin, Blumstein, & Shorek, 2005), there is a gender-based resilience pattern. Programs to reduce mortality should include physical activity, attendance of religious services, maintenance or improvement of ADL, and engaging in solitary leisure activities. For women smoke cessation programs and cognitive activities are very important and for men maintaining or increasing emotional ties will be beneficial.

In parallel with positive emotions, social relations seem to be very important for the survival and quality of life of very old people. Lyyra and Heikkinen (2006) studied 80-year-old Finns and found that the risk of death was 2.5 times higher in women with infrequent experiences of reassurance of worth, emotional closeness, sense of belonging, and opportunity for nurturance than women highest in these measures. This association remains even when controlling for sociodemographics and psychological and physiological health and functioning. None of these dimensions of social support seems to be relevant for men's mortality.

In summary, adaptation and its results in very old age can be predicted by some psychological characteristics of individuals, such as fatalism or self-confidence. These characteristics may positively influence illness and disability and even mortality by means of preventive behaviors or by making people more vulnerable to stress and subsequent disease.

Conclusion and Future Trends

This review of recent data about very old age shows that, as Marmot, Banks, Blundell, Lessof, and Nazroo (2004, p. 4) stated:

"Middle age is no paradise; old age is not hell. The challenge for the future is to understand what leads some 80-years-olds to high levels of functioning and some 50-year-olds already to show signs of decline."

It seems that cross-sectional studies show more decline than longitudinal ones, pointing to the importance of having more longitudinal research on aging and particularly following individuals for as long as possible. It is almost consensual that despite the decline observed in all studies heterogeneity is the rule and individual trajectories differ considerably and are quite stable at their own level. Apparently personality does not change significantly over time, and cognition suffers decline in some areas, mainly speed of information processing but differs enormously between individuals and to some extent with gender, wealth, and health status. The period near death seems to evidence a general decline in most old people. Health is a very important factor related to autonomy and well-being but once again there is still a significant amount of people (between 30% and 50%) who manage their lives independently and even continue to help others. Recent studies on health trends show that levels of disability are decreasing even though health continues to be a challenge. The pessimistic view conveyed by Baltes and Smith (2003) does not seem to be corroborated by many other papers reviewed here. In fact, at the individual level, the fourth age appears to be the continuation of the third age, enlarging the heterogeneity of aging results, and at least for one third of old people, living longer lives seems to be a positive and successful experience, until very close to dead.

We believe that on the whole, aging is a positive experience for the majority of people, even those in their 80s. In fact, optimism and positive emotions toward the self, others, and the world appear to be critical aspects of longevity and quality of life. Future research should seek to understand how these factors come to influence health and well-being in very old age.

Although people aged 80 years and older are the most vulnerable to loneliness and deprivation, the future trend for less literacy impairments in these cohorts is quite positive and makes us expect a better future for this growing group of very old people.

References

Anstey, K., Hofer, S., & Luszcz, M. (2003). A latent growth curve analysis of late-life sensory and cognitive function over 8 years: Evidence for specific and common factors underlying change. *Psychology and Aging, 18*, 714–726.

Baltes, P. (1997). On the incomplete architecture of human ontogeny: Selection optimization and compensation as foundation of developmental theory. *American Psychologist, 52*, 366–380.

Baltes, P., Cornelius, S., Spiro, A., Nesselroade, J., & Willis, S. (1980). Integration vs. differentiation of fluid-crystallized intelligence in old age. *Developmental Psychology, 16*, 625–635.

Baltes, P., & Mayer, K. (Eds.). (2001). *The Berlin aging study: Aging from 70 to 100.* Cambridge, UK: Cambridge University Press.

Baltes, P., & Smith, J. (2003). New frontiers in the future of aging: From successful aging of the young-old to the dilemmas of the fourth age. *Gerontology, 49*, 123–135.

Baltes P., & Staudinger, U. (2000). Wisdom: A metaheuristic (pragmatic) to orchestrate mind and virtue toward excellence. *American Psychologist, 55*, 122–136.

Banks, J., Breeze, E., Lessof, C., & Nazroo, J. (2006). *Retirement, health, and relationships of the older population in England. The 2004 English longitudinal study of ageing (Wave 2).* London: The Institute for Fiscal Studies.

Beekman, A.T., Deeg, D.J., van Tilburg, T., Smit, J.H., Hooijer, C., & van Tilburg, W. (1995). Major and minor depression in later life: A study of prevalence and risk factors. *Journal of Affective Disorders, 36*, 65–75.

Ben-Ezra, M., & Shmotkin, D. (2006). Predictors of mortality in the old-old in Israel: The cross-sectional and longitudinal aging study. *Journal of the American Geriatric Society, 54*, 906–911.

Benyamini, Y., Blumstein, T., Lusky, A., & Modan, B. (2003). Gender differences in the self-rated health-mortality association: Is it poor self-rated health that predicts mortality or excellent self-rated health that predicts survival? *Gerontologist, 43*, 396–405.

Brayne, C., Huppert, F., Paykel, E., & Gill, C (1992). The Cambridge project for later life: Design and preliminary results. *Neuroepidemiology, 11*(Suppl. 1), 71–75.

Breeze, E., Cheshire, H., & Zaninotto, P. (2006). Self-reported physical health. In J. Banks, E. Breeze, C. Lessof, & J. Nazroo (Eds.), *Retirement, health, and relationships of the older population in England. The 2004 English Longitudinal Study of Ageing (Wave 2).* London: The Institute for Fiscal Studies.

Callen, B.L., & Wells, T.J. (2003). Views of community-dwelling, old-old people on barriers and aids to nutritional health. *Journal of Nursing Scholarship, 35*, 257–262.

Caplan, L., & Schooler, C. (2003). The roles of fatalism, self-confidence, and intellectual resources in the disablement process in older adults. *Psychology and Aging, 18*, 551–561.

Chou, K.-L., & Chi, I (2005). Prevalence and correlates of depression in Chinese oldest-old. *International Journal of Geriatric Psychiatry, 20*, 41–50.

Crimmins, E. (2004). Trends in the health of the elderly. *Annual Reviews Public Health, 25*, 79–98.

Deep, C., & Jeste, D. (2006). Definitions and predictors of successful aging: A comprehensive review of larger quantitative studies. *American Journal of Geriatric Psychiatry, 14*, 6–20.

Duberstein, P., Sörensen, S., Lyness, J., King, D., Conwell, Y., Seidlitz, L. et al. (2003). Personality is associated with perceived health and functional status in older primary care patients. *Psychology and Aging, 18*, 25–37.

Field, D. (1997). "Looking back, what period of your life brought you the most satisfaction." *International Journal of Aging and Human Development, 45*, 169–194.

Freund, A., & Baltes, P. (1998). Selection, optimization, and compensation as strategies of life-management: Correlations with subjective indicators of successful aging. *Psychology and Aging, 13*, 531–543.

Fries, J. (1980). Aging, natural death, and the compression of morbidity. *New England Journal of Medicine, 303*, 130–135.

Ghisletta, P., Bickel J.-F., & Lovden, M. (2006). Does activity engagement protect against cognitive decline in old age? Methodological and analytical considerations. *Journal of Gerontology: Psychological Sciences, 61B*, P253–P261.

Hayward, M., & Zhang, Z. (2001). Demography of aging. A century of global change, 1950–2050. In R. Binstock & L. George (Eds.), *Handbook of aging and the social sciences* (pp. 69–85). San Diego, CA: Academic Press.

Hofman, A., Jong, P., van Duijn, C., & Breteler, M. (2006). Epidemiology of neurological diseases in elderly people: What did we learn from the Rotterdam Study? *Lancet, Neurology, 5*(6), 545–550.

Hong, T.B., Zarit, S.H., & Johansson, B. (2003). Mild cognitive impairment in the oldest old: A comparison of two approaches. *Aging and Mental Health, 7*, 271–276.

Howieson, D.B., Camicioli, R., Quinn, J., Silbert, L.C., Care, B., Moore, M.M. et al. (2003). Natural history of cognitive decline in the old old. *Neurology, 60*, 1491–1496.

Huppert, F., Gardener, E., & McWilliams, B. (2006). Cognitive function. In J. Banks, E. Breeze, C. Lessof, & J. Nazroo (Eds), *Retirement, health, and relationships of the older population in England. The 2004 English Longitudinal Study of Ageing (Wave 2)*. London: The Institute for Fiscal Studies.

Johansson, B., Hofer, S., Allaire, J.C., Maldonado-Molina, M., Piccinin, A., Berg, S. et al. (2004). Change in cognitive capabilities in the oldest old: The effects of proximity to death in genetically related individuals over a 6-year period. *Psychology and Aging, 19*, 145–156.

Jopp, D., & Rott, C. (2006). Adaptation in very old age: Exploring the role of resources, beliefs, and attitudes for centenarians' happiness. *Psychology and Aging, 21*, 266–280.

Jopp, D., & Smith, J., (2006). Resources and life-management strategies as determinants of successful aging: On the protective effect of selection, optimization, and compensation. *Psychology and Aging, 21*, 253–265.

Kramer, M. (1980). The rising pandemic of mental disorders and associated chronic diseases and disabilities. *Acta Psychiatrica Scandinavia, 62*, 282–297.

Krause, N., Shaw, B., & Cairney, J. (2004). A descriptive epidemiology of lifetime trauma and the physical health status of older adults. *Psychology and Aging, 19*, 637–648.

Lalive d'Espinay, C., Pin, S., & Spini, D. (2001). Présentation de SWILSO-O, une étude longitudinale suisse sur le grand âge: L'exemple de la dynamique de la santé fonctionnelle [Presentation of SWILSO-O, a Swiss longitudinal study of old age]. *L'Année Gérontologique, 15*, 78–96.

Lampinen, P., Heikkinen, R-L., Kauppinen M., & Heikkinen E. (2006). Activity as predictor of mental well-being among older adults. *Aging and Mental Health, 10*, 454–466

Lyketsos, C., Chen, L., & Anthony, J. (1999). Cognitive decline in adulthood: An 11.5-year follow-up of the Baltimore Epidemiologic Catchment Area Study. *American Journal of Psychiatry, 156*, 58–65.

Lyyra, T.-M., & Heikkinen, R.-L. (2006). Perceived social support and mortality in older people. *Journal of Gerontology: Social Sciences, 61B*, S147–S152.

MacDonald, S., Hultsch, D., & Dixon, R. (2003). Performance variability is related to change in cognition: Evidence from the Victoria Longitudinal Study. *Psychology and Aging, 18*, 510–523.

Maiden, R.J., Peterson, S.A., Caya, M., & Hayslip, B. Jr. (2003). Personality changes in the old-old: A longitudinal study. *Journal of Adult Development, 10*, 31–39.

Marmot, M. (2006). Introduction. In J. Banks, E. Breeze, C. Lessof, & J. Nazroo (Eds), *Retire-*

ment, health, and relationships of the older population in England. The 2004 English Longitudinal Study of Ageing (Wave 2). London: The Institute for Fiscal Studies.

Marmot, M., Banks, J., Blundell, R., Lessof, C., & Nazroo, J. (2004). Health, wealth, and lifestyles of the older population in England: The 2002 English Longitudinal Study of Ageing. London: Institute of Fiscal Studies.

McCrae, C., Wilson, N., Lichstein, K., Durrence, H., Taylor, D., Bush, A. et al. (2003). "Young old" and "old old" poor sleepers with and without insomnia complaints. Journal of Psychosomatic Research, 54, 11–19.

McGinnis, D., & Zelinski, E. (2003). Understanding unfamiliar words in young, young-old, and old-old adults: Inferential processing and the abstraction-deficit hypothesis. Psychology and Aging, 18, 497–509.

Newson, R.S., & Kemps, E.B. (2006a). Cardiorespiratory fitness as a predictor of successful cognitive aging. Journal of Clinical and Experimental Neuropsychology, 28, 949–967.

Newson, R.S., & Kemps, E.B. (2006b). The influence of physical and cognitive activities on simple and complex cognitive tasks in older adults. Experimental Aging Research, 32, 341–362.

Olshanansky, S., Carnes, B., & Desesquelles, A. (2001). Prospects for human longevity. Science, 291, 1491–1492.

Onder, G., Cesari, M., Russo, A., Zamboni, V., Bernabei, R., & Landi, F. (2006). Association between daily pain and physical function among old-old adults living in the community: Results from the ilSIRENTE study. Pain, 121, 53–59.

Park, H., O'Connell, J., & Thomson, R. (2003). A systematic review of cognitive decline in the general elderly population. International Journal of Geriatric Psychiatry, 18, 1121–1134.

Paúl, C., Ayes, S., & Abrahim, S. (2006). Psychological distress loneliness and disability in old age. Psychology Health and Medicine, 11, 221–232.

Paúl, C. Ayes, S., & Ebrahim, S. (in press). Fourth age challenges: Exploring adaptation mechanisms. Health and Aging.

Poon, L., Jang, Y., Reynolds, S., & McCarthy, E. (2005). Profiles of the oldest-old. In M.L. Johnson (Eds.), The Cambridge handbook of age and aging (pp. 346–353). Cambridge, UK: Cambridge University Press.

Read, S., Vogler, G., Pederson, N., & Johansson, B. (2006). Stability and change in genetic and environmental components of personality in old age. Personality and Individual Differences, 40, 1637–1647.

Resnick, B. (2003). Health promotion practices of older adults: Model testing. Public Health Nursing, 20, 2–12.

Rothermund, K., & Brandtstädter, J. (2003). Depression in later life: Cross-sequential patterns and possible determinants. Psychology and Aging, 18, 80–90.

Salthouse T. (1998). Cognitive perspectives on aging. In I. Nordhus, G. VandenBos, S. Berg, & P. Fromholt (Eds.), Clinical geropsychology. Washington, DC: American Psychological Association.

Samuelsson, SM., Alfredson, BB., Hagberg, B., Samuelsson, G., Nordbeck, B., Brun, A. et al. (1997). The Swedish centenarian study: A multidisciplinary study of five consecutive cohorts at the age of 100. International Journal of Aging and Human Development, 45, 223–253.

Shaie, K. (2000). The impact of longitudinal studies on understanding development from young adulthood to old age. International Journal of Behavior Development, 24, 257–266.

Singer, T., Lindenberger, U., & Baltes, P. (2003). Plasticity of memory for new learning in very old age: A story of major loss? Psychology and Aging, 18, 306–317.

Singer, T., Verhaeghen, P., Ghisletta, P., Lindenberger, U., & Baltes, P. (2003). The fate of cognition in very old age: Six-year longitudinal findings in the Berlin Aging Study (BASE). Psychology and Aging, 18, 318–331.

Small, B., Fratiglioni, L., von Strauss, E., & Bäckman, L. (2003). Terminal decline and cognitive performance in very old age: Does cause of death matter? *Psychology and Aging, 18*, 193–202.

Svensson, T., Dehlin, O. Hagberg, B., & Samuelsson, G. (1993). The Lund 80+ study: Some general findings. In J.J.F. Schroots (Ed.), *Aging health and competence* (pp. 345–354). Amsterdam: Elsevier.

Takkinen, S., & Suutama, T. (2004). Life-lines of Finnish people aged 83–87. *International Journal of Aging and Human Development, 59*, 339–362.

United Nations. (1996a). *World population prospects: The 1996 revision. Annex I: Demographic indicators*. New York: Department for Economics and Social Information and Policy Analysis, Population Division.

United Nations. (1996b). *World population prospects: The 1996 revision. Annex II and III: Demographic indicators by major area, region, and country*. New York: Department for Economics and Social Information and Policy Analysis, Population Division.

Walter-Ginzburg, A., Shmotkin, D., Blumstein, T., & Shorek, A. (2005). A gender-based dynamic multidimensional longitudinal analysis of resilience and mortality in the old-old in Israel: The Cross-Sectional and Longitudinal Aging Study (CALAS). *Social Science and Medicine, 60*, 1705–1715.

Weiss, A., Costa, P.T. Jr., Karuza, J., Duberstein, P.R., Friedman, B., & McCrae, R.R. (2005). Cross-sectional age differences in personality among medicare patients aged 65 to 100. *Psychology and Aging, 20*, 182–185.

WHO/NMH/NPH/02.8 (2002). *Active aging a policy framework*. Available online at http://whqlibdoc.who.int/hq/2002/WHO_NMH_NPH_02.8.pdf.

Wilms, H.-U., Riedel-Heller, S., & Angermeyer, M. (in press). Limitations in activities of daily living and instrumental activities of daily living capacity in a representative sample: Disentangling dementia- and mobility-related effects. *Comprehensive Psychiatry*.

Zhang, J., Ho, S., & Woo, J. (2005). Assessing mental health and its association with income and resource utilization in the old-old Chinese in Hong Kong. *American Journal of Geriatric Psychiatry, 13*, 236–243.

Zanjani, F., Shaie K-W., & Willis, S. (2006). Age group and health status effects on health behavior change. *Behavioral Medicine, 32*, 36–46.

Zelinski, E., & Lewis, K. (2003). Adult age differences in multiple cognitive functions: Differentiation, dedifferentiation, or process-specific change? *Psychology and Aging, 18*, 727–745.

9. Cognitive Plasticity and Cognitive Impairment

Rocío Fernández-Ballesteros, María Dolores Zamarrón,
M. Dolores Calero, and Lluís Tárraga

Introduction

Cognitive plasticity, cognitive reserve, and *learning potential,* three closely related concepts used by several authors as synonymous, emerged from the field of developmental psychology and neuropsychology and were transferred to the field of geropsychology. In the seminal article by Baltes and Schaie (1974), it was emphasized that *cognitive plasticity* is supported by empirical evidence about interindividual differences and the multidimensionality, multidirectionality, and *modifiability* of cognitive functioning in adulthood and old age as a product of biocultural and historical trajectories (in addition to ontogenetic age change) (see also Baltes & Schaie, 1976).

Therefore, these concepts are supported by the observation that people can improve, one way or another, on baseline performances after training. They are briefly defined as within-person variability or cognitive performance modifiability under the most favorable circumstances (Baltes & Schaie, 1974, 1976; Baltes & Lindenberger, 1988; Baltes & Willis, 1982; Kliegl & Baltes, 1987) and they have been operationalized as the observed change in a task performance after training (e.g., Fernandez-Ballesteros, Juan-Espinosa, Colom, & Calero, 1997).

From a methodological point of view, research on cognitive plasticity is based on experimental designs adopting test-training-retest format. These methods are variously named: dynamic assessment, learning tests, interactive assessment, mediated assessment, or testing-the-limits. Several tasks from intelligence tests are used (figural relations, progressive matrices, Koh's blocks, letter series, etc.), as well as from memory training programs (such as mnemonics techniques for recalling diverse materials) (for a review, see Fernández-Ballesteros, Juan-Espinosa, Colom, & Calero, 1997; Fernández-Ballesteros & Calero, 2000; Verhaeghen, 2000; Verhaeghen & Marcoen, 1996). Finally, as Verhaeghen (2000) points out, research on cognitive plasticity has been focused on the nature of the training effects on performance; the effect, directionality, and generalizability of gain scores; individual differences in cognitive plasticity; and finally, the limits of plasticity.

But what is the relationship between cognitive plasticity (or similar concepts) and so-called "gerontological intelligence"? Cognitive plasticity, cognitive reserve, or learning potential have been considered better measures than standard cognitive tests, and better predictors of the subject's modifiability than intelligence measures (Fernández-Ballesteros et al., 1997; Fernández-Ballesteros & Calero, 2000). Cognitive performance at a given point in the life of an individual is, without doubt, a measure of his/her cognitive reserve, since it is the product of myriads of transactions between that individual (as a bio-psycho-social system) and his/her environment (Richard & Sacker, 2003).

Baltes and Willis (1982) suggested conceptual relationships between cognitive performance and cognitive reserve; while cognitive performance can be considered *active reserve* – in other words, the portion of intellectual potential that has been put into operation – *latent reserve* (or *learning potential)* "includes that portion of intellectual potential that could be activated if additional energy and time were invested... Most individuals, including the elderly, therefore, if they choose to do so or are exposed to supportive conditions, can improve their performance" (p. 383). Bearing in mind that older cohorts are exposed to lower levels of cultural and physical stimulation than young and middle-aged cohorts, and considering also that one of the most widespread stereotypes and self-stereotypes about old age is that "elders cannot learn," research on plasticity, cognitive reserve or learning potential is a relevant issue both for science and for society.

Most cognitive plasticity studies have been devoted to normal aging, and how plasticity or changes after training can compensate for "normal" cognitive decline in healthy elders. In recent decades, however, research interest has moved to elders with cognitive impairment. Thus, it is important to consider some relevant neurological concepts.

Within the field of neuropsychology can be found two parallel hypothetical constructs: *brain or neural plasticity* (BP) and *brain reserve* (BR). Let us briefly describe both. Brain plasticity or neuroplasticity is considered a general property of the central nervous system (CNS), and defined as the lifelong capacity to change in response to experience or sensory stimulation (see Neville & Bavelier, 2000). Neuroplasticity encompasses development plasticity – when changes in the immature brain are produced by the first reception of sensory information – to injury-induced plasticity – when damage or dysfunction occur producing changes in the brain as a compensation mechanism. Neuroplasticity is present over the entire life course when learning produces changes in the brain. According to Drunbach (2000), brain changes with learning can be in the internal structure of the neurons or in the number of synapses and, as Gould, Tanapat, Hastings, and Shors (1999) suggest, learning and memory can even act on adult hippocampal neurogenesis.

With regard to brain reserve, Stern (2002, 2003) pointed out that, as emerged from observation, there are *no direct relationships* between impaired performance on a given task or test (even in daily life) and neurobiological factors that disrupt or cause the brain damage. There are two models of BR: the *threshold* model and the *cognitive reserve* model. From the former it is assumed that differences in the effect of brain damage on cognitive performance are due to critical thresholds related to structural differences in brain parameters (such as brain size or synapse count) (e.g., Katzman, 1993). From the cognitive reserve model it is assumed that individuals use several mechanisms for compensating or coping with their pathology, disrupting the brain networks that normally underlie performance by using brain structures or networks not engaged when the brain is not damaged. In other words, the biological bases of *cognitive reserve* take the form of using new brain networks that are more efficient for a given task, as occurs in normal and successful aging. Also, we might understand as a *compensation mechanism* – in response to brain damage – the involvement of certain brain structures or networks for optimizing cognitive performance, but this could also be understood as a normal process used by healthy individuals for coping with task demands, and could be measured by cognitive performance (Stern, 2003).

It can be concluded that neuroplasticity is the basic principle for brain and cognitive reserve – in other words, that brain reserve and cognitive reserve are consequences of neuroplasticity. That is, both BR and CR are both product – expressed at two different levels – of a biological property of the CNS (its plasticity) acting through the transactions between the CNS and the environment throughout the life course of the individual. Lifelong aspects such as physical and social stimulation, schooling, professional career, lifelong training, and so on, are determinants of this reserve capacity (both brain and cognitive reserve). Furthermore, brain and cognitive reserve are both *products* and, at the same time, *sources* of the positive effects on older persons' cognitive functioning through cognitive fitness programs or memory training (e.g., Ball et al., 2002; Kramer, Bherer, Colcombe, Dong, & Greenough, 2004; Richard & Sacker, 2003).

A basic question concerns the extent to which performance improvements after cognitive training (cognitive plasticity) are associated with changes in functional brain activity. Nyberg, Sandblom, Stingdotter, Petersson, Ingvar, and Bäckman (2003) trained 8 younger and 16 older volunteers using visuospatial mnemonic materials. Subjects were scanned during several training phases to obtain 14 measures of cerebral blood flow (CBF) from PET for each subject. During memory encoding, younger adults increase brain activity in both frontal and occipito-parietal zones, while those older adults who increased their performance after mnemonic training showed only occipito-parietal activity. These results suggest the possibility that cognitive reserve capacity is different from a quantitative and qualitative point of view in young and old but, nonetheless plasticity is in both age groups.

In summary, brain plasticity and brain reserve are interrelated neuropsychological constructs, operationalized through brain parameters and through cognitive performance (active cognitive reserve capacity assessed through cognitive tests as well as latent cognitive reserve assessed through cognitive changes after training, Baltes & Willis, 1982). Cognitive plasticity (cognitive reserve capacity or learning potential) is a behavioral construct supported by experimental methodology (pretest/training/posttest designs) and measured both by behavioral changes in performance and by changes in functional brain activity after cognitive training. Both brain plasticity and brain reserve are relevant for normal functioning as well as brain-damage situations, and it can be assumed that to some extent, cognitive plasticity, cognitive reserve and learning potential are ever-present in cognitive functioning.

Figure 1 shows the four levels at which cognitive plasticity and related concepts can be identified: neurobiological, behavioral, methodological, and performance.

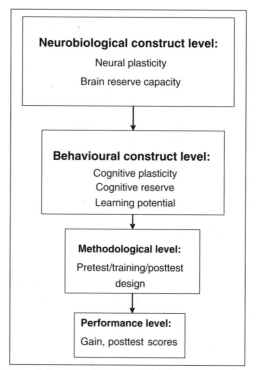

Figure 1 Cognitive plasticity and related constructs levels

Antecedents of Cognitive Plasticity and Cognitive Impairment Research

Cognitive plasticity has long been a main concern of European research. Its antecedents can be found in Vygotsky's concept of "proximal development" (Vygotsky, 1978). In the 1930s, considering that intelligence tests measure the product of the individual's past learning, Vygotsky tried to introduce an alternative concept expressing the current learning potential of the individual. Vygotsky's proposal refers to an experimental situation in which the subject is taught by a more capable adult or peer, leading to changes in his or her cognitive operations and observable behaviors. Vygotsky introduced all the elements present in cognitive plasticity: cognitive intervention or training and observed intraindividual change.

Research programs in cognitive plasticity have been developed mainly in healthy elders and it was not until the 1990s that the work of M.M. Baltes et al. (1992, 1995, 1996, 1997, 1998) triggered interest in cognitive impairment and reserve capacity. The most important findings from that research program and the results in cognitive plasticity in healthy elders can be summarized as follows (see also Baltes, Kliegl, & Dittman-Kohli, 1988; Baltes, Staudinger, & Lindenberger, 1999; Fernández-Ballesteros et al., 1997):

1. Healthy elders substantially improved their performance after training in cognitive as well as in memory tasks; these improvements compensate for "normal" decline between the ages of 50 and 70.
2. Improvements are similar in self-guided and tutor-guided training.
3. While generalizability over time is high, generalizability across tasks is quite limited; therefore, training is task-specific and there is minor generalizability at the level task or construct.
4. Cognitive plasticity is quite similar in those elders with many years of education and in those with very few (Fernández-Ballesteros & Calero, 1995).
5. There are individual differences in cognitive plasticity due to two factors: *age* and *illness*. Cognitive plasticity is substantially reduced in the oldest old and in those with any form of dementia or brain pathology (Baltes & Baltes, 1997).

These two sources of individual differences in cognitive plasticity (age and cognitive impairment due to brain pathology) have been the focus of interest over the last decade in Europe.

With regard to age as a determinant and limit in the reduction of cognitive plasticity, Singer, Lindenberger, and Baltes (2003) examined the longitudinal survivors of the Berlin Aging Study (range = 75–101), training them in a mnemonic skill (method of loci) to examine the plasticity of episodic memory performance in very old people. Plasticity (or within-person variability) is preserved in very old age, but to a greatly reduced degree. Analysis showed that 85% of these very old elders (75 to 101) were unable to improve their memory performance after training, even though 76% used mnemonic techniques. The authors concluded that "efforts at optimization in the domain of episodic memory functioning is severely restricted by age-related losses in very old age" (p. 315).

In a recent study on cognitive plasticity in the very old, Yang, Krampe, and Baltes (2006) compared two age groups (70- to 79-year-olds and 80- to 91-year-olds), screening each group for high and low level of cognitive functioning. They used a self-guided retest paradigm assessing improvement in psychometric abilities (reasoning, speed, and attention) after six standard training and a final posttest under the assumption that practice would "reactivate" or "refresh" skills still available. Results showed improvements in performance across practice in all cognitive tasks and in all samples, but improvements maintained those differences found at baseline (pretest).

In sum, it can be concluded that although age is strongly associated with decline in cognitive plasticity, old and very old individuals can benefit from deliberate practice.

The second source of individual differences in cognitive plasticity is cognitive impairment due to dementia. Two issues are of interest: the potential use of cognitive plasticity in the early diagnosis and in the course of dementia, and its use as a potential predictor of palliative treatment for dementia.

First, although there are tremendous differences between healthy subjects and subjects with dementia in cognitive functioning in all intellectual abilities assessed through intelligence tests, cognitive plasticity tests are very rarely in the field of cognitive impairment and dementia (Lindenberg & Baltes, 1997; Salthouse, 1991; Schaie, 1996). In clinical settings, screening procedures are usually mental status exams with very low sensitivity and specificity in the diagnosis at the first stage of cognitive impairment and dementia, and even in the prediction of the dementia course (Martínez Lage & Khachaturian, 2001). Could evaluating cognitive plasticity help in the diagnosis of cognitive impairment and dementia?

Secondly, although there is evidence from randomized controlled trials that cognitive training has a positive effect on cognitive functioning (Ball et al., 2002), it is a matter of discussion whether elders with dementia – as a chronic neurological disease – could benefit (with a reduction in impairment rates) from the administration of psycho-stimulation programs (Tárraga, 1992, 2001). Therefore, it is important to clarify whether cognitive training can palliate – at least to some extent – cognitive impairment over the dementia course. Most palliative psychostimulation programs do not have any empirical support, and have been developed from a prescientific perspective (Tárraga, 1992, 2001; Tárraga et al., 2006). Cognitive plasticity methodology could provide a source of empirical and theoretical support for these intervention efforts.

M.M. Baltes and associates have been pioneers in this field. Using the same procedures as those used by P.B. Baltes and associates in healthy elders, they demonstrated that little or no plasticity (minor intraindividual or no changes after training) could be interpreted as an early sign of cognitive impairment and dementia. Lack of plasticity also predict cognitive status at the 2-year follow-up (Baltes & Raykov, 1996). When the cognitive plasticity score was compared with other psychological measures, intraindividual change accounted for a unique 16.6% of variance in the prediction of mental status (Baltes et al., 1995; Raykov, Baltes, Neher, and Sowarka, 2002).

Also, Lindenberger and Reischies (1999) compared three age groups of nondemented elders and three groups of elders diagnosed with mild, moderate, and severe dementia in their performance in the Enhanced Cued Recall (ECR: it consists of pictorial items shown with and without category cues in both the encoding and recall phases). Comparisons between elders with and without diagnosis of dementia yielded differences both in performance at base line and in gains after trials (that is, in plasticity). When the three groups with dementia were compared to one another, the group with mild dementia significantly differed from the other two groups both in baseline performance and gains after trials. In conclusion, those individuals with moderate and severe dementia did not significantly improve their performance after trials.

Another important research program on cognitive plasticity and cognitive impairment was conducted by Bäckman (1992, 1996). Although he did not use the cognitive plasticity construct, his research with memory tasks supports the effect of training on episodic memory performance in Alzheimer's disease (AD) patients (Bäckman et al., 2001).

Finally, research on long-term cognitive training has been carried out in several European laboratories. For example, Zanetti et al. (1997) showed how AD patients can benefit from ADL (activity daily living) programs; Tárraga (1992, 1994, 2001) developed a psychostimulation program that reduces the cognitive impairment gradient in AD patients over three months – a reduction that is maintained through time during the course of dementia; several training programs for enhancing memory functioning in the elderly have been developed with positive results in healthy older individuals (Verhaeghen & Marcoen, 1996), while some positive effects with memory programs in elders with cognitive impairment have been reported (Bäckman, 1992, 1996; Tárraga et al., 2006, among others; see Hill, Bäckman, & Stigsdotter, 2000).

In conclusion, the concept of cognitive plasticity seems to be useful for the early detection as well as in the course of cognitive impairment and dementia.

Recent Studies on Cognitive Plasticity in Relation to Cognitive Impairment and Dementia

Assessment Procedures

A first step in any research program on cognitive plasticity and cognitive impairment is the development of assessment procedures for distinguishing between healthy subjects and those with cognitive impairment. These assessment procedures should fulfil two main conditions: (1) cognitive tasks should cover the impaired functions (verbal and visuo-spatial memory, executive function, verbal fluency, see Lezak, 1983); (2) in order to cover a broad range of cognitive competence, assessment materials (stimulus and training procedures) should have a very high ceiling and a very low floor.

Consistent with these conditions and taking into consideration that memory is one of the most vulnerable cognitive functions impaired in dementia, Calero and associates (Wiedl, Schöttke, & Calero, 2001; Calero, Navarro, Arnedo, García-Berben, & Robles, 2000; Calero & Navarro, 2003), selected two tasks assessing verbal and visuo-spatial memory. First, in order to assess verbal memory, they adapted the Auditory Verbal Learning Test for Learning Potential (AVLT-LP), following the version used in schizophrenic patients by Wiedl et al. (1999). The AVLT-LP consists of 15 words administered through 6 trials; the first two trials serve as baseline and the fifth and sixth as posttest, while the other four are administered with feedback and verbal reinforcement.

In order to assess cognitive plasticity through visuo-spatial memory tasks these researchers selected Feuerstein's adaptation of Rey's Positions Test (Feuerstein, Rand, & Hoffmann, 1979), designed to measure learning potential, but reduced and simplified for use in elderly persons (Calero & Navarro, 2003). In this test the subject is required to recall the different positions occupied by five marks on a 5 × 5 matrix across 8 trials.

Both tasks were evaluated in order to test their diagnostic capacity to distinguish between individuals with and without cognitive impairment obtaining positive results (see Calero et al., 2000; Calero & Navarro, 2003, 2004).

Fernández-Ballesteros, Zamarrón, Tárraga, Moya, and Iñiguez (2003; see also Fernández-Ballesteros, Zamarrón, Iñiguez, & Moya, in press) developed the Learning Potential Battery for Dementia (*BEPAD, Bateria de Potencial de Aprendizaje en Demencias*) In brief, the BEPAD contains *four tasks* selected from those reported by experts as having the greatest discriminative power for cognitive impairment: (1) visuo-spatial task (Position Learning Potential Test (PLPt, adapted from Rey – using matrices of 6 × 6, 5 × 5, 4 × 4, 3 × 3, or 2 × 2 and 5 trials, with a pretest and posttest, 3 training trials); verbal recall task, including delayed verbal recall, the Verbal Learning Memory Potential Test (VLMPt, adapted from Rey, 1964; Lezak, 1983; Calero & Lozano, 1994), in which 15 words are presented through 7 trials, of which the first and sixth have, respectively, pre- and posttest roles – in order to test interference – the seventh is administered after the HTPLt); executive control task (Hanoi Tower Potential Learning Test (HTPLt); and verbal fluency task (Verbal Fluency Learning Potential Test (VFLPt: words in 1 minute, two trials, Fernández-Ballesteros, 1968). Following criteria for developing learning potential tests, series of standardized *training procedures* were developed for each task from: practice (present through all trials), feedback (PLPt, VLMt, HTPA, VFPA), reinforcement (AVLT-PA, HTPA, VFPA), visual imagery (PLPt, VFLPt), and verbal coding (PTPA). A complete description of the battery (task and training procedures) was published elsewhere (Fernández-Ballesteros et al., in press), and a first report on learning results can be found in Fernández-Ballesteros et al. (2003).

Cognitive Plasticity in the Diagnosis of Cognitive Impairment and Dementia

Based on the studies by M.M. Baltes and group, by Lindenberger and Reischies, and by Bäckman and group, with the assessment procedures above described, several studies have been carried out for distinguishing between healthy subjects to those who are cognitively impaired and those with AD.

Fernández-Ballesteros et al. (2003) examined whether learning potential (measured in different tasks assessing different aspects of cognitive functioning) can discriminate between healthy people and those diagnosed with mild cognitive impairment (MCI) and with mild AD. With this purpose, 200 subjects were examined: 100 healthy elders (51 women, 49 men, mean age 73.13), 50 diagnosed with MCI (30 women, 20 men, mean age 74.89) and 50 diagnosed with mild AD (36 women, 14 men, mean age 75.07). Educational level was controlled across groups. Inclusion criteria for healthy subjects were absence of functional deficits in daily life activities and absence of cognitive deficits assessed by the MMSE (Folstein, Folstein, & Mc-Hugh, 1975) (scores of more than 24), absence of medical conditions and psychiatric disorders. Mild cognitive impairment subjects were included according to the Petersen, Smith, Waring, Ivnik, Tangalos, and Kokmen (1999) and Reisberg, Ferris, de Leon, and Crook (1982) criteria, and with MMSE scores of between 21 and 27. Finally, AD patients were diagnosed according to all standard criteria, including neuropsychological examination results[1]. In order to assess cognitive plasticity in healthy, MCI and AD subjects, the Battery of Learning Potential Assessment for Dementia (BEPAD) was administered.

Three main results were obtained from learning curves obtained for each subtest and each group, from discriminant analysis of each subtest in each group, and from discriminant analysis of the BEPAD.

---

1 Criteria from the Diagnostic and Statistical Manual of Mental Disorders (DSM-IV) (APA, 1994), criteria from the National Institute of Neurological and Communicative Disorders and Stroke – Alzheimer's Disease and Related Disorders Association (NINCDS-ADRDA), an MMSE score of 18 to 26 or a level 4 score on the Global Deterioration Scale (GDS, Reisberg et al., 1982), and a Hachinski Scale (Rosen, Mohs, & Davis, 1984) score of 4 or less.

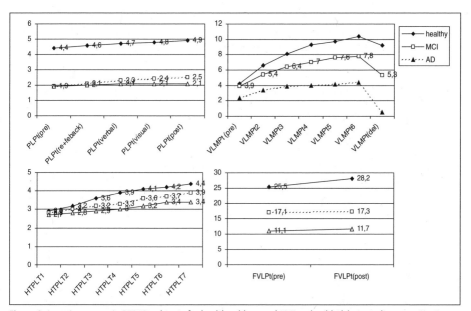

Figure 2 Learning curves in BEPAD subtests for healthy elders, and MCI and mild Alzheimer disease patients

1. Learning curves from all subtests for the three groups are shown in **Figure 2**, and permit us to draw the following conclusions: (a) In the four tasks of the BEPAD, all three groups improved their performance when training was administered; that is, posttest results are significantly better than pretest results in all subtests; (b) Healthy subjects obtained significantly higher scores in the pretest and the posttest, and higher gain scores than MCI and AD patients in all BEPAD Subtests; (c) There is a gradient of modifiability from Healthy to MCI and from MCI to AD. We should stress that although the AD group obtained the lowest scores in all subtests, this group also benefits from training in all BEPAD Subtests (Fernández-Ballesteros et al., 2003).

2. As **Table 1** shows, all cognitive plasticity measures (posttest or performance after training) classify healthy and MCI individuals and AD patients better than all pretest measures. The best posttest for classifying, independently, the three groups, was the posttest of the PLPt, which correctly classified 76.1% of our cases. It was also the best test for classifying healthy (92.8%) and MCI (50%); furthermore, it classified 64.1% of AD patients. The best tests for classifying AD patients were the cognitive plasticity measure of the Verbal Learning Test and delayed recall, both of them correctly classifying 93.8% of AD patients. Moreover, as found by several authors (Fliker, Ferris, & Reisberg, 1999; Welsh, Butters, Hughes, Mohs, & Heyman, 1992), delayed recall is the most powerful test for the diagnosis of severe cognitive impairment. In our data it is possible to interpret that VLMPt delayed recall as an almost pathognomonic symptom for dementia. Analyzing our descriptive data, while 93% of AD patients had a negative score (that is, Delayed Recall lower than pretest), only 3% of healthy and 42% of MCI subjects yielded such negative performance (Fernández-Ballesteros, Zamarrón, & Tárraga, 2005).

Table 1. Static ("pre") versus plasticity ("post") measures and original and estimated classification of healthy and mild cognitive impairment (MCI) subjects and Alzheimer's disease (AD) patients

			Estimated group				
		Groups	Healthy	MCI	AD	Total	Correctly classified
PLPt "pre"	Original	Healthy	96	4	0	100	
		MCI	0	20	28	48	
		AD	0	17	24	41	140
	%	Healthy	96	4	0	100	
		MCI	0	41.7	58.3	100	
		AD	0	41.5	58.5	100	74.1
PLPt "post"	Original	Healthy	90	7	0	97	
		MCI	4	22	18	44	
		AD	1	13	25	39	137
	%	Healthy	92.8	7.2	0	100	
		MCI	9.1	50	40.9	100	
		AD	2.6	33.3	64.1	100	76.1
VLMPt "pre"	Original	Healthy	38	25	37	100	
		MCI	15	15	20	50	
		AD	3	6	39	48	92
	%	Healthy	38	25	37	100	
		MCI	30	30	40	100	
		AD	6.3	12.5	81.3	100	46.5
VLMPt "post"	Original	Healthy	67	27	6	100	
		MCI	17	11	22	50	
		AD	0	3	45	48	123
	%	Healthy	67	27	6	100	
		MCI	34	22	44	100	
		AD	0	6.3	93.8	100	62.1
VLMPt "de-layed"	Original	Healthy	70	29	1	100	
		MCI	16	19	14	49	
		AD	0	3	45	48	134
	%	Healthy	70	29	1	100	
		MCI	32.7	38.8	28.6	100	
		AD	0	6.3	93.8	100	68
HTLPt "pre"	Original	Healthy	71	12	16	99	
		MCI	28	7	15	50	
		AD	24	9	13	46	91
	%	Healthy	71.7	12.1	16.2	100	
		MCI	56	14	30	100	
		AD	52.2	19.6	28.3	100	46.7

Table 1 continued

			Estimated group				
		Groups	Healthy	MCI	AD	Total	Correctly classified
HTLPt "post"	Original	Healthy	52	36	9	97	
		MCI	10	21	13	44	
		AD	1	16	23	40	96
	%	Healthy	53.6	37.1	9.3	100	
		MCI	22.7	47.7	29.5	100	
		AD	2.5	40	57.5	100	53
VFLPt "pre"	Original	Healthy	73	22	5	100	
		MCI	10	18	21	49	
		AD	4	6	39	49	130
	%	Healthy	73	22	5	100	
		MCI	20.4	36.7	42.9	100	
		AD	8.2	12.2	79.6	100	65.7
VFLPt "post"	Original	Healthy	82	17	1	100	
		MCI	11	19	19	49	
		AD	4	6	39	49	140

3. For testing the BEPAD classification power a discriminant analysis was carried out (Fernández-Ballesteros et al., 2005). A total of 89% of cases are correctly classified by the BEPAD: 95.7% of the healthy subjects, 94.9% of the AD patients and 71.1% of the MCI subjects were correctly classified. Nevertheless, 4.3% of healthy subjects were classified as MCI, 2.6% of MCI subjects were classified as healthy, 9.4% of AD patients were classified as MCI, and 26.3% of MCI subjects were classified as AD.

In sum, cognitive plasticity measures (posttest performance), deriving from four different tasks, are better diagnostic tools than their corresponding static measures (pretest or baseline) in classifying healthy, MCI, and AD patients. Or, in the words of Baltes and Willis (1982), measures of *activated reserve capacity* classify better healthy individuals than those with cognitive impairment than any other measure of *active reserve capacity* (or static measure). In sum, as argued by Baltes et al. (1992, 1995), and in the same line as the findings of Calero et al. (2000), cognitive reserve or cognitive plasticity should be considered as a diagnostic indicator of cognitive impairment. Moreover, latent reserve capacity, assessed through multiple tasks measuring multiple functioning, increases the predictive power of cognitive plasticity. Finally, not only can the cognitively impaired individuals learn, but (in accordance with Bäckman and his group), when trained through specific procedures, so can AD patients do. This finding is in support of efforts to develop psycho-stimulation and memory interventions as palliative programs for dementia patients.

Cognitive Plasticity in the Course of Cognitive Impairment

Subsequent studies were carried out for establishing the predictive power of cognitive plasticity through the course from normal mental status to cognitive impairment and MCI to dementia. Let us consider two studies.

Calero and Navarro (2004) conducted a 2-year follow-up in a sample of 203 elderly persons aged between 60 and 93 (mean = 74.74). They were screened through the MEC[2] (Minimental Examen Cognoscitivo, Lobo et al., 1979); 102 individuals were classified as "healthy" according to the MEC score (above the cut-off of 24), while 101 scored below the MEC cut-off (24–16) and fulfilled Petersen's criteria for MCI (Petersen, 2000). All subjects were assessed through the AVLT-LP to evaluate cognitive plasticity, and also through the MEC for assessing mental status at baseline and after two years.

Results already reported showed that the group of elderly persons who presented higher cognitive plasticity (1.5 SD above mean gain score) in the AVLT-LP pretest evaluation maintained their mental status in the MEC at the 2-year follow-up, while those who scored lower in cognitive plasticity showed significant cognitive impairment, regardless of their initial mental status.

In order to test whether cognitive plasticity could predict the course of dementia, Fernández-Ballesteros et al. (2005) followed up a group of elders diagnosed with mild cognitive impairment (Petersen, 2000) one year after this diagnosis. The main goal of this study was to test the extent to which cognitive plasticity measures, assessed through the BEPAD, can predict after one year the subjects whose diagnosis changes from MCI to AD, by comparison with a standard mental exam such as the MMSE.

Twenty-seven individuals diagnosed with MCI (as described above), 13 women and 14 men (mean age = 73.5) were followed up. At this 1-year follow-up, 6 subjects (4 women and 2 men) had changed their diagnosis to AD. The BEPAD discriminant analysis yielded an overall discrimination power of 96.2%; sensitivity was 85.7% and specificity was 100%. On the other hand, the MMSE – usually employed in screening – correctly classified only 71.4% of those MCI subjects diagnosed after one year as AD patients.

The conclusion is that cognitive plasticity (learning) scores are good predictors for assessing those individuals whose status will in the coming years change from mental health to cognitive impairment, or from mild cognitive impairment to AD. It can also be stated that measures of plasticity are better predictors than measures from mental status exams in predicting to future cognitive impairment.

---

2   The MEC (Mini-Examen Congnoscitivo; Lobo, Ezquerra, Gómez, Sala, & Seva, 1979) is a modified version of the MMSE by Folstein et al. (1975). It yields a maximum score of 35 rather than 30, and the cut-off score is 23/24 (sensitivity 89.8%, specificity 89.8%).

Cognitive Plasticity and Cognitive Intervention Programs

In recent decades, considerable efforts have been made in support of so-called "non-pharmacological" or "palliative" intervention programs, most of them attempting to reduce the speed of cognitive impairment in dementia patients or to ameliorate memory problems. Therefore, our third concern has been to explore the relation between plasticity and the effectiveness of long-term cognitive training programs in the same line we already tested in other populations (Fernández-Ballesteros & Calero, 1993), and in accordance with other European research programs conducted by Bäckman et al. (2001), Zanetti et al. (1996), and Badelli et al. (1993).

Two main hypotheses were tested: first, whether cognitive plasticity (measured through intra-individual change after short-term training) could be a good predictor of people's level of cognitive modifiability after long-term cognitive intervention, and second, whether cognitive plasticity or cognitive reserve capacity can be improved through long-term cognitive intervention programs – or in other words, whether cognitive training can increase reserve capacity also in persons with dementia.

Calero and Navarro (2006a) focused on the extent to which plasticity scores could predict improvements obtained in a long-term memory training program. In this case, the sample consisted of 133 voluntary subjects with low educational background (mean age = 76.87 years) attending senior citizens' clubs. Memory training programs were offered to senior citizens' clubs in the city of Granada (Spain). A quasi-experimental design was used with the following procedure: In each club, after a set of cognitive instruments had been administered, subjects were divided into an experimental and a control group. Experimental groups received a memory training program, while control groups were put on a waiting list for receiving the same training after the experimental groups had finished.

In the study summarized here, 78 subjects (mean age = 76.85) participated in a small-group memory training program, and 55 subjects were in the control (waiting list) group (mean age = 74.80). Before training all subjects were tested through a set of cognitive instruments. Cognitive plasticity was assessed through the Position Test-LP and the AVLT-LP. Also, all subjects were assessed for mental status with the MEC (Lobo et al., 1979) and Wechsler Digit Span (from the WAIS-III; Wechsler, 2004). Finally, working memory was measured by the Oakhill, Yuill, and Parkin (1989) experimental task. Memory training consisted of 15 one-hour sessions distributed over three months (after Dively & Cadavid, 1999; see Calero & Navarro, 2006a,b).

The results indicate that all the elderly persons who participated in the memory training program achieved a significant improvement in cognitive performance (measured by the MEC), short-term memory (measured by a digits test) and working memory, while the control group did not improve their scores in the various tests. Moreover, experimental subjects maintained their improvement at the follow-up nine months after the training. Most importantly, significant interaction between plasticity as measured in the initial evaluation and improvements maintained after participation in the memory training program were found. Thus, the elderly persons who showed greater plasticity in the AVLT-PA also obtained greater improvements after the memory training program and at the nine-month follow-up, as measured by the MEC, digit span and working

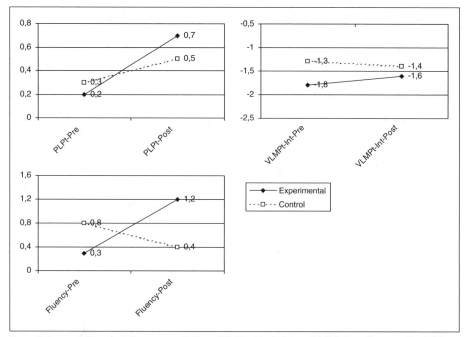

Figure 3 Four cognitive plasticity measures in three BEPAD subtests from mild Alzheimer disease patients following cognitive intervention programs and controls

memory tests. In sum, the results show that cognitive plasticity can act as an important predictor of cognitive modificability in elderly persons, as was found in children and adolescents (Fernández-Ballesteros & Calero, 1993).

To test the hypothesis that cognitive plasticity or reserve capacity can be improved through cognitive training programs even in dementia patients, Zamarrón, Tárraga, and Fernández-Ballesteros (in press) conducted a first *pilot* study with the participation of 27 mild Alzheimer's patients (19 women and 8 men; mean age = 75.30) recruited in two different clinical settings: the diagnostic unit of the ACE Foundation and the Alzheimer Educational Center. From the total sample, in line with specific requirements from these clinical units, 17 mild AD patients (13 women, 4 men) were attending cognitive intervention programs at the Alzheimer Educational Center (after diagnosis in the Diagnosis Unit), while 9 patients, constituting the control group, were recently diagnosed with mild AD from the Diagnosis Unit of the Catalan Institute of Applied Neurosciences. All patients were receiving the same medication throughout the experimental process.

All subjects were assessed with the assessment methodology described above and in Fernández-Ballesteros et al. (2005). Their mean MMSE score in the experimental condition was 20, and in the control condition, 23. Differences in pretest MMSE scores were due to the clinical process from diagnosis at the diagnosis unit to the receipt of treatment at the Alzheimer Educational Center, which led to differences in participants' mental status. Nevertheless, the fact that the control group scored higher on the MMSE can be considered as a factor in favor of the null hypothesis.

The cognitive intervention programs for mild AD patients lasted 6 months. The intervention consisted of 90-minute sessions 3 to 5 days per week[3]. These cognitive interventions were evaluated, and their effectiveness was tested in AD patients and MCI individuals (Tárraga, 1992, 1994, 2001). All subjects were assessed before and after the intervention through the BEPAD.

The results should be considered as provisional because they come from a pilot study with very small samples taken from the clinical setting. As **Figure 3** shows, mild AD patients following cognitive interventions improved their gain scores in the Position Learning Potential test (PLPt), improved their gain and interference scores on the Verbal Learning Memory Potential test (VLMPt), and finally, improved their verbal fluency. At the same time, the control group participants, even if in the pretest they had higher scores in all BEPAD subtests[4], obtained reduced scores after six months. Although these differences show the same clear trend in our four cognitive plasticity measures and in the differences between experimental and control groups, they still do not attain statistical significance.

Conclusions and Future Perspectives

Cognitive plasticity (cognitive reserve capacity or learning potential) is a behavioral construct supported by experimental methodology (pretest/training/posttest designs) and measured both by behavioral changes in performance and by changes in functional brain activity, both types of change being produced after short cognitive training programs. Also, brain plasticity and reserve capacity are relevant to normal functioning as well as for situations of brain damage, and it can be assumed that, to some extent, cognitive plasticity, cognitive reserve and learning potential are ever-present in cognitive functioning throughout the life cycle.

Research on cognitive plasticity in the field of cognitive impairment requires measurement instruments with a high ceiling as well as a low floor, in order to capture broad differences in cognitive functioning in healthy and pathological aging.

Cognitive plasticity measures constitute good tools for classifying individuals with different levels of cognitive functioning and cognitive impairment. Measures of cognitive plasticity or cognitive change – as dynamic measures – are better indicators than common measures from mental exams or static measures of cognitive functioning. Also, cognitive plasticity is a good predictor of the course from normality to cognitive impairment, and also of the course from cognitive impairment to dementia. These findings are important in relation to the early detection of cognitive impairment and dementia and for implementing preventive measures for the postponement of dementia.

Cognitive plasticity is a good predictor of cognitive modifiability after cognitive intervention programs and the stability of the modifications over time. Finally, some evidence has been found of the modifiability of cognitive plasticity or cognitive reserve through cognitive intervention programs in mild AD patients. Most importantly, there

---

3   No direct training on BEPAD subtests was preformed during the intervention sessions.
4   Results from the HTLP test are not included here because many people did not finish the test.

is also evidence that patients not receiving cognitive interventions increase their cognitive impairment, while those who are treated can improve their cognitive functioning. Future perspectives are as follows:

1. The study of cognitive plasticity assessed through cognitive change after short training programs should be complemented with other bio-neurological examinations in order to improve our knowledge about normal and pathological cognitive functioning and their neurobiological correlates.
2. Much more evidence is required with broader and more representative samples of healthy and cognitive impaired individuals and patients at different stages of dementia.
3. Much more progress is needed regarding the evaluation of cognitive interventions in cognitive functioning – including cognitive plasticity – in healthy as well as in pathological aging. This is essential in order to support active palliative policies for dementia and efforts to remove the "nihilistic" positions frequently found in health professionals working in the field of dementia.
4. Finally, cost-benefit analyses are also required with regard to (a) the early diagnosis of cognitive impairment and dementia, and (b) the protective or preventive effect of cognitive interventions in increasing cognitive reserve for those with cognitive impairment and dementia.

References

American Psychiatric Association. (1994). *Diagnostic and statistical manual of mental sisorders DSM-IV. Fourth edition.* Washington, DC: Author.

Bäckman, L. (1992). Memory training and memory improvement in Alzheimer's disease: Rules and exceptions. *Acta Neurologica Scandinavica, 139,* 84–89.

Bäckman, L. (1996). Utilizing compensatory task conditions for episodic memory in Alzheimer's disease. *Acta Neurologica Scandinavia, 165,* 109–113.

Bäckman, L., Small, B.J., & Fraiglioni, L. (2001). Stability of the preclinical episodic memory deficit in Alzheimer disease. *Brain, 124,* 96–102.

Badelli, M.V., Pirano, A., Motta, M., Abati, E., Mariano, E., & Manzi, V. (1993). Effect of reality orientation therapy on elderly patients in the community. *Archives of Gerontology and Geriatrics, 17,* 211–218.

Ball, K., Berch, D.B., Helmers, K.F., Johe, J.B., Leveck, M.D., Marsiske, M. et al. (2002). Effects of cognitive training interventions with older adults. *Journal of the American Medical Association, 288,* 2271–2281.

Baltes, M.M., & Baltes, P.B. (1997). Normal versus pathological cognitive functioning in old-age: Plasticity and testing-the-limits of cognitive/brain reserve capacity. In P. Baltes, F. Forette, Y. Christen, & F. Boller (Eds.), *Démences et longvité.* Paris: Foundation IPSEN.

Baltes, M.M., Kühl, K.P., & Sowarka, D. (1992). Testing for limits of cognitive reserve capacity: A promising strategy for early diagnosis of dementia? *Journal of Gerontology, 47,* 165–167.

Baltes, M.M., Külh, K.P., Sowarka, D., & Gutzman, H. (1995). Potential of cognitive plasticity as a diagnostic instrument: A cross-validation and extension. *Psychology and Aging, 10,* 167–172.

Baltes, M.M., & Raykov, T. (1996). Prospective validity of cognitive plasticity in the diagnosis of mental status: A structural equation model. *Neuropsychology, 10,* 549–556.

Baltes, P.B. (1987). Theoretical propositions of lifespan developmental psychology: on the dynamics between growth and decline. *Developmental Psychology, 23,* 611–626.

Baltes, P.B., & Schaie, K.W. (1974). The myth of the twilight years. *Psychology Today, 40,* 35–38.

Baltes, P.B., & Schaie, K.W. (1976). On the plasticity of intelligence in adulthood and old age. *American Psychologist, 31,* 720–725.

Baltes, P.B., Kliegl, R., & Dittman-Kohli, R. (1988). On the locus of training gains in research on the plasticity of fluid intelligence in old age. *Educational Psychology, 80,* 392–400.

Baltes, P.B., & Lindenberger, U. (1988). On the range of cognitive plasticity in old age as a function of experience: 15 years of intervention research. *Behavior Therapy, 19,* 283–300.

Baltes, P.B., Staudinger, U., & Lindenberger, U. (1999). Lifespan psychology: Theory and application to intellectual functioning. *Annual Review of Psychology, 50,* 471–507.

Baltes P.B., & Willis, S. (1982). Plasticity and enhancement of intellectual functioning in old age. Penn State's adult development and enrichment project (ADEPT). In F.I.M. Craik & S.E. Treud (Eds.), *Aging and cognitive processes* (pp. 353–389). New York: Plenum Press.

Calero, M.D., & Lozano M.A. (1994): La evaluación del potencial de aprendizaje en ancianos [The assessment of learning potential in the elderly]. *Revista de Psicología General y Aplicada, 44,* 89–100.

Calero, M.D., & Navarro, E. (2003). Test de posiciones: Un instrumento de medida de la plasticidad cognitiva en el anciano con deterioro cognitivo leve [Position test: An instrument for measuring cognitive plasticity in elders with cognitive impairment]. *Revista de Neurología, 36,* 619–624.

Calero, M.D., & Navarro, E. (2004). Relationship between plasticity, mild cognitive impairment and cognitive decline. *Archives of Clinical Neuropsychology, 19,* 653–60.

Calero, M.D., & Navarro, E. (2006a). Cognitive plasticity as a modulating variable on the effects of memory training in elderly persons. *Archives of Clinical Neuropsychology* (in press).

Calero, M.D., & Navarro, E. (2006b). Influence of level of activity on cognitive performance and cognitive plasticity in elderly persons. *Archives of Gerontology and Geriatrics* (in press).

Calero, M.D., Navarro, E., Arnedó, M.L., García-Berben, T.M., & Robles, P. (2000). Estimación del potencial de rehabilitación en ancianos con y sin deterioro cognitivo asociado a demencias [Estimating the potential rehabilitation of elderly with and without mild cognitive defects associated with dementia]. *Revista Española de Geriatría y Gerontología, 35*(2), 44–50.

Dively, M., & Cadavid, C. (1999). *Memoria + 65. Programa de mejora de la memoria en personas mayores* [Memory 65+. Program of memory improvement for old people]. Madrid, Spain: Grupo Albor-Cohs.

Drunbach, D. (2000). *The brain explained.* Upper Saddle River, NJ: Prentice Hall.

Fernández-Ballesteros, R. (1968). *Entrenamiento de la fluidez verbal en el Terman-Merrill* [Training verbal fluency from the Terman Merrill text]. Madrid, Spain: Autonoma University of Madrid.

Fernández-Ballesteros, R., & Calero, M.D. (1993). Measuring learning potential. *International Journal of Cognitive Education and Mediated Learning, 3,* 9–20.

Fernández-Ballesteros, R., & Calero, M.D. (1995). Training effects on intelligence of older persons. *Archives of Gerontology and Geriatrics, 20,* 135–148.

Fernández-Ballesteros, R., & Calero, M.D. (2000). The assessment of learning potential. The EPA instrument. In C.S. Lidz & J. Elliot (Eds.), *Dynamic assessment: Prevailing models and applications* [pp. 293–324]. Greenwich, CT: JAI.

Fernández-Ballesteros, R., Juan-Espinosa, M., Colom, R., & Calero, M.D. (1997). Contextual and personal sources of individual differences in intelligence: Empirical results. In W. Tomic & J. Kingman (Eds.), *Advances in cognition and educational practice* (Vol. 4, pp. 221–274). New York: JAI.

Fernández-Ballesteros, R., Zamarrón, M.D., Tárraga, L., Moya, R., & Iñiguez, J. (2003). Cognitive plasticity in healthy, mild cognitive impairment (MCI) subjects and Alzheimer's disease patients: A research project in Spain. *European Psychologist, 8*, 148–159.

Fernández-Ballesteros, R., Zamarrón, M.D., & Tárraga, L (2005). Learning potencial: A new method for assessing cognitive impairment. *International Psychogeriatrics, 17*, 119–128.

Fernández-Ballesteros, R. Zamarrón, M.D., Tárraga, L., Iñiguez, J., & Moya, R. (in press). *Batería de Evaluación de Potencial de Aprendizaje en Demencias (BEPAD)* [Learning potential assessment for dementia battery]. Madrid, Spain: TEA.

Fliker, C., Ferris, S.H., & Reisberg, B. (1999). Mild cognitive impairment in the elderly: Predictors of dementia. *Neurology, 41*, 1006–1009.

Feuerstein, R., Rand, Y., & Hoffman, M.B. (1979). *The dynamic assessment of retarded performers. The learning potential assessment device: Theory, Instrument and techniques.* Baltimore: U.P.P.

Folstein, M.F., Folstein., S.E., & McHugh, P.R. (1975). Mini-Mental-State. A practical method for grading the cognitive state of patients for the clinician. *Journal of Psychiatric Research, 12*, 189–198.

Gould, E., Tanapat, P. Hastings, N.B., & Shors, T.J. (1999). Neurogenesis in adulthood: A possible role in learning. *Trends in Cognitive Sciences, 3*, 187–191.

Hill, R.D. Bäckman, L., & Stigsdotter, A. (Eds.). (2000). *Cognitive rehabilitation in old age.* New York: Oxford University Press.

Katzman, R. (1993). Education and the prevalence of dementia and Alzheimer's disease. *Neurology, 43*, 13–20.

Kliegl, R., & Baltes, P.B. (1987). Theory-guided analysis of mechanisms of development and aging through testing-the-limits and research on expertise. In C. Schooler & K.W. Schaie (Eds.), *Cognitive functioning and social structure over the life course* (pp. 95–119). Norwood, NJ: Ablex.

Kramer, A.F., Bherer, L., Colcombe, S.J., Dong, W., & Greenough, W.T. (2004). Environmental influences on cognitive and brain plasticity during aging. *Journal of Gerontology: Medical Sciences, 59-A,* 940–957.

Lezak M.D. (1983). *Neuropsychological assessment* (2nd ed.) New York: Oxford University Press.

Lindenberg, U., & Baltes, P.B. (1997). Intellectual functioning in old and very old age: Cross-sectional results from Berlin Aging Study. *Psychology and Aging, 12*, 410–432.

Lindenberger, U., & Reischies, F.M. (1999). Limits and potentials of intellectual functioning in old age. In P.B. Baltes & K.U. Mayer (Eds.), *The Berlin Study. Aging from 70 to 100.* Cambridge, UK: Cambridge University Press.

Lobo, A., Ezquerra, J., Gómez, F., Sala, J., & Seva, A. (1979). El Mini Examen cognoscitivo. Un test sencillo y práctico para detectar alteraciones intelectuales en pacientes médicos [Cognitive Mini-Exam: An easy and practical test for screening intellectual impairment in medical patients]. *Actas Luso Españolas de Neurología y Psiquiatría, 7*, 189–201.

Martínez Lage, M., & Khachaturian, Z.S. (Eds.). (2001). *Alzheimer XXI. Ciencia y Sociedad* [Alzheimer XXI. Science and society]. Barcelona, Spain: Masson.

Neville H.J., & Bavelier, D. (2000). Specificity and plasticity in neurocognitive development in humans. In M.S. Gazzaniga (Ed.), *The new cognitive neurosciences* (2nd ed., pp. 83–99). Cambridge, MA: MIT.

Nyberg, L., Sandblom, J., Stingdotter, A., Petersson, J.M., Ingvar, M., & Bäckman, L. (2003). Neural correlates of training-related memory improvement in adulthood and aging. *Proceedings of the National Academic of Sciences USA, 100*, 1328–1333.

Oakhill, J., Yuill, N., & Parkin, A. (1989). Working memory, comprehension ability and the resolution of text anomaly. *British Journal of Psychology, 80,* 351–361.

Petersen, R.C. (2000). Mild cognitive impairment or questionable dementia? *Archives of Neurology*, *57*, 643–644.

Petersen, R.C., Smith, G., Waring, S.C., Ivnik, R.J., Tangalos, E.G., Kokmen, E. (1999). Mild cognitive impairment. Clinical characterization and outcome. *Archives of Neurology*, *56*, 303–308.

Raykov, T., Baltes, M.M, Neher, K., & Sowarka, D. (2002). A comparative study of two psychometric approaches to detect risk status for dementia. *Gerontology*, *48*, 185–193.

Reisberg, B., Ferris, S.H., de Leon, M.J., Crook, T. (1982). The Global Deterioration Scale for assessment of primary degenerative dementia. *American Journal of Psychiatry*, *139*, 1136–1139.

Rey, A. (1964). *L'examen clinique en psychologie* [Clinical examination in psychology]. Paris: Presses Universitaires de France.

Richard, M., & Sacker, A. (2003). Lifetime antecedents of cognitive reserve. *Journal of Clinical and Experimental Neuropsychology*, *25*, 614–624.

Rosen, W.G., Mohs, R.C., & Davis, K.L. (1984) A new rating scale for Alzheimer's disease. *American Journal of Psychiatry*, *141*, 1356–1364.

Salthouse, T.A. (1991). *Theoretical perspective on cognitive aging*. Hillsdale, NJ: Erlbaum.

Schaie, K.W. (1996). *Adult intellectual development: The Seattle longitudinal study*. New York: Cambridge University Press.

Singer, T., Lindenberger, U., & Baltes, P.B. (2003). Plasticity of memory for new learning in very old age: A story of major loss?. *Psychology and Aging*, *18*, 306–317.

Stern, Y. (2002). What is cognitive reserve?. Theory and research application of the reserve concept. *Journal of the International Neuropsychological Society*, *8*, 448–460.

Stern, Y. (2003) The concept of cognitive reserve: A catalyst for research. *Journal of Clinical and Experimental Neuropsychology*, *25*, 589–593.

Tárraga, L. (1992). La Stimulation Cognitive, intérêt et limites [Cognitive Stimulation, interest, and limits]. *Gerontologie et Societé*, *62*, 91–101.

Tárraga, L. (1994). Cognitive psychostimulation: A nonpharmacological therapeutic strategy in Alzheimer's disease. In M. Selmes & M.A. Selmes (Eds.), *Updating of Alzheimer's disease. III Rd. Annual Meeting Alzheimer Europe*. (pp. 72–80). Madrid, Spain: Alzheimer Europe.

Tárraga, L. (2001). Tratamientos de psicoestimulación [Psycho-stimulation treatment]. In R. Fernández-Ballesteros & J. Díez-Nicolás (Eds.), *La enfermedad de Alzheimer y trastornos afines* [Alzheimer's disease and related disorders]. Madrid, Spain: Obra Social Caja de Madrid

Tárraga, L., Boada, M., Modinos, G., Espinosa, A., Diego, S., Morera, A. et al. (2006). A randomized pilot study to assess the efficacy of Smartbrain®, an interactive, multimedia tool of cognitive stimulation in Alzheimer's disease. *Journal of Neurology, Neurosurgery and Psychiatry*, *77*, 1116–1121.

Verhaeghen, P. (2000). The interplay of growth and decline. Theoretical and empirical aspects of plasticity of intellectual and memory performance in normal old age. In R.D. Hill, L. Bäckman, & A. Stigsdotter-Neely (Eds.), *Cognitive rehabilitation in old age* (pp. 3–22). New York: Oxford University Press.

Verhaeghen, P., & Marcoen, A. (1996). On the mechanisms of plasticity in young and older adults after instruction in the method of loci: Evidence for an amplification model. *Psychology and Aging*, *11*, 164–178.

Vygotsky, L.S. (1978). *El desarrollo de los procesos psicológicos superiores* [The development of high psychological process]. Barcelona, Spain: Grijalbo (first edition in Russian in 1934).

Wechsler, D. (2004). *Escala Wechsler de Medida de la Inteligencia-III* [Wechsler Adult Intelligence Scale-III]. Madrid, Spain: TEA Ediciones.

Welsh, K.A., Butters, N., Hughes, J.P., Mohs, R.C., & Heyman, A. (1992). Detection and staging of dementia in Alzheimer's disease. *Archives of Neurology*, *49*, 448–452.

Wiedl, K.H., Wienöbst, J., & Schöttke, H. (1999) Estimating rehabilitation potential in schizophrenic subjects. In H.D. Brenner, W. Böker, & R. Gennes (Eds.), *The treatment of schizophrenia: Status and emerging trends* (pp. 185–208). Bern, Switzerland: Verlag Hans Huber.

Wiedl, K.H., Schöttke, H., & Calero, M.D. (2001). Dynamic assessment of cognitive rehabilitation potential in schizophrenic persons and in old people with and without dementia. *International Journal of Psychological Assessment, 17,* 112–119.

Yang, L., Krampe, R.T., & Baltes, P.B. (2006). Basic forms of cognitive plasticity extended into the oldest-old: Retest learning, age, and cognitive functioning. *Psychology and Aging, 21,* 372–378.

Zamarrón, M.D., Tárraga, L., & Fernández-Ballesteros, R. (in press). Cambios en reserva cognitiva de pacientes de la enfermedad de Alzheimer que asisten a programas de estimulación cognitiva [Cognitive reserve capacity in Alzheimer's patients following cognitive psychostimulation programs]. *Psicothema.*

Zanetti, O., Binetti, G., Magni, E., Rozzini, L., Bianchetti, A., & Trabucchi, M. (1996). Procedural memory stimulation in Alzheimer's disease: Impact of a training program. *Acta Neurologica Scandinavia, 95,* 152–157.

10. Cognitive Decline and Dementia

Stig Berg, Anna Dahl, and Sven Nilsson

Introduction

Cognition can be described as those functions of the mind that are used for processing information and knowledge. Fundamental to cognition are memory and intelligence, including functions such as problem solving, learning, and decision making. Very broadly, it can be seen as the human ability to think. Cognitive functioning is central to the aging process, and intact cognitive functioning is without doubt the single most important factor for successful aging, including retained health, functioning, and quality of life. Many elderly are scared of memory problems and dementia, there being a common belief among both young and old that aging is equal to cognitive decline. However, there is a great span of cognitive functioning in old age. Some elderly are able to solve the most difficult crossword puzzles while others do not remember the names of their children. These striking differences have made cognitive aging a key area in psychogerontology.

Since the beginning of the modern psychology of aging during the 1950s, a very large number of studies on cognitive functioning have been undertaken. Both life-span perspectives and shorter perspectives, usually studying the last decades of life, have been applied. A main theme in this research has been to what extent there is a cognitive decline with increasing age and what factors are associated with this negative development. It is a truly international research area with different research groups all over the world. There is no special European perspective on the study of cognitive functioning. However, in two areas Europe has special assets: One is the large number of longitudinal research projects and the other is the possibility to do quantitative genetic gerontological research using the large twin registers in Denmark, Finland, Sweden, and Norway. These large population-based registers contain unique information on cognitive functioning and health during the aging process.

There is no general definition of what is meant by *cognitive decline*. However, generally cognitive decline is defined as a decrease in the performance in different cognitive abilities measured by a neuropsychological test, dementia symptoms, or a diagnosed dementia illness. Cognitive aging research tries to disentangle decline associated with nonnormative events such as disease and distance to death and change due to normal aging processes. Several factors, such as general developmental processes, various illnesses, and other pathological conditions as well as different external environmental influences are proposed to cause cognitive decline in old age. Still, it is rather unclear what is really meant by normal aging, but in general it is seen as caused by different environmental, genetic, or stochastic chance processes (Finch & Kirkwood, 2000).

In medically oriented studies cognitive decline is usually synonymous with dementia illness or dementia symptoms, and the decline is nearly always measured by some broad scale, most often the Mini Mental State Examination [MMSE] (Folstein, Folstein, & Mc-Hugh, 1975). Very often these investigations have a prospective design trying to identify those with or without decline after a certain amount of time, from a few years up to 10 or more years. Various kinds of event history analyses, such as Cox regression models, are frequently used to find predictors for cognitive dysfunction and dementia.

In psychologically oriented studies the methodological and statistical approach is similar to the one used in medically oriented studies. However, cognitive decline usually implies changes from relatively mild deficits in memory and intelligence to severe dementia. These studies are usually based on cognitive theories and models using different intelligence and memory tests looking at intra- and inter-individual variations and changes in test scores. In a developmental perspective it is important to note that different cognitive abilities change at different rates; some will decline early in life while other cognitive areas are stable into old age. There are also inter-individual differences, which mean that people differ from one another in the rate of change of the same ability. Intra-individually, individuals might decline in some cognitive functions while they remain stable or even improve in other abilities; and this might also vary over time due to such factors as the present mental and physiological status of the individual at the time the measurement is done.

Studies of Normal Aging

During the last decades more than 40 large longitudinal studies, many of them based on European samples, have been undertaken world-wide (Schaie & Hofer, 2001). These studies have examined cognitive change in a life-span perspective from young adulthood to old age, or during longer periods in middle or old age. The explicit purpose of these studies is to map the normal cognitive change with increasing age, and they are usually based on population-based samples. The focus is on the normal aging processes, and the problem with changes due to nonnormative events is not addressed or is related to in a rather general way.

The results from the intelligence studies have mainly been analyzed using the model of two high-order factors: "crystallized" and "fluid" intelligence (Horn & Cattell, 1967). The general results are that fluid abilities such as reasoning, visuo-spatial functioning, and processing speed decline with increasing age. Crystallized abilities, like knowledge and verbal meaning, remain relatively stable in late life. The fluid abilities are used in novel cognitive tasks and are considered more biologically based while crystallized abilities are more related to learning and culture.

The Seattle Longitudinal Study was the first large longitudinal study investigating cognitive function. It started already in 1956 with adults between 22 and 70 years of age, and the subjects have been retested every 7 years (Schaie, Willis, & Caskie, 2004).

The study shows a different change pattern for various abilities. Most age-sensitive is processing speed, which has its peak at age 25 and slowly declines after that age. Spatial and numerical ability is highest when people are in their 40s, declining after that. The most age-insensitive functions are verbal meaning, which has its peak among the 60s, and verbal memory, which is highest in late 50s. In general, before the age of 60 the decline is less than 0.2 standard deviations, but at age 81 the average decline is around one standard deviation for most abilities. Consequently, these results imply that there is a curvilinear decline with increasing age although the start of the change is different for different abilities.

There are several factors, according to the Seattle Longitudinal Study, that lead to early decline in cognitive functions for some persons and maintenance of high functioning up to high ages for others. Half a century of research indicates that factors that reduce the risk of cognitive decline include absence of chronic diseases, a favorable environment mediated by high socioeconomic status and living in a complex and intellectually stimulating milieu. Psychological factors like a flexible personality style at midlife and maintenance of high information processing speed are also important for keeping up good cognitive functioning, according to the Seattle Longitudinal Study.

One of the European longitudinal research projects, the Berlin Aging Study, is a 6-year longitudinal population-based study of individuals aged 70 to 103 at the start of the project. It includes both fluid and crystallized intelligence measures. Longitudinally the results are similar to those found in the Seattle Longitudinal Study; that is, fluid measures like perceptual speed and word fluency show a clear decline while a crystallized function like verbal ability showed less negative change relative to other abilities, with stability in performance up to about the age of 90. The rate of decline did not differ between men and women. The study indicates that after age 70 cognitive change varies mainly by distance to death, age, and type of intellectual ability domain (Singer, Verhaegen, Ghisletta, Lindenberger, & Baltes, 2003).

Another European investigation is the Gothenburg Gerontological and Geriatric Population Study (H70). It is a single-age cohort study that started already in 1971 with a sample of 70-year-olds, who were followed for the next 30 years. Later, other single-age cohorts were added to the project. The results from the H70 study show large inter-individual differences in various tests and to some extent also intra-individual variations. There is a clear decline in different cognitive functions with increasing age, but the change is to a great extent due to health problems and distance to death (Roth, 2005; Thorvaldsson, 2005).

The development of growth curve models has made it possible to estimate the rate of decline for various cognitive abilities with greater precision. One investigation that has applied a growth curve model is the Swedish Twin Study of Aging (SATSA) based on the Swedish Twin Registry. In one of the sub-categories of this study only nondemented twins were included and were examined 4 times during a 13-year period. At the investigation's start the participants were aged 50 and above. The results showed a small but increasing decline with increasing age in both crystallized and fluid abilities as well as in memory (Reynolds, Finkel, McArdle, Gatz, Berg, & Pedersen, 2005).

Very few longitudinal studies have focused on memory, though one such project is the Betula Study from the northern part of Sweden. Also using a growth curve model, it shows relatively limited but significant decline in semantic (verbal knowledge) and episodic (memory of events) memory over a 5-year period. The studied group consisted of a random sample of the population with an age range between 60 and 80 years of age at the start of the study. There was less change in semantic memory than in episodic memory. Chronological age was related to both baseline level and change in memory performance (Lövdén, Rönnlund, Wahlin, Bäckman, Nyberg, & Nilsson, 2004).

There are many factors that can explain the cognitive decline observed in longitudinal normal aging investigations, on both the individual level and the group level. However, the different studies often have rather scant information on different nonnormative events such as physical illnesses or dementia. They usually take an epidemiological approach, which makes it difficult to include more advanced health examinations and/or psychiatric assessments within the test protocols. Sometimes, but not always, studies of normal cognitive aging exclude individuals with signs of dementia. There are also only very few studies that have a design that makes it possible to estimate the relative importance of genes and environment to the variation in cognitive function in old age using quantitative genetic statistical models.

In population-based twin studies it is possible to estimate the relative contribution of genetic or environmental influences to the variation in a trait or a disorder, or to what extent the change in different traits with increasing age (e.g., cognitive decline) is related to these influences. The model is based on the fact that identical or monozygotic twins share all of their genes while fraternal or dizygotic twins on average share 50% of their segregating genes. In the main twin model environmental effects are subdivided into genetic effects, shared rearing environment effects and nonshared environment effects. Shared environment relates to experiences shared by twins in the uterus and when they grew up together. Nonshared environment are experiences that are unique to individuals and therefore contribute only to differences within twin pairs. The genetic effect is estimated by a statistic called heritability, which is usually expressed as the proportion of the variance in a trait or disorder that can be accounted for by genetic differences among individuals. The environmental effects are also expressed as proportions of the total variance.

There are relatively few quantitative genetic studies on cognition and aging, but most of them are based on European populations. Existing cross-sectional twin studies show that genetic factors explain a large proportion of the variation in cognitive functioning among adults. For general cognitive ability, the SATSA study reported heritability around 80% for middle-aged and young old individuals, while measures of more specific intelligence abilities, both crystallized and fluid, showed slightly lower heritability figures, usually between 50 and 75% of the variation (Pedersen, Plomin, Nesselroade, & McClearn, 1992). The Swedish OCTO-Twin Study of twins 80 years old and above reported a somewhat lower heritability for general cognitive ability and specific abilities indicating more influence from environmental factors in the latter part of old age (McClearn et al., 1997). The genetic influence on different memory functions seems to explain 50% or less of the variation. Most of the environmental effects on cognitive functioning in middle and old age are related to nonshared environmental factors – experiences that are unique to the individual.

In cross-sectional studies the variation of the level of cognitive function is closely related to genetic factors while in longitudinal studies the genetic factors seem to be of much less importance for the change or decline in the cognitive scores. As mentioned earlier, twin studies are of great importance when it comes to the evaluation of the influence of genes and environment on cognitive change. In a 13-year longitudinal analysis from the SATSA study using latent growth-curve models, it was found that the change scores were much less influenced by genetic factors compared to the relatively high genetic influence on the level of different cognitive abilities. For general cognitive ability the heritability of the level was 91%, but for the longitudinal change the heritability was only 43%. The results were similar for most of the different cognitive tests in the study. The results also imply a change in the proportion of genetic and environmental sources of variation with increasing age. The genetic effects decrease and the nonshared environmental factors increase with age. This is an indication that in later life cognitive decline to a great extent is driven by environmental influences (Reynolds et al., 2005)

A central factor for general cognitive decline is the slowing of basic information processing speed, which can be seen both in intelligence and memory functions. It was reported already in the 1960s, and various cross-sectional studies have since shown that processing speed can explain 50 to 90% of the age difference in some learning and memory measures (Verhaegen & Salthouse, 1997). However, longitudinally the speed of information processing seems to be less important for cognitive change (Lempke & Zimprich, 2005). The exact underlying mechanisms at work in slowing information processing speed are still unclear although there are studies that suggest changes in anatomic structures and transmittor systems in the brain. However, several studies, both cross-sectional and longitudinal, indicate that the correlations between processing speed and various measures of cognitive ability are almost entirely genetically mediated. A longitudinal analysis of twin data from the SATSA study also shows that in the second half of the life-span it is mainly the accelerating age changes in the fluid test scores that share the genetic variance with processing speed (Finkel, Reynolds, McArdle, & Pedersen, 2005).

Another explanation of cognitive decline in longitudinal studies is terminal decline or terminal drop (Berg, 1996). The general terminal decline hypothesis states that changes in many functions are not correlated primarily with chronological age as such but are instead related to distance to death. According to this hypothesis, most people maintain stable or only slightly declining functions into old age, and more marked accelerating cognitive decline is an indication of impending death. Terminal decline can be seen in many different functions, for example grip strength, but the term has most frequently been used for changes in cognitive abilities. The terminal decline effect can be seen in both fluid and crystallized abilities as well as memory and seems to be more prominent in the young old rather than among the oldest old. Some longitudinal studies show a decline 3 to 6 years before death, but there are also examples of 10 years or more (Figure 1).

The terminal decline phenomenon has been used as an explanation for the frequently observed discrepancies in cognitive test scores between cross-sectional and longitudinal studies; that is, a clear decline in cognitive test scores with increasing age can be seen in the cross-sectional designs compared to the usually more stable levels of functioning in longitudinal studies. The decrease in the cross-sectional scores can according

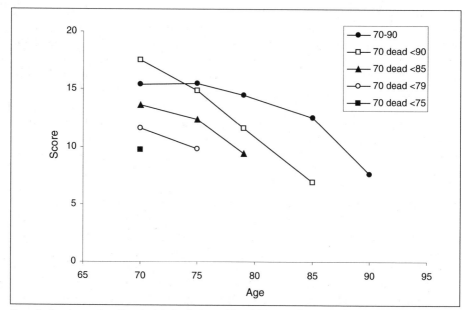

Figure 1. Development and terminal decline between 70 and 90 years of age in spatial ability measured through the block design test. Longitudinal data from the Gothenburg Gerontological and Geriatric Population Study (H70) database

to the terminal decline hypothesis be explained by the fact that there were a greater proportion of people in a kind of terminal phase who therefore have poor test scores and not by aging itself. The same kind of logic also explains the dip that can be seen at the last measurement point in many longitudinal studies. What factors lay behind terminal decline have been discussed, but mostly decline is considered to be due to basic biological aging factors and different kinds of illnesses and health problems. However, in the reports from the different survival and terminal decline studies there has been very little discussion about the roles of general health and specific illnesses. Many studies do not include health variables or use only different self-reports on health and do not have independent health assessments.

Dementia

The major causes of cognitive decline in old age are different dementia illnesses, of which the most common are Alzheimer's disease and vascular dementia. They are characterized by a relatively similar behavioral pattern with wide negative effects on various cognitive abilities although there are also specific traits for various diseases. Dementia in general is a syndrome with progressive memory loss as the key symptom, but it also includes one or several disturbances like aphasia, apraxia, agnosia, and disturbances in executive functioning. To be diagnosed as demented the disturbances must

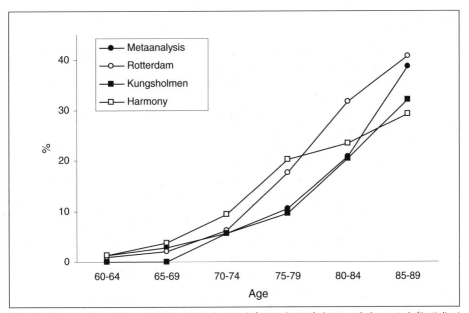

Figure 2. The prevalence of dementia in the Rotterdam study (Ottet al., 1995), the Kungsholmen study (Fratiglioni et al., 1991), the HARMONY study (Gatz et al., 2005) and a meta-analysis of 47 different studies (Jorm et al., 1987)

significantly affect the daily life and sometimes personality changes. Dementia is a threshold diagnosis, which means that before the dementia diagnosis there might be a very long sub-clinical period.

Dementia is an age-related condition. The prevalence of dementia varies between different populations but it usually is around 1% at the age of 65 and 40 to 50% at the age of 90 and over. As the average age is increasing in Europe, dementia is becoming a major health concern equally for individuals, families, and health care systems. For example, in Sweden about around half of the people living in different old-age care institutions have severe cognitive problems. Demented elderly are also more prone to be hospitalized and in need of other resources such as home healthcare visits, medication, and so on. Some studies indicate that dementia is somewhat more frequent among women than among men even when the longer life expectancy among women is taken into consideration. The association between gender and risk of dementia is still disputed, and in some studies the gender difference is not seen.

The most frequent neurodegenerative dementia illness is Alzheimer's disease with around 50 to 60% of all dementia cases. It is probably not a specific disease but a group of illnesses with similar symptoms and stemming from various environmental and genetic factors. Vascular dementia is the second most common dementia illness with around 20 to 30% of all cases. It is often a part of a more general vascular disease with severe implications for the central nervous system. Comorbidity of Alzheimer's disease and vascular dementia is not unusual. There are also several other dementia illnesses, for example dementia related to Parkinson's disease but also dementia due to effects from different physical illnesses (Figure 2).

Genetic Factors

Twin studies make it possible to evaluate in a broader way the genetic and environmental influences on Alzheimer's disease. The most basic information in a twin study is whether a twin pair is concordant or discordant. Concordant means that both twins have the disorder while discordant means that only one of the twins is affected. If the monozygotic twin pairs are concordant to a greater extent than the dizygotic twin pairs, there is an indication of genetic influences.

To date, the largest population twin study of Alzheimer's disease is based on the Swedish Twin Registry. In this project, called the HARMONY study, all twins in the registry aged 65 years or older were screened for cognitive dysfunction and suspected cases of dementia, and their co-twins received a complete clinical diagnostic evaluation for Alzheimer's disease. The study included 11,844 twin pairs, and there were 392 pairs in which one or both members had Alzheimer's disease (Gatz et al., 2006). The results showed that the rate of disease was higher in older groups compared to younger groups. The average age of onset for Alzheimer's disease was 78 years for both monozygotic and dizygotic twins. However, for the monozygotic pairs the average difference in age at onset was 3.7 years while the same difference for dizygotic pairs was 8.1 years. This means that the timing of the onset of Alzheimer's disease probably is under genetic control. In addition, the concordance rate was greater for monozygotic pairs than for dizygotic pairs, suggesting a genetic influence. Using statistical modeling, the heritability for Alzheimer's disease was estimated at 79%, and the remaining 21% was explained by nonshared environmental influences. There were no significant differences between men and women in prevalence or heritability after controlling for age. The same genetic effect seems to be operating in both men and women. The concordance rate for vascular dementia was very low, which means that the illness is influenced by shared and nonshared environmental factors without evidence of genetic influence.

So far, studies have indicated only one specific gene that seems to have some influence on cognitive decline and the risk of developing Alzheimer's disease. It is the APO-E gene that codes for apolipoprotein E and which is the major cholesterol transporter in the brain. A large number of studies have demonstrated that specifically the APO-E ε4 allele increases the risk of cognitive decline and Alzheimer's disease. For example, in the SATSA study the presence of the ε4 allele increased the risk of Alzheimer's disease 3.6 times (Pedersen, Gatz, Berg, & Johansson, 2004).

Risk Factors

For many people old age means an increased risk of different illnesses, especially chronic diseases that are related to vascular functioning, nutrition, and metabolism. This kind of unhealthiness is a problem among young adults and middle-aged people, especially in Western Europe and North America. During recent years a large number of studies have indicated that these kinds of problems might increase the risk of cognitive decline and sometimes different types of dementia. The predictive period varies among different studies; in some cases the perspective is only a few years while others might have their starting point in midlife or even earlier. Recently there have also been indications of long-time effects of fetal malnutrition. An interesting possibility is that many of these disorders can be prevented or mitigated by changes in lifestyle factors and/or medicines, which means that an eventual related cognitive decline might be reversed or stopped. There have been studies relating cognitive decline to a vast number of different illnesses, symptoms, and syndromes as well as different kinds of biochemical indicators, but only a few frequent conditions will be presented here.

One of the most common disorders among elderly people is diabetes. In Europe the prevalence among the 70–74-year-old range varies from about 5% in Poland to 25% in Finland. Including both diabetes and impaired fasting plasma glucose about one third of all Europeans in this age group have impaired glucose metabolism, many without being aware of it (Teuscher, Reinli, & Teuscher, 2001). The number of people with diabetes is also likely to increase in all age groups due to such factors as aging and the increasing prevalence of obesity and sedentary lifestyles. However, the current burden is greatest among the elderly: 1 out of every 2 of all diabetics is 65 years of age and above. Furthermore, the greatest increase is expected in this age group.

Diabetes is a complex metabolic disorder associated with severe complications such as stroke, hypertension, and reduced life expectancy. It has also been proposed that cognitive decline should be added to the list of chronic complications of diabetes (Cuikerman, Gerstein, & Williamsson, 2005), since there is a growing body of evidence that diabetics have lower cognitive function in addition to greater risk and greater rate of decline compared to nondiabetic controls. The relation been confirmed in meta-analyses of case-control and large population studies. (Strachan, Ewing, Deary, & Frier, 1997; Cukierman, Gerstein, & Williamsson, 2005). In all of the reviewed studies, subjects with diabetes had lower cognitive results than nondiabetic subjects, even if not always significant. Most researchers agree that learning and memory abilities are especially affected in individuals with type diabetes (Ryan & Geckle, 2000). These abilities are measured by neuropsychological tests that are known to be sensitive to small cognitive changes. However, cognitive decline can almost always also be seen with the more insensitive MMSE (Cukierman et al., 2005).

In a review about memory and learning dysfunctions in type 2 diabetics, Ryan and Geckle (2000) state that these impairments are only seen in diabetics older than 60–65 years of age. A group seldom included in this definition and researched is the oldest old. A Swedish study which focuses on this age group is the previously mentioned OCTO-Twin study. A broad test battery was used both at the baseline of the investigation as well at the follow-up investigations. The test battery included crystallized and fluid intelligence tests as well as short-term memory, semantic memory, episodic memory, and the MMSE (Hassing, Hofer, Nilsson, Berg, Pedersen, & McClearn, 2004). At baseline, there were no significant differences in the neuropsychological tests related to diabetes when older twins with dementia were excluded. The longitudinal analyses, however, showed that diabetes was a significant predictor of decline for many of the tests 6 years later.

Most studies report an increased risk of all-cause dementia, Alzheimer's disease, and vascular dementia for diabetics compared to nondiabetics (Cukierman et al. 2005). Although these results have to be evaluated according to the fact that there is a high comorbidity of Alzheimer's disease and vascular dementia, it can be very hard to differentiate them from each other, and the diagnoses are dependent on the definitions and diagnostic criteria. Using longitudinal data from the Rotterdam study, Ott, Stolk, van Harskamp, Pols, Hofmann, & Breteler (1999) found individuals with diabetes had a 2 times increased risk for getting all-cause dementia. In the Swedish OCTO-Twin Study, it was found that subjects with type 2 diabetes, adjusted for age, gender, education, smoking habits, and circulatory disease, had a more than two times higher risk of getting vascular dementia. There was no increased risk for Alzheimer's disease (Hassing, Johansson, Nilsson, Berg, Pedersen, & Gratz, 2002).

In type 1 diabetes the beta cells of the pancreas have lost their ability to produce insulin. In type 2 diabetes the body still produces insulin. However, the production is not sufficient for two reasons. The first reason is insulin resistance, which is a defect in the insulin action where insulin progressively loses its ability to promote glucose transport into the cells. The other reason is that the body doesn't have the ability to produce enough insulin after a meal when the glucose level increases. This defect is called impaired glucose tolerance. When the insulin resistance increases, the pancreas is unable to compensate by elevated insulin secretion, which results in elevated fasting insulin, which is called hyperinsulinemia. There is ample evidence suggesting that these disturbances in glucose metabolism always precede the development of type 2 diabetes.

In a Finnish case-control study, elderly people with only slightly disturbed glucose metabolism had worse scores on tests measuring memory, attention, perceptual speed, and verbal fluency than normoglycaemic elderly people (Vanhanen, Koivisto, Karjalainen, Soininen, & Riekkinen, 1997). Moreover, there were no significant differences on any cognitive test between those elderly with impaired glucose tolerance and those with noninsulin-dependent diabetes mellitus. Additionally, at least one prospective study among elderly women has shown that prediabetic elderly have impaired cognitive function and increased risk of developing cognitive impairments compared with elderly with normal glucose metabolism. These findings are also supported by several cross-sectional studies even if it is not possible to draw conclusion from these (Yaffe, Blackwell, Kanaya, Davidowitz, Barret-Connor, & Kreuger, 2004a). The association between Alzheimer's disease as well as other kinds of dementia and impaired glucose tolerance needs to be further explored, since there are few studies and inconclusive results on this topic.

The conclusion is that there is strong evidence for an association between type 2 diabetes and cognitive impairment. It has also been proposed that the association is stronger in diabetics who have been diagnosed for a longer time, in persons who have poor glycemic control and in those who are on insulin therapy (Ryan & Geckle, 2000). However, there are still few reliable studies relating better diabetic control or specific treatments to prevention of cognitive dysfunction.

Another very common disease in the population and especially among the elderly is hypertension. About 50% of all people aged 60 and above have hypertension (Van Rossum, van de Mheen, Witteman, Hofman, Mackenbach, & Grobbee, 2000). Hyper-

tension, in this age group, is commonly defined as a systolic blood pressure of
> 140 mm Hg and/or a diastolic blood pressure of > 90 mm Hg (Rigaud & Forette,
2001). There are numerous articles on the association between blood pressure and cognitive functions. Despite this, the association is not clearly understood. Longitudinal
studies yield mixed results due to such factors as the age at which blood pressure is
measured and the time interval. An early meta-analysis (Waldstein, Manuck, Ryan, &
Muldoon, 1991) showed that there is an evident association between hypertension and
reduced performance on neuropsychological tests measuring memory, attention, and
abstract reasoning. Weaker associations were reported for tests measuring perception,
constructional ability, and psychomotor speed.

There is a growing body of evidence for an association between midlife high blood
pressure and cognitive dysfunction in old age. For example, a Swedish population
study of men followed from 50 to 70 years of age showed that high diastolic blood
pressure at baseline predicted later impairment in the scores for the cognitive tests
MMSE and the Trail-Making Test (Kilander, Nyman, Boberg, Hansson, & Lithell,
1998). Moreover, midlife hypertension seems to be the strongest risk factor for all
forms of vascular dementia (Rigaud & Forette, 2001) and probably for Alzheimer's
disease (Qui, Winblad, & Fratiglioni, 2005). A Finnish population-based longitudinal
study by Kivipelto et al. (2001) found that raised systolic blood pressure in midlife was
significantly associated with Alzheimer's disease in old age, even after controlling for
age, body mass index, education, vascular events, smoking, and alcohol consumption.
In contrast there was no relationship between diastolic blood pressure and cognitive
dysfunction.

Systolic blood pressure rises progressively until the age of 70 or 80, while diastolic
blood pressure rises until the age of 50 or 60. However, the definition of hypertension
does not change with age. The increase in blood pressure seen with normal aging might
have other implications for cognitive functions than midlife hypertension. In fact, the
results from longitudinal studies of late-life blood pressure and cognition are inconsistent. In the Swedish population study "Men Born in 1914," it was shown that high
diastolic blood pressure at age 68 was inversely related to verbal, spatial, and speed
performance at age 81 (Reinprecht, Elmsthål, Janzon, & André-Petersson, 2003). The
OCTO-Twin Study reported that over a 4-year period a medical history of arterial hypertension was associated with a decline in baseline MMSE scores. Intact cognition
through the observation period however, was associated with higher baseline systolic
blood pressure, and conversely declining cognition was related to diminishing systolic
blood pressure. The longitudinal relationship also remained when frailty indicated by
time to death was considered (Nilsson, Read, Berg, Johansson, Melander, & Lindblad,
2007).

The association between high blood pressure in late life and all-cause dementia is
also not clear, for several reasons. One reason is that low blood pressure is associated
with the pathogenesis of Alzheimer's disease, meaning that a low blood pressure might
be a prestage of Alzheimer's disease. Moreover, it is seldom distinguished between
those elderly with a history of hypertension and those with late-life onset hypertension.
Consequently, the most relevant way to study the association in late life is with a longitudinal approach preferably from midlife and throughout late life. There are several

studies which not report any association between hypertension and different kinds of dementia, while some do (Qiu et al., 2005). From the H70 it has for example been reported that elevated diastolic blood pressure at age 70 predicted Alzheimer's disease 10 to 15 years later (Skoog et al., 1996).

The potential positive effects for cognitive functioning of lowering blood pressure through medication have been discussed. In a randomized investigation of the antihypertensive substance candesartan, MMSE scores were stable when blood pressure was lowered, and the authors suggested that effective antihypertensive therapy might reduce cognitive decline (Skoog et al., 2005). The introduction of diuretics and other antihypertensive medicines definitely has improved the cardiac prognosis, but in aging subjects brain circulation might be depressed with harmful side effects on cognitive functioning, especially in the oldest old (Nilsson et al., 2007).

Often elderly individuals have both hypertension and type 2 diabetes. A couple of studies have investigated the effect of this comorbidity on cognitive functioning. In the OCTO-Twin Study a decrease in MMSE scores longitudinally was associated with type 2 diabetes, but there was no such relation for hypertension. However, there was an interaction between hypertension and diabetes, which means that those with both illnesses had a more pronounced cognitive decline (Hassing et al., 2004). From a Finnish cross-sectional investigation it has been reported that patients with comorbid hypertension and hyperinsulinemia performed more poorly on complex cognitive tasks which required abstraction, problem solving skills, and semantic memory (Kuusisto et al., 1993). Additionally, the Framingham Heart Study reported a synergistically interactive effect of hypertension and type 2 diabetes on learning and memory skills (Elias et al., 1997). Presence of both hypertension and type 2 diabetes has also been reported to increase the risk of vascular dementia six-fold (Posner, Tang, Luchsinger, Lantigua, Stern, & Mayeux, 2002).

Obesity is a progressively increasing major public health problem in Europe. During the last decade obesity has not only been identified as a significant risk factor for cardiovascular disease but has been for cognitive impairment as well. Kivipelto et al. (2001) reported an association between midlife obesity and dementia in old age. In the H70 Gustafsson, Rothenberg, Blennow, Steen, and Kuller (2003) showed that obesity indicated by a high body mass index among women in their 70s was positively correlated with the development of dementia 10 to 18 years later, especially Alzheimer's disease. The relation was not found among men. However, the Framingham Heart Study among healthy nondemented individuals without cardiovascular disease indicated that there was a negative effect between obesity and measures of learning and memory but only for men (Elias, Elias, Sullivan, Wolf, & D'Agostino, 2003).

Even if severe vitamin deficiencies are rare among the elderly in the developed countries, milder vitamin deficiencies are not uncommon. There are several studies that have linked low vitamin status with low cognitive function. It seems that especially low levels of vitamin B_{12} are related to cognitive dysfunction. Homocysteine is regarded as a marker of the function of B_6, B_{12}, and folate, and high levels of plasma homocysteine can be attributed to inadequate status of B vitamins. Elevated levels of homocysteine have been related to decline in different cognitive abilities and MMSE scores and an increased risk for cerebrovascular disease and dementia. However, the results are conflicting as there are studies that show no relation between homocysteine and cognitive decline.

There are some suggestions that higher total serum cholesterol may be associated with an increased risk of Alzheimer's disease although the results are mixed. Kivipelto et al. (2001) reported that over a 21-year period high serum cholesterol was associated with a greater risk for mild cognitive impairment.

Even if the above-mentioned risk factors often are considered to be single risk factors independent from each other, this is not actually the case. For example, as much as one third of the variability in the insulin action can be explained by age and obesity alone (Kalmijn et al., 2000). Type 2 diabetes is associated with an increased risk of hypertension and so forth. Comorbidity of different cardiovascular risk factors such as type 2 diabetes or insulin resistance, hypertension, obesity, or lipid abnormalities is often referred to as the metabolic syndrome. Surprisingly, only a few studies have reported on the joint effect of the metabolic syndrome on cognitive functions. However, the available studies report an association between the metabolic syndrome and cognitive impairment (Yaffe et al., 2004b; Vanhanen et al., 2006; Kalmijn et al., 2000). To our knowledge, only the Framingham Heart Study has evaluated the cumulative impact of multiple risk factors including hypertension, type 2 diabetes, cigarette smoking, and obesity (Elias, Elias, Robbins, Wolf, & D'Agostino, 2001). For every additional risk factor, the risk to be in the lowest quartile of the test scores for learning and memory increased with 39%.

Many epidemiological studies indicate a relation between depression and cognitive dysfunction. Generally, patients with depression score lower on cognitive tests than nondepressed individuals (Palsson, Johansson, Berg, & Skoog, 2000). A history of psychiatric illness, especially depression, may also be associated with an elevated risk of Alzheimer's disease. Here, the depressive symptoms are seen as early markers of the illness (Wetherall, Gatz, Johansson, & Pedersen, 1999)

Lifestyle

In recent years there has been a clear interest in different lifestyle factors protecting against cognitive decline and dementia. The results from a number of studies have been presented, but lifestyle has also attracted much attention in media. In one of the largest Swedish newspapers there was recently an article that stated that a high level of education, solving crossword puzzles, playing cards, and a daily walk would help protect against Alzheimer's disease, while watching TV would be harmful.

Higher education has been proposed as a protective factor against cognitive decline and Alzheimer's disease. The nature of this association is unclear as educational attainment might be influenced by both genetic and environmental factors. A lengthy education might lead to greater cognitive reserves that delay the clinical onset of dementia. As education is an indicator of socioeconomic status, individuals with higher education might also have more mentally stimulating work and better access to resources that lead to a healthier lifestyle and better physical health. In an analysis of potentially modifiable risk factors, the HARMONY twin study showed that low education was a significant risk factor for Alzheimer's disease and that this association was not mediated by genetic influences shared by education and Alzheimer's disease. Risk factors that partially accounted for the association between education and Alzheimer's disease included unfavorable early life development and low socioeconomic status as an adult. The risk factors were assessed from questionnaires sent to the twins three decades before, and the results indicate that environmental factors that may be modifiable during the life span contribute to cognitive dysfunction (Gatz et al., in press).

As mentioned above, physical or mental activities at midlife have been pointed out as factors that might decrease the risk of cognitive decline and dementia. A general problem with the epidemiological studies of lifestyle and cognitive decline is that the participants cannot be randomly assigned to the different levels of activities, for example high or low leisure-time physical activities. Instead, the researchers have to identify confounders and try to take them into account using statistical methods, something that often can be difficult, especially finding the right confounders. The lifestyle measures used are often rather crude and self-reported, which increases the uncertainty of many studies.

There are relatively few studies on mental exercise and cognitive function, and many of them showing conflicting results. The mechanisms are unclear, and the relatively short follow-up times in many studies make it possible that the effects are confounded by early cognitive decline or sub-clinical dementia. So far, the longest study is based on Finnish cohorts with a mean follow-up time of 21 years (Rovio et al., 2005). They found that leisure-time physical activity at midlife at least twice a week was associated with a reduced risk of dementia after adjustments for a number of background factors. In a similar way there are studies that show that participating in different kinds of regular social activities also lowers the risk of dementia (Fratiglioni, Paillard-Borg, & Winblad, 2004). On the other hand, it has been difficult to show that different kinds of mental training or "puzzle solving" programs prevent cognitive decline. When improvements are found, they are often modest and are not maintained over time and do not generalize to other abilities than those trained.

Concluding Remarks and Future Perspectives

Very generally the results from all of the longitudinal studies of cognitive development can be summarized in the following way:
– The average performance on most cognitive tasks declines with increasing age.
– There are large variations; some individuals may change very little whereas others deteriorate dramatically.
– There are differences in at what age different cognitive abilities start to decline.
– Dementia illnesses are major threats to functioning and well-being in late life.

For most people healthy aging means relatively small changes in cognitive functioning. Some of these changes are related to genetic factors, but most are influenced by nonshared environmental factors. Alzheimer's disease can to a large extent be explained by genetic factors while vascular dementia mainly seems to be related to environmental factors. Cognitive decline and dementia are influenced by a large number of nonnormative events such as physical illnesses and possibly different lifestyle factors. It is also possible that preclinical dementia might account for a large proportion of the "normal" cognitive decline in late life.

Today, the general pattern of cognitive change during the life span is relatively well known through a number of longitudinal studies. However, the effects of different nonnormative events such as chronic diseases and life styles are to a great extent unknown. Many of the studies show divergent results and the research designs are often relatively unsophisticated. Often only a single risk factor is examined although many of the health variables are interrelated or part of a syndrome. Future research should to a greater extent concentrate on risk factors for cognitive decline and dementia, both in a life span perspective and in old age.

References

Berg, S. (2001). Aging, behavior and terminal decline. In J.E. Birren & K.W. Schaie (Eds.), *Handbook of the psychology of aging* (4th ed.). San Diego, CA: Academic Press.

Cuikerman, T., Gerstein, H.C., & Williamsson, J.D. (2005). Cognitive decline and dementia in diabetes – Systematic overview of prospective observational studies. *Diabetologia, 48,* 2460–2469.

Elias, P.K., Elias, M.F., D'Agostino, R.B., Cupples, L., Wilson, P., Silberhatz, H. et al. (1997). NIDDM and blood pressure as risk factors for poor cognitive performance. *Diabetes Care, 20,* 1388–1395.

Elias, M.F., Elias, P.K., Robbins, M.A., Wolf, P.A., & D'Agostino, R.B. (2001). Cardiovascular risk factors and cognitive functioning: An epidemiologic perspective. In S.R. Waldstein & M.F. Elias (Eds.), *Neuropsychology of cardiovascular disease* (pp. 83–104). Mahwah, NJ: Erlbaum.

Elias, M.F., Elias, P.K., Sullivan, L., Wolf, P., & D'Agostino, R.B. (2003). Lower cognitive function in the presence of obesity and hypertension: The Framingham heart study. *International Journal of Obesity, 27,* 260–268.

Finch, C.E., & Kirkwood, T.B.L. (2000). *Chance, development and aging.* New York: Oxford University Press.

Finkel, D., Reynolds, C.A., McArdle, J.P., & Pedersen, N.L. (2005). The longitudinal relationship between processing speed and cognitive ability: Genetic and environmental influences. *Behavior Genetics, 35,* 535–549.

Folstein, M., Folstein, S., & McHugh, P. (1975). Mini-mental-state: A practical method for grading the cognitive state of patients for the clinician. *Journal of Psychiatry Research, 12,* 189–198.

Fratiglioni, L., Grut, M., Forsell, Y., Viitanen, M., Grafström, M., Holmén, K. et al. (1991). Prevalence of Alzheimer's disease and other dementias in an elderly urban population: Relationship with age, sex, and education. *Neurology, 41,* 1886–1892.

Fratiglioni, L., Paillard-Borg, S., & Winblad, B. (2004). An active and socially integrated lifestyle in late life might protect against dementia. *Lancet Neurology, 3,* 343–353.

Gatz, M., Frataglioni, L., Johansson, B., Berg, S., Mortimer, J.A., Reynolds, C.A. et al. (2005).

Complete ascertainment of dementia in the Swedish Twin Registry: The Harmony Study. *Neurobiology of Aging, 26,* 439–447.

Gatz, M., Reynolds, C.A., Fratiglioni, L., Johansson, B., Mortimer, J.A., Berg, S. et al. (2006). Role of genes and environments for explaining Alzheimer's disease. *Archives of General Psychiatry, 63,* 168–174.

Gatz, M., Mortimer, J.A., Fratiglioni, L., Johansson, B., Andel, R., Berg, S. et al. (in press). Accounting for the relationship between low education and Alzheimer's disease. *The Journal of the Alzheimer Association.*

Gustafsson, D., Rothenberg, E., Blennow, K., Steen, B., & Kuller, L. (2003). An 18-year follow-up of overweight and risk of Alzheimer's disease. *Archives of Internal Medicine, 163,* 1524–1528.

Hassing, L., Hofer, S., Nilsson, S., Berg, S., Pedersen, N., McClearn, G. et al. (2004). Comorbid type 2 diabetes mellitus and hypertension exacerbates cognitive decline. *Age and Ageing, 33,* 355–361.

Hassing, L., Johansson, B., Nilsson, S.-E., Berg, S., Pedersen, N., Gatz, M. et al. (2002). Diabetes mellitus is a risk factor for vascular dementia, but not for Alzheimer's disease: A population-based study of the oldest old. *International Psychogeriatrics, 3,* 239–248.

Horn, J.L., & Cattell, R.B. (1967). Age differences in fluid and crystallized intelligence. *Acta Psychologica, 26,* 107–129.

Kalmijn, S., Foley, L., White, C., Burchfield, J., Curb, H., Petrovich, H. et al. (2000). Metabolic cardiovascular syndrome and risk of dementia in Japanese-American elderly men. *Arteriosclerosis Thrombosis Vascular Biology, 20,* 2255–2260.

Kilander, L., Nyman, H., Boberg, M., Hansson, L., & Lithell, H. (1998). Hypertension is related to cognitive impairment – A 20-year follow-up of 999 men. *Hypertension, 31,* 780–786.

Kivipelto, M., Helkala, E.-L., Laakso, M.P., Hänninen, T., Hallikainen, M., Alhainen, K. et al. (2001). Midlife vascular risk factors and Alzheimer's disease in later life: Longitudinal, population based study. *British Medical Journal, 322,* 1447–1451.

Kuusisto, J., Koivisto, K., Helkala, E.-L,, Vanhanen, M., Hänninen, T., Pyörälä, K. et al. (1993). Essential hypertension and cognitive function – The role of hyperinsulinemia. *Hypertension, 22,* 771–779.

Lempke, U., & Zimprich, D. (2005). Longitudinal changes in memory performance and processing speed in old age. *Aging, Neuropsychology, and Cognition, 12,* 57–77.

Lövdén, M., Rönnlund, M., Wahlin, A., Bäckman, L., Nyberg, L., & Nilsson, L.-G. (2004). The extent of stability and change in episodic and semantic memory in old age: Demographic predictors of level and change. *Journal of Gerontology: Psychological Sciences, 59B,* P130–P134.

McClearn, G., Johansson, B., Berg, S., Ahern, F., Nesselroade, J., Pedersen, N. et al. (1997). Substantial genetic influence on cognitive abilities in twins 80+ years old. *Science, 276,* 1560–1563.

Nilsson, S.E., Read, S., Berg, S., Johansson, B., Melander, A., & Lindblad, U. (in press). Low systolic blood pressure is associated with impaired cognitive function. *Aging: Clinical and Experimental Studies.*

Ott, A., Breteler, M.M.B., van Harskamp, F., Claus, J.J., van der Cammen, T.J.M., Grobbe, D.E. et al. (1995). Prevalence of Alzheimer's disease and vascular dementia: Association with education. The Rotterdam study. *British Medical Journal, 310,* 970–973.

Ott, A., Stolk, R., van Harskamp, F., Pols, H., Hofman, A., & Breteler, M. (1999). Diabetes mellitus and risk of dementia: The Rotterdam study. *Neurology, 53,* 1937–1942.

Palsson, S., Johansson, B., Berg, S., & Skoog, I. (2000). A population study on the influence of depression on neuropsychological functioning in 85-year-olds. *Acta Psychiatrica Scandinavica, 101,* 185–193.

Pedersen, N.L., Plomin, R., Nesselroade, J., & McClearn, G.E. (1992). A quantitative genetic analysis of cognitive abilities during the second half of the life span. *Psychological Science, 3,* 346–353.

Pedersen, N.L., Gatz, M., Berg, S., & Johansson, B. (2004). How heritable is Alzheimer's disease in later life? Findings from Swedish twins. *Annals of Neurology, 55,* 180–185.

Posner, H., Tang, M., Luchsinger, J., Lantigua, R., Stern, Y., & Mayeux, R. (2002). The relationship of hypertension in the elderly to AD, vascular dementia, and cognitive function. *Neurology, 58,* 1175–1181.

Qui, C., Winblad, B., & Fratiglioni, L. (2005). The age-dependent relation of blood pressure to cognitive function and dementia. *Lancet Neurology, 4,* 487–499.

Reinprecht, F., Elmståhl, S., Janzon, L., & André-Petersson, L. (2003). Hypertension and changes of cognitive function in 81-year-old men: A 13-year follow-up of the population study "Men born in 1914," Sweden. *Journal of Hypertension, 21,* 57–66.

Reynolds, C.A., Finkel, D., McArdle, J.J., Gatz, M., Berg, S., & Pedersen, N.L. (2005). Quantitative genetic analysis of latent growth curve models of cognitive abilities in adulthood. *Developmental Psychology, 41,* 3–16.

Rigaud, A.S., & Forette, B. (2001). Hypertension in older adults. *Journal of Gerontology: Medical Sciences, 56,* M217–M225.

Roth, A. (2005). *Sources of individual differences in cognitive functioning.* PhD thesis in Human Development and Family Studies. University Park, PA: Pennsylvania State University.

Rovio, S., Kåreholt, I., Helkala, E.-L., Virtanen, M., Winblad, B., Tuomilehto, J. et al. (2005). Leisure-time physical activity at midlife and the risk of dementia and Alzheimer's disease. *Lancet Neurology, 4,* 705–711.

Ryan, C., & Geckle, M. (2000). Why is learning and memory dysfunction in type 2 diabetes limited to older adults? *Diabetes/Metabolism Research and Review, 16,* 308–315.

Schaie, K.W., & Hofer, S.M. (2001). Longitudinal studies in aging research. In J.E. Birren & K.W. Schaie (Eds.), *Handbook of the psychology of aging* (5th ed.). San Diego, CA: Academic Press.

Schaie, K.W., Willis, S.L., & Caskie, G.I.L. (2004). The Seattle Longitudinal Study: Relationship between personality and cognition. *Aging, Neuropsychology, and Cognition, 11,* 304–324.

Singer, T., Verhaegen, P., Ghisletta, P., Lindenberger, U., & Baltes, P.B. (2003). The fate of cognition in old age: Six-year longitudinal findings in the Berlin Aging Study (BASE). *Psychology and Aging, 18,* 218–231.

Skoog, I., Lernfelt, B., Landahl, S., Palmertz, B., Andreasson, L.-A., Nilsson, L. et al. (1996). 15-year longitudinal study of blood pressure and dementia. *Lancet, 347,* 1141–1145.

Skoog, I., Lithell, H., Hansson, L., Elmfeldt, D., Hofman, A., Olofsson, B. et al. (2005). Effects of baseline cognitive function and antihypertensive treatment on cognitive and cardiovascular outcomes: Study on cognition and prognosis in the elderly (SCOPE). *American Journal of Hypertension, 18,* 1052–1059.

Strachan, M., Ewing, F., Deary, I., & Frier, B. (1997). Is type 2 diabetes associated with an increased risk of cognitive dysfunction? *Diabetes Care, 20,* 438–445.

Teuscher, A.U., Reinli, K., & Teuscher, A. (2001). Glycemia and insulinemia in elderly European subjects (70–75 years). *Diabetic Medicine, 18,* 150–153.

Thorvaldsson, V. (2005). *Late-life terminal decline and independence among cognitive changes as a function of age and mortality.* Department of Psychology, Göteborg University.

Vanhanen, M., Hoivisto, K., Moilanen, L., Helkala, E.L., Hanninen, T., Soininen, H. et al. (2006). Association of metabolic syndrome with Alzheimer's disease: A population-based study. *Neurology, 67,* 843–847.

Vanhanen, M., Koivisto, K., Karjalainen, L., Soininen, H., & Riekkinen, P. (1997). Risk for noninsulin-dependent diabetes in the normoglycaemic elderly is associated with cognitive impairment. *Neuroreport, 8,* 1527–1530.

Van Rossum, C., van de Mheen, H., Witteman, J., Hofman, A., Mackenbach, J., & Grobbee, D. (2000). Prevalence, treatment, and control of hypertension by sociodemographic factors among the Dutch elderly. *Hypertension, 35,* 814–821.

Verheagen, P., & Salthouse, T.A. (1997). Meta-analyses of age-cognition relations in adulthood: Estimates of linear and nonlinear age effects and structural models. *Psychological Bulletin, 122,* 231–249.

Waldstein, S., Manuck, S., Ryan, C., & Muldoon, M. (1991). Neuropsychological correlates of hypertension: Review and methodological considerations. *Psychological Bulletin, 110,* 451–468.

Wetherall, J.L., Gatz, M., Johansson, B., & Pedersen, N.L. (1999). History of depression and other psychiatric illnesses as risk factors for Alzheimer's disease in a twin sample. *Alzheimer Disease and Related Disorders, 13,* 47–52.

Yaffe, K., Blackwell, T., Kanaya, A.M., Davidowitz, N., Barret-Connor, E., & Kreuger, K. (2004a). Diabetes, impaired fasting glucose, and development of cognitive impairment in older women. *Neurology, 63,* 658–663.

Yaffe, K., Kanaya, A., Lindquist, K., Simonsick, E., Harris, T., Shorr, R. et al. (2004b). The metabolic syndrome, inflammation, and risk of cognitive decline. *Journal of the American Medical Association, 292,* 2237–2242.

11. Demographic Change, the Need for Care, and the Role of the Elderly

Ursula Lehr, Susanna Re, and Joachim Wilbers

Has Europe Prepared Enough for the Demographic Change?

We are living in an aging world. Never before could so many persons reach an advanced age in Europe. There is an enormous extension of the life span in all European countries. This is a result of the progress of modern medicine, the improvement of socioeconomic living conditions, and it is also influenced by lifestyles (preventive behavior: nutrition, physical and mental activities, etc.).

However, it is not only important to add years to life, but also to add life to years. Many years ago Hans Schäfer, an expert in social medicine and professor at the University of Heidelberg stated:

> Our life expectancy depends on our lifestyle. Life expectancy does not only mean length of life, but also quality of life. It does not only count how old one will be, but how one will get old (Schaefer, 1975).

Aging has many different faces. Aging itself is not only a biological process. It is a process determined by a number of biological, social, and ecological factors. Sometimes there are great differences between people of the same chronological age within the same country (Thomae, 1976, 1983, 1993).

Aging in the beginning of the 21st century is completely different from what is used to be in the beginning and the middle of the last century. Far more people reach the age of 60, 80, or even 100 years. Lifestyles have changed; everyday life is easier in many aspects. A better education, more knowledge of foreign languages, and a better status of health is typical for the old of today in comparison to the old of yesterday in many countries of the world.

Technical innovations make communication much easier. They facilitate social contacts by phone, by internet-chat, or email; traveling is easier and cheaper. This also helps to keep families together, because in the more industrialized countries the extended family is not living together – which was the case 100 years ago and which is also true today in developing countries, but even there it is changing. Globalization needs mobility. Fewer adult children will live in the neighborhood of their parents and in the near future this trend will increase. The "multilocal multigeneration family" emerges.

The Demographic Changes

Europe is turning grey in the 21st century. Five aspects of demographic change seem to be especially important:

The Rise of Individual Life Expectancy

The life expectancy of newborns in Europe is among the highest in the world: nearly 76.0 years for males and more than 82 years for females (Statistisches Bundesamt, 2006).

In most of the European countries a 60-year-old person can expect 20 to 23 more years. That means that a person will live one-fourth of his/her life after retirement. Many of the persons of today are not prepared for such a long period in a postoccupational – and additionally postparental – stage (UN, 2002).

The Aging Population – The Graying Society

15.5% of the European population in 1996 were older than 65. If the figures for the development of the elderly population from 1995 to 2025 in Europe, Latin America, and Asia are compared there is relatively little change in Europe, but an enormous increase in Latin America and Asia (UN, 2002).

Scientists of all disciplines and faculties, administrators, and practitioners, and politicians, too, must discuss the question of longevity combined with a state of psychophysical well-being. What can be done to assure healthy aging? What can be done to assure the quality of life in old age?

The demographic change has two important underlying trends: the increase in life expectancy and the decrease in the birth rate, which can be found in all European countries. It is not likely that the fertility rate will increase in the European countries and even if it does it will not lead to a remarkably altered demographic situation than calculated now (European Commission, 2004).

The Proportion Between the Different Age Groups, and Between the Generations

One hundred years ago the proportion of persons beyond and below 75 years of age in Germany was 1:79; in 1925 the ratio was 1:67; in 1936 it was 1:45, in 1950 1:35, in 1970 1:25, in 1994 1:14.8, in the year 2000 it was 1:12.8, and in 2040 it will be 1:6.2 (Lehr, 2003).

These figures make clear that every effort for a healthy and competent aging is necessary. Physical, mental, and social activities as well as healthy nutrition should be promoted strongly to enable a life in old age with less necessity of treatment and care.

Additionally, there has been an important change in the structure of households. We have a trend from the three-generation household, to the two-generation household, to the one-generation household – and finally to the one-person household. In Germany only 0.8% of all the nearly 40 million households are three-generation households. In 1900 only 7% of all households were one-person households – today it is 36%! In 1900, 44.4% of all the households were five- and more person households – today 5 or more persons are living in less than 5 of 100 households. Of all the people 65 years and older, about 40% are living in one-person households, and in the age group 75 and older, 68% of the women and 26% of the men live in one-person households. The situation may vary in different European countries but the trend seems to be the same: Living-arrangements of the elderly together with their children will be reduced in the future; the number of two- and one-person households will increase. This has consequences for potential caregivers, if they are needed.

According to a number of studies conducted in many European countries the change in household structure should not be identified with loneliness or isolation of the elderly, as frequent intergenerational contacts are reported independently from the household structure. On the contrary: In European countries where the elderly have the highest score of contacts with family members – like Greece, Portugal, and Italy – Walker and Maltby (1997) found in their studies the highest percentage of loneliness (36% in Greece, more than 20% in Portugal, and 15–19% in Italy), whereas in Denmark, where most of the elderly are not living with their family, less than 5% had the feeling of loneliness; in Germany, the Netherlands, and the UK it was 5–9%; in Belgium, France, Ireland, Luxembourg, and Spain 10–14%. The family integration of the elderly is quite different in each European country. While most of the elderly prefer "intimate relations by distance" as the ideal situation – in particular in Denmark, in the Netherlands and in England, where less than 20% stated that they had daily contact – the daily contact within the family structure in Italy, Greece, Portugal, and Spain (60–70%) is much stronger.

There is also a trend from the three-generation family to the four- or five-generation family. In former times a newborn child very seldom had the opportunity to get to know all four grandparents. Today this is quite frequent, and often one or two great-grandparents as well. However, it is also quite common that persons 60 years and older care for their own parents. In the Interdisciplinary Longitudinal Study of Adulthood and Aging (ILSE) 36% of the persons in their mid-60s (born 1930–1932) have living parents or parents-in-law (Martin, Ettrich, Lehr, Roether, Martin, & Fischer-Cyrulies, 2000). The grandparent generation of today is a "sandwich generation," helping children and grandchildren and also helping and caring for their own parents.

From the Three-Generation Contract to the Five-Generation Contract

The three-generation contract was introduced in Germany by Bismarck, who created the pension system more than 110 years ago. The idea of the three-generation contract is that those persons in the labor force have to provide (via insurance contributions and taxes) for those who are not yet working and those who have finished working, who are retired. Around the turn of the last century, the 15–70-year-olds were in the labor market and provided for the age group under 15 and the over 70 in this way. At that time just 2% of the population were 70 years and older. Today young people in Germany are beginning their occupational life at an average age of 25 years and – because of the situation at the labor force as well as because of the high unemployment rate – people in Germany are ending their occupational life when they are 59/60 years of age, and many gave up work much earlier because of attractive early pension schemes. This situation is different in other countries: In the age group 55–65 years in Germany 43% of the males are in the labor force but in Switzerland it is 77%, and in Norway 72% (European Commission, 2004).

The early retirement age creates many problems in the retirement system and the health insurance business. The group of employed persons between 25–58 years of age has to provide for those who are not yet working and for those who have already finished their occupational work – and these are 26% of the population, often two generations. This has consequences for the pension system: The employed in Germany have to pay 19.9% of their earnings for the pension insurance.

Once again: This is not primarily a problem of the extended life span; it is a problem of the economic situation, because many of those 55 years and older would be able to work, are healthy and willing to do a job, but the critical situation in the labor force makes it impossible (Lehr & Kruse, 2006).

Aging Does Not Necessarily Mean Getting Frail and Dependent

Most elderly people, even those 80 and older, are competent and able to manage their daily life. In the age group of 60–80 years only 3–4% are dependent and need help. In the age group of 80 years and over 31% are dependent, indicating that nearly 70% of this group are competent to master their daily life (Bundesministerium für Familie, Senioren, Frauen und Jugend, 2001).

The number of people over the age of 80 will continue to rise in all the European countries so the number of people needing help and care could increase. However, it is expected that dependency and helplessness will start at a later age. According to research findings of Svanborg (Svanburg, Landahl, & Meilstroem, 1982), Göteborg, Sweden, of Manton (Manton, Stallard, & Corder, 1998) from Duke University in the United States, the aged of today are in a much better health status than the aged of 15 or 20 years ago. The estimated number of persons needing care in the future could be lower if the increase in life expectancy is caused by longer lasting health, fostered by a healthier lifestyle, prevention, and rehabilitation.

A Policy for Healthy Aging – An Answer to the Demographic Change

Today a policy for the elderly has to be more than just a policy for pension systems and a policy for care. It also has to include other aspects than the financial. In order to cope with the challenges of a graying world three issues should be stressed.

1. The first issue is maintaining and increasing the competence of the elderly in order to prevent dependency, and to secure healthy aging with a high degree of quality of life.
2. The second one is the extension and the improvement of rehabilitation measures in order to reenable the elderly for an independent life. It is quite necessary to promote rehabilitation programs for the aged and to qualify medical doctors and nurses in geriatric medicine and gerontology.
3. The third issue asks for the solution of the problem of the dependent and frail elderly, and the problems of caring.

There are many studies that confirm that physical activity is a prerequisite for successful aging. Age-determined physical changes – such as functional impairments of the organs, changes in the motor system and muscular system, as well as changes in the respiratory organs (which of course, depending on the individual, can appear at any age) are similar to the effects of lack of exercise (Meusel, 1996). The young physically inactive individual seems old, just as the old but active individual seems young. Physical activity also affects psychic well-being in regard to certain mental abilities, subjective well-being, social skills, and self-concept.

Mental activity is a prerequisite of successful aging, too. Many studies have found that people who are mentally more active, individuals with a higher range of interests, a farther reaching future time perspective and a greater number of social contacts reach old age with greater feelings of psychophysical well-being. It has been established that cognitive activity is essential for healthy aging. An older person must be given mental tasks; she/he must be furnished with (new) information and be challenged to mental activity. Reduction in mental activity can speed up the process of aging. This can also work in reverse: Mental challenge can result in older people acting spontaneously in ways one would only expect from younger people (see Lehr, 1982, 2003).

Motivation for mental, physical, and social activity has to be increased. Numerous possibilities must be offered in order to make this goal attractive to each individual and many of the barriers in our societies (such as a negative image of older people, ecological conditions) must be reduced or done away with completely.

A policy for the aged is a policy for healthy aging, combined with a state of psychophysical well-being. We know that aging is affected by biological heredity as well as by individual behavior and a wide range of social, environmental, cultural, and political factors. Healthy aging is the result of a lifelong process. So it is necessary to optimize the development of the individual. We know that a variety of influences in early childhood, adolescence, during early and middle adulthood, but also the present life situation of the aged determine the process of aging and well-being in old age.

Interdisciplinary cooperation is needed, to which the biology of aging, geriatrics, and behavioral as well as social sciences should contribute. Healthy aging is a challenge for all gerontologists and geriatricians, a challenge for scientists of many disciplines, a challenge for politicians, and a challenge for all practitioners, for all persons, working with the aged.

Demographic change, an aging Europe, and an aging world is a challenge for all of us. A policy for the aged, however, should not be determined only by the question: "What can we do for the aged?" One should also ask: "What can the aged do for the society?" For this we need to revise the negative image of the aged, which can be found in some countries. Most of the elderly are competent and wish to involve themselves with other people, with society. Societies, communities, churches, clubs, etc. should promote this readiness for voluntary public engagement and be prepared to provide the framework and to utilize the potential and services elderly people have to offer.

Caregiving: Psychological Implications

Since E. Brody's (1981) appeal for consideration of those "women in the middle" who are burnt out by their conflicting roles as mothers of young or adolescent children, as wives, and as caregivers for an elderly family member, the number of studies on this situation increased steadily. Pearlin et al. (1990) state that research into care-giving has become "a flourishing enterprise." Again and again the association between caregiving for a demented family member and a higher prevalence of depression in caregivers has been demonstrated (Bruder, Klusmann, Lauter, & Lüders, 1981; Bruder, 1990, 1993; Gallagher, Rose, Rivera, Lovett, & Thompson, 1989; Schulz, 1990; Schulz, O'Brian, Bookwala, & Fleissner, 1995). On the other hand, the theory of a necessary burn-out effect of the multiple role conflict of the "women in the middle" has been questioned by Bowman, Mukherjee, and Fortinsky (1998). They argue that the presence of children in the household of a caregiving person can reduce caregiver stress and that outside employment enhances the well-being of these women.

Regulations like these require, however, the availability of some kind of social support for the care-giving person. The absence of social support, especially if other family members were not able to provide it, was a major stressor in the situation of caregivers (Kruse, 1988, 1995).

Kruse (1988) found interrelationships between the response styles of the patients and their caregivers. A higher prevalence of depressive reaction in the patients correlated with a prevalence of depressive reaction in the caregiver. A tendency in the patient to cope actively with the situation or to accept it cognitively and emotionally was associated with a response style of the caregiver in which achievement-related behavior, prosocial behavior and emotions, and high amount of identification with the fate of the patient were present. This aspect certainly needs further clarification.

Evaluating the effects of certain ways of caregiver coping is another aspect that deserves more attention. Some findings indicate that some caregivers do well with stress. Knight (1992) showed that coping styles like "accepting the situation" and "finding some good in it" predicted lower stress in caregivers, whereas escapism or attributing responsibility to oneself for the problem led to higher degree of distress in the caregiver.

Data like these indicate that a reorientation of research on caregiving is needed emphasizing interindividual, social, and situation-specific differences. In addition, the decreasing availability of support from family members, which is to be expected by demographic and social changes, should encourage more research on institutional care and factors leading to stress and burden.

Caregiving: Results of Empirical Research

Caring for a dependent and frail parent or grandparent may be valuable and helpful for all family members, and may contribute to an increase of intergenerational understanding and enrichment to the younger generation. However,empirical studies have shown that the same situation may lead to many problems within the family (Lehr & Wand, 1986):

1. It may lead to the separation of the adolescent children from their caring parents and to conflicts in the relationship between husband and wife.
2. "Family care" is almost exclusively identical with "daughter care," assigning the responsibilities for the dependent person to women. This can result in adverse effects in the personality development of these women and can sometimes result in a negative aging process. Because of the stereotype that caring and nurturing are inborn needs of women, society assigns to them an additional burden, which makes it more difficult for them to adjust to their own aging and make themselves more independent. This aspect has to be stressed especially as there are some indications that the aging daughter has to take over the care of parents at an age when she would otherwise have a last chance to reenter the labor force or to take over extrafamilial roles in social organizations, political organizations, church, community, etc. These extrafamilial roles would extend her own life-space and would offer her the stimulation necessary for her mental development and her psychophysical well-being in old age. Research has shown that "family-centered" women deteriorate earlier and achieve a lower degree of quality of life (see Maas & Kuypers, 1974; Fooken, 1980, 1985; Minnemann, 1994).
3. Family care also has demographic limitations as there exists a growing number of single elderly persons who do not have children.
4. With fewer children per family, caring for dependent, older parents cannot be shared by several siblings, respectively, by several daughters and granddaughters.
5. More and more women are in the labor force, which does not allow for intensive care of a dependent family member.
6. There are some indications that some elderly people, especially those who faced the grandparent-role in their late forties or early fifties, are not too enthusiastic about living in a three-generation household.

All these factors make it more difficult for the frail elderly to rely on family care. This is also true if one considers the increase in numbers of four- or five-generation families. About 50% of the caretaking persons in Germany are women 65 years and older – 25% are women 75 years and older.

In the years 1984/1985, 55- to 70-year-old daughters were interviewed who had to take care of their 78–98-year-old parents or parents-in-law. Life histories were recorded as well as data on the present life situation. Quantitative and well as qualitative aspects of the intergenerational relationships were studied. Generally, a very strong and mostly positive interaction was found. Some of the main findings were (Lehr & Wand, 1986):

1. Single daughters more frequently cared for a parent than married ones.
2. Daughters who did not have any sibling were caring for a parent more often than those who had brothers and sisters. On the one hand it seems that the common decision for

institutionalization of a parent is much easier as soon as the responsibility is taken over by more children. On the other hand, there is also some evidence that very old parents with many children prefer living in homes for the aged.

3. The quality of housing did not influence the decision to live together, i.e., of home-care vs. institutional care. Some 70% of the elderly daughters found it generally possible to have their parents in their own home, but for personal reasons (e.g., fear of restriction of their own life space, conflicts with husband or other family members, or stressful relationships with the older family member in the past and present time) they did not want it.

4. Financial problems of the aged parents promote living in the same household, whereas old parents with enough income preferred to live in their own apartment independently, or, if necessary, in homes for the aged.

5. Conflict and stress in the daughter-parent relationship has many causes both past and present. Different components for increased stress experience became evident. "Being restricted in one's own mobility" and "renouncement of many private activities in leisure time and vacation" were reported most often as causes for perceived stress, followed by "heavy physical work."

6. Biographical variables such as mother-daughter interactions during adolescence, early, and middle adulthood were important for the perception of being responsible for very aged parents, especially mothers. The most crucial situation arises if a daughter-in-law has to care for a parent-in-law who had been against the marriage. The extent of conflicts during these former life-stages influenced the present situation of caregiving and made it extremely stressful – especially if the daughters did not have any other social contacts.

7. There are some factors of positive influence on the situation of the elderly daughter/caregiver. The mutual exchange of help as well as the existence of extrafamilial social interaction is perceived as helpful in the situation of caring for old parents. Furthermore, it became evident that willingness to care for a very old parent is also influenced by positive biographical determinants rooted far back in the past. Those daughters who perceived their parents as promoting their own development during adolescence and young adulthood had a more positive attitude to caring for their old parents. It was easier for them to accept the restriction of their lifespace, remembering the wonderful years they had together with their parents in former times.

8. Personality-factors are also important. A high degree of independence and autonomy, of self-confidence and higher scores in activity as well as special coping styles such as "accepting the situation as it is, but making the best of it," achievement-oriented behavior and cultivating social contacts combined with assertive behavior are correlated with higher life-satisfaction for the caretaking daughter.

Daughters who are able to fulfill their own needs, develop their own interests, and who are ready to maintain their own space in relationship to their parents (a feature of "filial maturity" as Blenkner, 1965, called it) are more successful at coping with the family situation than daughters who are not able to affirm their autonomy against their parents. Caregiving children must realize the limits of responsibility for their older parents. Without acceptance of the limits effective coping is not possible. It is not only aging children who are confronted with the developmental task of accepting limits; the old parents, too, have to accept that children have the right and obligation to lead their own lives and to reduce their help in some degree. Otherwise the personality development of these children would be endangered. Daughters have to realize the limit of their own power; otherwise they would stress themselves to a high degree resulting in conflicting family relationships. Filial maturity in the sense of accepting the limits is a task for both: the aging children and their aged parents.

The Need of Care For the Caregiver

It is necessary to rethink, to differentiate, and to widen the existing support systems. Because of lack of information or of resistance on behalf of the very old parents who did not want to "have so many strangers around them," ambulatory social services are frequently not asked for help.

Consequences for the care for the aged to be drawn from these findings include first, organization of support-systems for the caring daughter, which should consist of more than short-term visits. Visit-services, two or three times a week for 2 to 3 h, which would allow the daughter to go out (for shopping or to meet friends) would be helpful ("elderly sitting"). Another point would be the organization of expert-led group work with family members. Families with frail elder relatives need some counseling. "It is a prerequisite for adequate coping strategies to reduce the attendant relative's burden, e.g., for the relief available using professional help" (Bruder et al., 1981; Bruder, 1990, 1993).

A last finding of the study may be of interest: Almost all of the elderly caring women said that they would not expect or accept help like this from their own children.

The Competence of the Elderly in Intra- and Extrafamilial Intergenerational Relationships

We should avoid seeing the aged only as an object of nursing who is dependent on the family. Family roles in old age are not only defined by receiving help but also by giving help. This help is offered not only to the older generation, it is offered also to the grown-up children and grandchildren.

Although there are many intrafamilial roles in old age it would be wrong to regard these as a substitute for extrafamilial social participation. Our studies show that extrafamilial social participation may produce decreasing quantity but increasing quality of intrafamilial contacts. In these cases a higher degree of life-satisfaction is given. Lack of extrafamilial social participation correlates with a higher quantity but a lower quality of familial contacts and with less life-satisfaction.

The need for increased family contacts with children is expressed more frequently in those aged:

- who have some problems in the spouse-role (especially in women),
- or who have lost their partners (widowhood),
- who have a poorer health and are physically dependent,
- who have economic strains,
- who have a lack of extrafamilial participation,
- who have restricted interests and a lower degree of mental activity,
- in those aged women who were living their whole lives only for their family and their children and who did not find any other meaningful sense of their life.

Focusing attention on the children is very often related to a negative perception of age or to life situations that are defined by deprivations and stress. One should regard this kind of extreme family centeredness in old age as neither normal nor ideal.

The need for increased family contact with old parents also occurs in situations involving problems of the children (e.g., health or economic problems or need for help with homework). The relationship with one's parents is regarded more often as a source of conflict during the whole life-cycle than the relationship with one's children.

Intrafamilial participation is seen in a very positive way, is rewarding and contributes to the quality of life in old age if it is based on common interests and mutual stimulation and enrichment – rather than on mutual dependency. Resources for mutual stimulation and enrichment are very often given in extrafamilial participation, which should be cultivated throughout the whole life.

A strong degree of family centeredness (as suggested by traditional role expectations) causes adjustment problems for women in old age. The extreme job-centeredness of men also causes adjustment-problems in old age: very often it makes them helpless and dependent on help from a homemaker.

What is needed is a family policy that looks at all members of the family from a lifelong perspective, which encourages women already in young adulthood in extrafamilial orientation and which encourages in men a more intrafamilial orientation. Only in this way will a real partnership be established, which is not based on mutual dependency, but on a high degree of community and on mutual interests and tasks. Such a partnership will be decisive for life satisfaction in old age.

Intrafamilial as well as extrafamilial social participation is necessary for quality of life in old age. Interests and social contacts within and outside the family should not be regarded as compensatory functions or as substitutes. Intrafamilial and extrafamilial interests and participation should be regarded as necessary completion or supplement for husbands and wives, for parents and children during their whole life-cycle.

Intervention to Avoid Frailty

The main goal of all kind of intervention measures is to live a long life with psycho-physical well-being. There are a variety of determinants, each influencing longevity and well-being in old age.

The Multidimensional Determinants of Longevity

The results of many studies show that no single variable can independently explain longevity. As influential as genetic and physical factors may be, they are not sufficient in explaining longevity (Lehr 1982; Martin, Poon, Kim, & Johnson, 1996).

The results of international longevity research point to a number of interesting relationships. Yet, considering the present state of research, it still seems premature to derive theories or even relationships that may be related to long life expectancy. It should especially be stressed that a series of factors that can possibly influence increased life expectancy interact with each other. This interaction points to a complicated, reciprocal causal network.

Genetic, physical, and biological factors can be regarded as having a direct influence upon longevity and also upon the personality development of an individual (personality, intelligence, activity, morale, adaption, self-esteem, etc.). Personality development, moreover, is determined by socialization processes.

Child-rearing methods, teachers, significant others, and the social environment in general determine the experience and behavior of an individual; historical factors also play a role in this socialization process. In addition, ecological determinants such as physical environment, living in urban or rural areas with their specific stimulations, and climatic conditions have an impact on personality development. A number of studies have determined direct connections between personality and longevity. Correlations between ecological factors and longevity are frequently indicate also, especially in studies about centenarians. Personality variables, on the other hand, have an impact on education and occupational training, on occupational activities, and on socioeconomic status (SES). Correlations between social status and longevity have been determined primarily from vital statistics and demographic analyses and also by follow-up and longitudinal studies finding increased life expectancy for persons with high SES.

Social status and personality as well as ecological factors influence nutritional habits and a direct correlation between nutrition and longevity is claimed to exist. The role of nutrition for diabetes in relation to age and nutritional aspects of atherosclerosis and stroke is important. Smoking and use of alcohol must also be mentioned here.

Genetic and biological factors, personality, ecological variables, and SES have been found to influence physical activities and sports, and also preventive medical care, and hygiene. Correlations of all these variables with longevity have also been demonstrated.

This model by no means includes all variables that may possibly influence longevity. It is merely meant to stimulate further empirical studies and to provide encouragement for future modification, elaboration, and differentiation (see Lehr 1982.)

In the WHO program "Health For All," the issue of prevention is stressed. Aside from regular medical checkups, problems of nutrition (including problems of alcohol and nicotine abuse), and physical activity as well as coping with stress are mentioned. Whereas the issues of nutrition and physical activity receive much attention, the aspect of coping with stress is neglected although many studies point to the decisive role of these coping processes.

Aging is not only a biological, physiological, and psychological process. Aging is a social fate, too. Society, scientists, and policy makers have to learn that a decline of mental competence is not necessarily associated with increasing age. It is possible to avoid or attenuate decline if there was an optimal stimulation of mental growth in childhood and adolescence and if there were also chances for stimulation in middle age. Furthermore, decline can be avoided if a reactivation of the activity and competencies is initiated immediately after some breakdowns or crisis situations in old age.

For physical activities the theory of atrophy by inactivity has demonstrated the reduction of unused competencies. In the same way, a disuse hypothesis of mental decline points to correlations between disuse of mental abilities and mental impairment. There is an old German saying "Fange nie an, aufzuhören – höre nie auf, anzufangen" or "Never start stopping – never stop starting."

In our societies many negative stereotypes about the aged exist, including those held by doctors, nurses, and hospital staff. Many people regard the decline of abilities in old age as unavoidable and irreversible.

In this context one should remember that the expectancies of others will determine the self-concept and, thus, the behavior of the individual. By virtue of negative stereotyping the old very often become a problem case in society. If we want to deal with the aged in an adequate way we have to revise our image of the aged.

Old age, longevity, should not be seen as a problem but as a chance and challenge – a challenge for everyone: for the aging individual, for his family, and for our society. We should not settle for only the problems and deficits of aging and old age. Aging from birth to dying and death is development. We have to ask for, to open our eyes to, and initiate research on the new potentials of the aged, and the competencies and contributions of very old persons.

References

Blenkner, M. (1965). Social work and family relationships in later life. In E. Shanas & G.F. Streib (Eds.), *Social structure and the family: Generational relations* (pp. 46–59). Englewood Cliffs, NJ: Prentice Hall.

Bowman, K.F., Mukherjee, S., & Fortinsky R.H. (1998). Exploring strain in community and nursing home family caregivers. *Journal of Applied Gerontology, 17,* 371–392.

Brody, E.(1981). The "women in the middle" and family help to older people. *The Gerontologist, 21,* 471–480.

Bruder, J. (1990). Alterspsychotherapie und Angehörigenarbeit [Psychotherapy in old age and caregivers]. In R.D. Hirsch (Ed.), *Psychotherapie im Alter* [Psychotherapy in old age] (pp. 73–82) Bern, Switzerland: Verlag Hans Huber.

Bruder, J. (1993). Beratung von pflegenden Angehörigen psychisch kranker alter Menschen [Counselling caregivers of old persons with a psychiatric disease]. In C. Kulenkampff & S. Kanowski (Eds.), *Die Versorgung psychisch kranker alter Menschen* [Care of old persons with a psychiatric disease] (p. 146–159). Cologne, Germany: Rheinland.

Bruder, J., Klusmann, D., Lauter, H., & Lüders, L. (1981). *Beziehungen zwischen Patienten und ihren Familienangehörigen bei chronischen Erkrankungen des höheren Lebensalters* [Relations between patients with chronic disease and their caregivers]. Bonn, Germany: Deutsche Forschungsgemeinschaft.

Bundesministerium für Familie, Senioren, Frauen und Jugend. (2001). Dritter Altenbericht [Third report on the situation of the elderly]. Berlin, Germany: Author.

European Commission (Ed.) (2004). *2004 Eurostat Jahrbuch* [2004 Eurostat yearbook]. Luxembourg: Author.

Fooken, I. (1980). *Frauen im Alter. Intra- und interindividuelle Differenzen* [Women in old age: Intra- and inerindividual differences]. Frankfurt, Germany: Lang.

Fooken, I. (1985). Old and female: Psychological concomitants of the aging process in a group of older women. In J.M.A. Munnichs, P. Mussen, E. Olbrich, & P. Coleman (Eds.), *Life span and change in a gerontological perspective* (pp. 77–102). Orlando, FL: Academic Press.

Gallagher, D., Rose, J., Rivera, P., Lovett, S., & Thompson, L.W. (1989). Prevalence of depression in family caregivers. *The Gerontologist, 29,* 449–456.

Knight, B. (1992). Emotional distress and diagnosis among helpseekers: A comparison of dementia caregivers and depressed older adults. *Journal of Applied Gerontology, 11,* 361–372.

Kruse, A. (1988) Die Auseinandersetzung älterer Menschen mit chronischer Krankheit, Sterben und Tod [Coping with chronic disease, dying, and death in old age]. In A. Kruse, U. Lehr, F. Oswald, & C. Rott (Eds.), *Gerontologie: Wissenschaftliche Erkenntnisse und Folgerungen für die Praxis* [Gerontology: Scientific results and practical impact] (pp. 384–426) Munich, Germany: Bayerischer Monatsspiegel.

Kruse, A. (1995). Menschen im Terminalstadium und ihre betreuenden Angehörigen als "Dyade" [Persons in terminal stage and their caregivers as dyad]. *Zeitschrift für Gerotologie und Geriatrie, 28,* 264–272.

Lehr, U. (1982). Socio-psychological correlates of longevity. *Annual Review of Gerontology and Geriatrics, 3,* 102–147.

Lehr, U. (2003). *Psychologie des Alterns* [Psychology of aging] (10th ed.). Wiebelsheim, Germany: Quelle & Meyer.

Lehr, U., & Kruse, A. (2006). Verlängerung der Lebensarbeitszeit – Eine realistische Perspektive [Prolongation of working life – a realistic perspective]? *Zeitschrift für Arbeits- und Organizationspsychologie, 50,* 240–247.

Lehr, U., & Wand, E. (1986). *Ältere Töchter alter Eltern* [Aging daughters of elderly parents]. Stuttgart, Germany: Kohlhammer Verlag.

Maas, H.S., & Kuypers, J.A. (1974) *From thirty to seventy.* San Francisco: Bass.

Manton, K., Stallard, E., & Corder, L.(1998). The dynamics of dimensions of age-related disability 1982–1994 in the U.S. elderly population. *Journal of Gerontology, Biological Sciences, 53A,* B59–B70.

Martin, P., Ettrich, K.U, Lehr, U., Roether, D., Martin, M., & Fischer-Cyrulies (Eds.). (2000). *Aspekte der Entwicklung im mittleren und höheren Lebensalter* [Aspects of development in midlife and old age]. Darmstadt, Germany: Steinkopff.

Martin, P., Poon, L.W., Kim, E., & Johnson, M.A. (1996). Centenarians. *Experimental Aging Research, 22,* 121–139.

Meusel, H. (1996). *Bewegung, Sport und Gesundheit im Alter* [Exercise, fitness, and health in old age]. Wiesbaden, Germany: Quelle und Meyer.

Minnemann, E. (1994). *Die Bedeutung sozialer Beziehungen für eine Lebenszufriedenheit im Alter* [The importance of social relations for life satisfaction in old age]. Regensburg, Germany: Roderer.

Pearlin, L.I., Mulan, J.T., Semple, S.J., & Skaff, M.M. (1990). Caregiving and the stress process. *The Gerontologist, 19,* 583–594.

Schaefer, H. (1975). *Plädoyer für eine neue Medizin* [A plea for a new medicine]. Munich, Germany: Piper.

Schulz, R. (1990). Theoretical perspectives on caregiving. In D.E. Biegel & A. Blum (Eds), *Aging and caregiving* (pp. 9–52). Newbury Park, CA: Sage.

Schulz, R., O'Brian, A.T., Bookwala, J., & Fleissner, K. (1995). Psychiatric and physical morbidity effects on dementia caregiving. *The Gerontologist, 35,* 771–791.

Statistisches Bundesamt. (2006). *Statistisches Jahrbuch für die Bundesrepublik Deutschland* [Statistical yearbook for the Federal Republic of Germany]. Wiesbaden, Germany: Metzler-Poeschel.

Svanburg, A., Landahl, S., & Meilstroem, D. (1982). Basic issues in health care. In H. Thomae & G.L. Maddox (Eds.), *New perspectives in old age* (pp. 53–75) New York: Springer Publishing.

Thomae, H. (1976). *Patterns of aging – Findings from the Bonn Longitudinal Study (BOLSA).* Basel, Switzerland: Karger.

Thomae, H. (1983). Alternsstile und Altersschicksale. Ein Beitrag zur Differentiellen Gerontologie [Aging style and aging fate. A contribution to differential gerontology]. Bern, Switzerland: Verlag Hans Huber.

Thomae, H. (1998). Probleme der Konzeptualisierung von Altersformen [Problems of conceptualizing styles of aging]. In A. Kruse (Ed.), *Psychosoziale Gerontologie* [Psychosocial gerontology] (Vol. 1, pp. 35–50). Göttingen, Germany: Hogrefe.

United Nations. (Ed.). (2002). *World population ageing 1950–2050.* New York: Author.

Walker, A., & Maltby, T. (1997). *Ageing Europe.* Buckingham, UK: Open University Press.

12. Quality of Life, Life Satisfaction, and Positive Aging

Rocío Fernández-Ballesteros, Andreas Kruse, María Dolores Zamarrón, and Mariagiovanna Caprara

Introduction

In recent decades, a new positive perspective, we might even say a paradigm, has emerged in gerontology (Fernández-Ballesteros, 2002a). Throughout the history of humanity there have been two traditions in the study of aging: the positive perspective of Plato and Aristotle's negative view. In the recent history of gerontology (see first chapter in this volume) – as the science of aging, age, and the aged (see Birren, 1996) – work on aging has been chiefly devoted to the study of negative (pathological) conditions emphasizing those human systems, functions, or characteristics that decline, are impaired, or are lost across the process of aging.

It is in this recent period that new scientific concepts in the field of aging have emerged: quality of life (QoL), successful (optimal, productive, active, adaptive) aging, wisdom, positive affect, and so on have been emblematic concepts in gerontology as we enter the 21st century. These concepts differ in their characteristics: They may refer to the population or to the individual; they may require multilevel and multidisciplinary approaches (such as QoL and successful aging) or, also, they may be psychological concepts (such as wisdom, life satisfaction[LS], or subjective well-being). However, even if they require multilevel assessment many authors have reduced them to subjective conditions (such is the case for QoL and successful aging).

All of these concepts are relevant in the applied field because they are goals in most policies, programs, and actions for elders in our aging world. As Walker (2005b) stressed, the growth in scientific research is most likely related to policymakers' concern with the extension of health to the aging population, as well as its social costs. A good global example is the Second International Plan of Action on Ageing (UN, 2002), whose priority directions, issues, and objectives include the following: to promote active and productive aging, to extend well-being in old age, and to improve quality of life among the elderly.

This new positive perspective has two main characteristics: (1) It emerged at the same time that gerontology is being "psychologized" or "subjectivized" and that psychology is being "positivized" (or approached with a positive view). (2) It deals with complex, amorphous, and overlapping concepts. This is not the place to deal with the growing importance of psychology for gerontology and geriatrics, except to note that this growth can traced back to 1947, when the World Health Organization changed the conceptualization of health from the "absence of illness" to the total physical, mental, and social well-being of the individual. Nor is it our brief here to elaborate on the emergence of a "positive" psychology, both as an applied field (e.g., Fernández-Ballesteros, 2002c) and as a basic or general discipline (e.g., Kahneman, Diener, & Schwarz, 1999). Our most important objective in this chapter is to introduce some conceptual clarification of these positive concepts and to present some European empirical research on them.

Some European Research on QoL, LS and Well-Being, and Successful Aging

QoL emerged as a scientific concept in the final third of the 20th century within the social, psychological, and biomedical scientific literature (for a review, see Fernández-Ballesteros, 1998a). One of the best known theorists of this concept, Lawton (1983), defined QoL as the multidimensional evaluation, by both intrapersonal and social-normative criteria, of the person-environment system of an individual. From this broad definition he developed a model for QoL incorporating four major domains: well-being, behavioral competence, perceived QoL, and environmental or objective QoL. Most importantly, the multidimensional, multilevel concept of QoL embraces the subjective conditions of the individual (e.g., well-being or LS, perceived QoL), behavioral components (e.g., competence), and external or environmental circumstances.

The issue of QoL and aging has been one of the major concerns in gerontological research in Europe supported by the European Union (EU) Fifth Framework Program (PF-5), in which QoL was one of the key actions.

The multidimensional and multilevel conceptualization of QoL has been endorsed by most of the European researchers involved in the FORUM Project devoted to QoL, chaired by Walker (2005b) and supported by the EU. Examples of European research on QoL are the EQUAL and OASIS Projects, both supported by FP-5. From a population-aging perspective, the EQUAL Project covered five European countries (Germany, Italy, the Netherlands, Sweden, and the UK), and in each country a set of QoL conditions were reviewed from the existing aggregate data. These conditions were environmental (housing, neighborhood, transport, and new technology), physical and mental health, employment and networks, family and support networks, participation and social integration, health and social services, LS and subjective well-being, and inequality and variation in QoL (see Walker, 2005a).

From the individual perspective, the OASIS Project (Old Age and Autonomy: The Role of Service Systems in Intergenerational Family Solidarity; see Tesch-Römer, von Kindratowitz, & Motel-Klingebiel, 2001) is based on a stratified random sample of the urban population aged from 25 to 102 years, assessed in five European countries: Norway, England, Germany, Spain, and Israel (total $N = 6,106$). QoL was measured through the World Health Organization Quality of Life (WHOQOL) criteria, which considers the following conditions: physical health, psychological health, social relationships, and environment and living conditions.

Both research projects operationalized QoL through a set of factors, some of them unifactorial constructs (such as LS and well-being), and some of them involving other constructs (such as positive, active, or successful aging). Nevertheless, as Walker (2005b) and other authors pointed out, it should be stressed that QoL has a frame of reference that is broader than aging, and in most studies the environmental circumstances of the individuals are also present.

LS and subjective well-being are related emotional concepts considered as outcomes of regulatory processes of the individual (Higgins, Grant, & Shah, 1999) and, although they have expanded exponentially in recent decades, both are old constructs in psychology (see Fernández-Ballesteros, 2002a). Diener and Lucas (1999) specified three major components of subjective well-being: LS, the presence of frequent pleasant affect, and the infrequent presence of unpleasant affect. Diener considers LS as the cognitive component of subjective well-being, since it requires an evaluation process (comparisons between present and past situations), as well as expected and attained plans and goals. LS is usually assessed through a simple question or through multi-item scales; subjective well-being is assessed through positive and negative adjectives, as well as through simple questions about the extent to which the individual feels happy or unhappy. Although these nuances of definition between the two concepts are important, most authors use the terms almost interchangeably.

As reported by Ferring et al. (2004), there are several surveys on LS and well-being that set out to make cross-national comparisons. A single question about LS was administered using a harmonized Eurobarometer data set. Results showed minor differences between the EU-15 countries.

There are also many other European LS and well-being studies that attempt to identify the factors that contribute to LS for older people, assessing LS with a general measure (e.g., ESAW, Ferring et al., 2004). Furthermore, SHARE (Survey of Health, Ageing, and Retirement in Europe) examines relations between productivity, well-being, and health, assessing well-being through a measure of health-related QoL (Wahrendorf, von Knesebeck, & Siegrist, 2006) with the final purpose of examining the extent to which well-being can be managed and extended in old age for a considerable length of time (e.g., Steverink, Lindenberg, & Slaets, 2005). In sum, LS and well-being are central topics in European research on aging.

Successful aging, optimal aging, positive aging, productive aging, active aging, adaptive aging, or, simply, aging well are all concepts that emerged during the last decades of the 20th century without a commonly accepted definition, but embracing well-being and LS, as well as health and physical competence. Although some of the personal components of these concepts are shared with QoL and some authors emphasize the inclusion of person-environment adjustment (Lawton, 2001), the latter can be considered as a more comprehensive concept covering extrapersonal or external conditions. It is also important to add that some authors consider QoL as an outcome of successful aging. For example, the WHO (2002) defines active aging as the process of optimizing opportunities for health, participation, and security in order to enhance QoL as people age, and Walker (2005b) stressed that one of the key factors determining QoL in old age is successful aging.

Most of the European projects cited above, although primarily dealing with QoL,

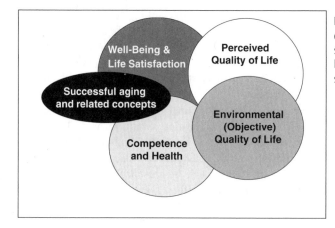

Figure 1. Relationships among quality of life, well-being and life satisfaction, and successful aging based on Lawton's (1983) four-sector theory of quality of life

subjective well-being, or LS, also consider successful aging as a key word or as a subproject or outcome of QoL. For example, the "Ageing Well" project, developed under the auspices of FP5, estimates the direct causal contribution of five key components of QOL (physical health and functioning, mental efficacy, life activity, material security, and social support) to the outcome of a variable called "aging well."

Furthermore, the EXCELSA-Pilot (Fernández-Ballesteros et al., 2003) has been planned as the first stage of a Cross-European Longitudinal Study on Ageing, under the auspices of FP-5, with the central research objective of arriving at an empirical definition of competence and its potential determinants (distal factors such as sociode-mographics and education, and proximal factors such as psychosocial and biophysical variables). In the next section we describe this research to some extent. Finally, the ENABLE-AGE Project, a cross-national (participant countries: Sweden, Germany, the UK, Latvia, and Hungary) project on "Enabling Autonomy, Participation, and Well-being in Old Age: The Home Environment as a Determinant for Healthy Ageing" (Iwarsson, Whal, & Nygren, 2004; see Chapter 4), illustrates well the importance and overlap of all these concepts.

Figure 1 summarizes the theoretical relations between QoL, well-being and LS, competence and health, and successful aging, and related concepts on the basis of Lawton's four-sector model. First of all, well-being and LS, and competence and health, are personal conditions both for successful aging (and related concepts) and for QoL. But while QoL also embraces environmental conditions (both perceived and objective), successful aging can be considered as an individual's multidimensional and multilevel conditions. As pointed out by Walker (2005a,b), QoL is an umbrella or meta-level concept embedding other conditions, both personal and environmental. Although there are authors who reduce QoL to some of its subjective or/and personal components (e.g., health-related QoL or perceived QoL), we emphasize here that the multidimensional – personal and environmental conditions – and multilevel – biophysical-psycho-social – conceptualization is considered as the main characteristics of research in QoL in Europe. Finally, while LS and subjective well-being are psychological constructs, successful aging is also a multidomain, multilevel concept referring mainly to the individual as bio-psycho-social but incapable of being reduced to any of its components (such as health, physical competence, or well-being).

Quality of Life

As pointed out elsewhere, QoL is a key concept emerging from the environmental, biomedical, social, and psychological sciences (Fernández-Ballesteros, 1998a); it is also current in public policy and among lay people. After a review of literature carried out in the early 1990s in the gerontology laboratory at the Autónoma University of Madrid, a research program on QoL (under the auspices of the Institute of Ageing and Social Services) began with the following theoretical assumptions:

1. Although QoL can be considered at a societal or population level, our interest is focused on older individuals and their life quality.
2. Since life has myriad constituents, QoL should be considered as a highly complex, multidimensional concept in which socioenvironmental factors (such as pension systems, housing, or access to health and social services), as well as personal conditions (health, functional abilities, etc.) interact.
3. Contextual and personal factors should not be confused with or considered equivalent to objective and subjective assessment procedures, in the sense that contextual factors are those objectively assessed and personal conditions are those subjectively considered. On the contrary, most of the contextual and personal ingredients of QoL can be appraised both objectively and subjectively[1], as pointed out by Lawton (1983). Nevertheless, LS and well-being are ever-present as subjective ingredients of QoL.
4. Although the concept of QoL is nomothetic or socionormative, it should be adapted to individual circumstances; in other words, before the utilization of a standard procedure for assessing QoL, this procedure must be carefully adapted to the particular context.
5. Finally, QoL is a cultural concept and its empirical definition should be carefully studied through cross-cultural comparisons.

Implicit Concept of Quality of Life

Since QoL is a new concept as yet without scientific consensus, a first step in QoL research should be the study of the implicit or "folk" concept in the population (see Sternberg, 1990). In the context of a population study on QoL in old age, the following question was asked: "Please indicate what you think are the *three* most important conditions for the quality of life of old persons (people over 65)." A list with nine ingredients (ever-present in QoL literature) and a final open question were included in the QoL questionnaire. The questionnaire was administered to a representative

---

1 For example, housing conditions can be assessed by standard observation as well as by the subject's appraisal, just as health can be assessed by means of physician's records or by subject's evaluation.

sample (by age and gender) of the Spanish population (over 18; N = 1,205, sampling error ±3%).

Results yielded the order (percentage of individuals selecting in 1st, 2nd, and 3rd place) of the most important conditions considered by Spaniards to be the constituent elements of QoL. First: to have good health (86%); second: to be independent (66%); third: to have a good pension or income (34%); fourth: to have good relationships with family members and friends (31%); fifth: to be active (26%); sixth: to have health and social services available (24%); seventh: to have a comfortable apartment or house (17%); eighth: to feel satisfied with life (11%); ninth: to have opportunities for learning (3%); no other conditions of QoL were reported by participants. Post hoc comparisons yielded no differences resulting from gender, age, or socioeconomic status (SES), but older subjects reporting poor health overestimated health, while subjects reporting low income considered "to have a good pension or income" more important (Fernández-Ballesteros, 1993, 1998b). Moreover, when these components of QoL were self-reported by elders or reported by relatives about their close elders, and factorial analysis was performed, a factorial structure according with these QoL components emerged in both subsamples (elders' self-reports and relatives' reports about their close elders).

At this stage of our project it was concluded that Spaniards' concept of elderly QoL is very close to the concept held within the scientific field, and that this conceptualization is in accordance with the factorial structure arising from independent data. This concept is also coincident with other population QoL conceptualizations defined in other European countries (Fernández-Ballesteros & Maciá, 1993; Fernández-Ballesteros, 2002a; Walker, 2005a). In sum, health and independence, wealth, and social relationships are the three essential constituents of QoL but other such aspects such as be activity, availability of health and social services, environmental quality, feeling satisfied with life, and opportunity for learning are also ingredients for QoL in old age.

Differential Conditions for QoL

Our second step had the main objective of examining the extent to which three contextual conditions – living in the community or in residences, living in rural or urban environments, and SES – are sources of variance of QoL among elders in Spain. Two representative (by age and gender) samples of Spanish elders aged 65 and over (mean age = 73.9, range = 65 to 95 years old) were selected by random routes in rural and urban habitats: 507 participants lived in the community (210 men and 297 women) and 507 participants (204 men and 303 women) lived in residences for the elderly (251 in private residences and 256 in public residences).

Taking into consideration our general assumption on QoL, we prepared a questionnaire on the nine selected personal and contextual dimensions of QoL, assessing them through objective and subjective questions. This questionnaire inquired about the following conditions: health (subjective health, number of illnesses, pains reported, and medicine being taken), functional abilities (ADL I and II), social integration (living alone or with others, social contact frequency, and social satisfaction), activity level (physical activity, leisure and cultural activities, and activity satisfaction), LS (the Philadelphia Geriatric Center Morale Scale-PGCMS, by Lawton [1975] was administered, as well as a direct and simple question and comparative appraisal on LS and satisfaction with age), social and health services (availability, utilization, and satisfaction with 19 types of service), environmental conditions (in-home facilities and outdoor conditions, self-reported and observed by the interviewer), and socioeconomics (income, other financial resources, education, marital status, age, and gender).

After several psychometric and descriptive analyses regarding our main objective – the extent to which contextual and personal variables influence QoL domains, – ANOVAs and z distributions of the 136 QoL items (continuous or nominal/ordinal variables, respectively) in the three contextual conditions (living in the community and in residences, living in rural or urban contexts, and SES) and the two personal variables (age and gender) were carried out. We shall now report the most important results.

Place of residence (in the community or in residences) had effects in 51.9% of the QoL elements. People that live in the community (in their own home) do not differ from those in public or private residences with regard to most of the health indicators, but the former reported better functional abilities (both in terms of their subjective appreciation and of the number of difficulties encountered in carrying out daily life activities). Furthermore, those living in the community (in their own home) reported carrying out more physical, cultural, and leisure activities (and being more satisfied with them) and reported greater social integration, a broader social network, and higher levels of satisfaction with these relationships. On the other hand, environmental quality (of both the place of residence and its surroundings) appears to be higher for those living in institutions (both public and private), compared to those living at home. This is the case according to both the subjects' own evaluations and those of the trained observers. In conclusion, social integration, activity level, and satisfaction are QoL ingredients favored by the community context, while environmental quality is a better condition in residences. Finally, the two contexts studied differ, essentially, in terms of satisfaction about one's activity and interpersonal relationships. Most important, from this study we derived a set of recommendations for the promotion of social relationships and sociorecreational activity in public residences.

Also, elders with different SES significantly differed in 46% of the QoL items. People with upper and middle SES, compared to those with low SES, had better health and functional abilities, performed more physical, cultural, and leisure activities, and had better environmental quality. Minor effects were seen for rural/urban habitat (32.2%), participants living in town (less than 10,000 inhabitants) with respect to those living in middle size cities (10,000 to 100,000) with those living in big cities (more than 100,000 inhabitants) reported more interpersonal relationships, less environmental quality (both self-reported and observed), lower income, and lower schooling.

Personal variables, age and gender, had important effects on QoL. Age was a source of variance in 49.3% of the QoL conditions – with the exception of environmental quality (both observed and self-reported) and availability of health and social services. That is, older participants in comparison to younger ones reported poorer health and functional abilities; fewer physical, cultural, and leisure activities; lower social integration; and lower schooling and income. Finally, gender is also a powerful differential condition for QoL in 48.35% of our QoL components. Men, with respect to women, had better subjective and objective health, had better functional abilities, and reported better LS, as well as higher education and income. No differences in activity level, environmental quality, and health and social services (availability, utilization, or satisfaction) were found.

Summarizing, a multidimensional concept of QoL was useful in the careful assessment of persons over 65 with different circumstances. In other words, QoL conditions were sensitive both to personal variables (age and gender) and to contextual or external conditions. Older elders, with respect to younger ones, men, with respect to women, those living in the community in comparison to those living in residences, and those from the upper and middle classes, with respect to those from lower classes, all reported higher levels in a range of QoL elements. It can be concluded that QoL is a differential and multidimensional construct useful for describing people, groups, and contexts.

The Role of LS Within QoL Conditions

As already pointed out, LS is an important construct in the psychosocial study of aging, and one of the commonly-accepted subjective conditions of QoL and of successful aging. In our studies on QoL, LS was measured using an aggregate instrument containing 13 items from Lawton's Morale Scale and other direct LS questions. However, in our analysis (as occurred in our study on positive aging) we did not find any contextual source of differences of LS; nor were any age differences found in relation to LS, though women did report less LS than men. Next, on the basis of an exploratory factor analysis conducted with all 136 of the QoL items, a path analysis was carried out. In order to reach our final

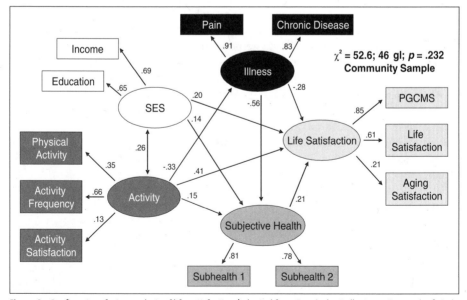

Figure 2. Confirmatory factor analysis of life satisfaction (adapted from Fernández-Ballesteros, Zamarrón, & Ruíz, 2001)

model we proceeded step-by-step, testing simple submodels (Zamarrón & Fernández-Ballesteros, 2000; Fernández-Ballesteros, Zamarrón, & Ruíz, 2001).

Figure 2 shows our final model, which explains 69% of life satisfaction variance. LS (measured by Lawton's Morale Scale and other direct LS questions) is explained by distal sociodemographic factors (income and education), both directly (.61, $p < .001$) and indirectly through physical illness ($-.50$, $p < .001$), and through perceived health (.44, $p < .001$). Social and leisure activities (physical activity level, satisfaction with leisure activities, and frequency of social relationships) have the strongest explanatory power in LS (.74, $p < .001$), both directly (.26, $p < .05$) and indirectly through perceived health (.39, $p < .001$), and physical illness has a negative effect on LS ($-.45$, $p < .001$). Among the psychosocial factors, social and leisure activities and health both contribute to explaining LS. Finally, physical illness has a negative influence on LS ($-.45$, $p < .000$), and perceived health has the lowest weight (.23, $p < .05$) ($\chi^2 = 52.6$; 46 gl; $p = .232$).

In sum, LS could be considered as a buffer variable of other QoL conditions. This model was replicated in two different contexts: in people living in the community and in people living in residences (Zamarrón & Fernández-Ballesteros, 2000; Fernández-Ballesteros, Zamarrón, & Ruiz, 2001).

Developing an Instrument for Assessing QoL: The CUBRECAVI

QoL is an important objective of most public policies, therefore, a standard measure for assessing comparisons within subjects or between subjects, or among programs or institutions, was an objective in our QoL research program. With this goal in mind, several psychometric studies have been conducted and reported elsewhere (Fernández-Ballesteros, Zamarrón, & Maciá, 1996; Fernández-Ballesteros & Zamarrón, 2007).

First of all, on the basis of our previous analysis, we considered nine QoL factors: health (subjective, objective, and mental), functional abilities, social integration, activity level and leisure, LS, environmental quality, health and social services, education, and income. From those domains, after performing several psychometric analyses (internal consistency, response set bias, and construct and criterion validity) the most sensitive items were selected.

In order to evaluate the reliability of these selected multi-item domains, internal consistency (through α coefficients) was calculated. With exception of social relationships Alpha coefficients were between moderate and high (from .70 to .92). The effect of impression management in our dependent variables was also examined through comparisons categorizing high and low impression management individuals. High impression management elders reported better subjective, objective, and mental health, higher income, better environmental quality (subjective), greater satisfaction with their home or residence, and greater LS. In summary, a source of bias of any self-report is impression management or faking, and it seems to be particularly important in old people (Fernández-Ballesteros & Zamarrón, 1996).

In order to examine the internal validity of our QoL domains, an exploratory factor analysis (principal components, oblimin rotation) was carried out, yielding seven factors that accounted for 71.26% of the total variance. The first factor was called social position (loaded by education and income, it accounts for 23% of variance), the second factor was health (loaded by all objective and subjective indicators of health and by LS, it accounts for 12.75% of the variance), the third factor was functional abilities (loaded by difficulties in performing daily life activities and level of dependency, and the frequency of health and social services utilization, it accounts for 9.6% of the variance), the fourth factor was called activity level (loaded by physical activity level, and frequency and satisfaction of performed activities, it accounts for 7.49% of the variance), the fifth factor was environment (loaded by environmental satisfaction, it accounts for 6.56% of variance), the sixth factor was called social relationships (loaded by frequency and satisfaction of social interaction, it accounts for 5.86% of variance), and the seventh factor was loaded by other items (accounting for 5.1% of variance). In summary, the factor structure closely reflects the selected QoL domains, with two exceptions: LS loaded on the health factor and social services loaded on the functional abilities factor.

In order to test criterion validity, several stepwise regression analyses were performed. At this point, we considered what might be the best criterion of QoL. Our criterion variables were two: subjective QoL constructed as a combined variable with the subjective appraisal of all elements of our protocol, called subjective QoL (S-QoL), and LS, formed by the total PGCMS score. Our first equation, taking S-QoL as criterion variable, contained the following dependent variables: chronic problems ($\beta = -.09$), pains ($\beta = -.12$), mental health complaints ($\beta = -.55$), functional disabilities ($\beta = -.084$), culture and leisure activities frequency ($\beta = .38$), physical activity ($\beta = .09$), and home repair ($-.06$). This equation explained 40% of the S-QoL variance. Our second equation, taking LS as criterion, contained the following dependent variables: satisfaction with home/apartment ($\beta = .39$), health satisfaction ($\beta = .31$), satisfaction with cultural and leisure activities ($\beta = .60$), and activities frequency ($\beta = .48$). This equation explained 43% of the LS variance. In sum, although the CUBRECAVI can predict satisfaction (both LS and satisfaction with QoL domains), this prediction does not manage, in any of the cases, to account for half of the total variance on LS. Therefore, our conclusion is that although LS is an important domain for QoL, it cannot be reduced to it (for a review, see Fernández-Ballesteros, Zamarrón, & Ruíz, 2001).

The CUBRECAVI contains 19 items organized in nine domains. It can be self-administered or applied by interview, requires primary educational level, and takes about 15–20 minutes. Scores in each domain have a range of 1–4, and there is no QoL total score, but a profile with all the QoL ingredients. Norms in percentiles for people living in the community and in residences for all QoL domains are also provided, giving the opportunity to make comparisons with a standard sample.

The CUBRECAVI has been applied in Spain and in other Latin-American countries for assessing the QoL of elders living both in institutions and in the community, as well as for the evaluation of programs or treatments. In Spain, a new sample of 234 (mean age = 80.45, range = 53–101; 150 women, 84 men) individuals living in residences was assessed by the CUBRECAVI. Internal structure was examined by means of exploratory factor analysis, producing a factorial structure that identified the main domains of CUBRECAVI: health, functional abilities, social relationships, activity, LS, and income.

In Latin America, the CUBRECAVI was found to be extremely useful for program evaluation, as reported by Fernández-Ballesteros and Zamarrón (2007). For example, in Colombia, significant differences were found in the expected direction in most CU-BRECAVI domains (with the exception of functional abilities) in two samples of over-60s ($N = 427$, selected at random) assigned to two programs for the elderly. In Venezuela, D'Alessandro and Peña Torbay (2004) found significant differences in six domains of CUBRECAVI (health, functional abilities, activity level, LS, social relationships, and environmental quality) in the expected direction in those people attending a program for promoting active aging ($N = 300$), compared to a control group ($N = 263$). Furthermore, in Uruguay, differences were found in five CUBRECAVI domains (health, functional abilities, LS, activity level, and social relationships) in over-70s doing volunteer work ($N = 100$), by comparison with a nonequivalent control group. All of these studies show that, with the exception of health and social services, education and income, the CUBRECAVI domains have a high level of generalizability across countries with the same language and a similar culture (Korotky, 2003).

Quality of Life in the Elderly in Specific Contexts

As already stated, QoL is context-based; up to now we have examined QoL in community and residence settings, but it has also become a key concept in comprehensive diagnosis of inpatients suffering from dementia (see Albert & Logsdon, 2000). On the assumption that the planning and implementation of intervention measures should not be based exclusively on an assessment of cognitive impairments, but should also consider individual aspirations and preferences in a given situation, the Heidelberg Instrument for the Assessment of Quality of Life in Dementia (HILDE) was developed as an option for more individualized care for patients in nursing homes. In a sample of 362 residents from 22 nursing homes, four patterns of competence could be identified and independently cross-validated (for details, see Becker, Kaspar, & Kruse, 2006). Each of these four different dementia-syndrome groups is characterized by specific needs and values. They can be used as points of reference within as well as between these competence groups, in order to plan individual interventions with competence-oriented expectations. The results of the HILDE study support the theoretical conception of Veenhooven (2000), which focuses particularly on the empirical relationships between the four dimensions suggested in the original Lawton model in terms of antecedent and outcome variables. In line with this theoretical position, QoL is again defined as a constellation of personal and environmental, material and nonmaterial resources, and subjective well-being. Recently, the Heidelberg research group began a further step of the project, aimed at enabling staff members in nursing homes to use the HILDE instrument independent of the supervision of researchers for assessing QoL and planning and evaluating individual intervention measures.

Positive Aging

Successful, healthy, optimal, active, productive aging, or simply positive aging or aging well, are concepts that emerged within the field of aging in the final decades of the

20th century, from three main observed facts supported by longitudinal, cross-sectional, experimental, and quasiexperimental studies: (1) the compression of morbidity; (2) the extreme variability of any bio-psycho-social condition in old age; (3) the plasticity of human beings, expressed through the modifiability of most declined or impaired conditions, and finally, (4) the assumption that aging involves not only decline, but also positive change and development.

These four main assumptions were set out by the pioneers of this approach, such as Fries and Crapo (1981) who in their seminal work "Vitality and Ageing" pointed to the "quadragulation" of the survival curve as the expression of the modifiability of most declining conditions associated with aging. In the same line, based on empirical data from the MacArthur Foundation Study of Successful Aging, Rowe and Khan (1998) provided both an empirical definition of and a set of strategies for promoting successful aging. Furthermore, Baltes and Baltes (1990) published "Successful Aging," which took a bio-psycho-social perspective and described the process of selective optimization and compensation (SOC) for aging with success (see Chapter 15); Heckhausen and Schultz (1993) proposed the theory of primary and secondary control; and finally, Carstensen (1993) introduced a developmental theory (the emotional selectivity theory) emphasizing the importance of emotions and the self-regulation process throughout the life span.

As stressed elsewhere, competence is a highly complex and not yet well-defined construct. Competence is considered as the person's ability to perform a broad range of activities (behavioral, cognitive, emotional, and social) considered essential for independent living (Dielh, 1998; Eisenberg & Fabes, 1992; Masterpasqua, 1989). Competence is a key concept for successful, active, productive, or optimal aging and, therefore, embraces a set of conditions such as health and physical fitness, good cognitive functioning, a high level of well-being and LS, and social participation and integration.

Recently, Depp and Jeste (2006) reported their review of major longitudinal studies on successful aging (most of them carried out in the U.S., Canada, and Australia, with only one from Europe), trying to identify the components in the empirical definitions of successful aging, as well as its predictors or determinants. From this list, 28 research articles fulfilled the inclusion criteria, and from these reports 29 definitions of successful aging contained 10 different domains present in a limited number of studies (in parentheses): disability/physical functioning (26), cognitive functioning (15), LS/well-being (9), social/productive engagement (8), presence of illness (6), longevity (4), self-rated health (3) personality (2), environment/finances (2), and self-rated successful aging (2). It is interesting to note that physical, cognitive, emotional, and social functioning are the four domains most often present in the studies reviewed.

Aging, Health, and Competence

In order to study mutual interactions between aging, health, and competence the multidisciplinary Cross-European Longitudinal Study on Ageing (EXCELSA) , under the auspices of the EU PF-5, was planned with the participation of seven European countries (Austria, Finland, Germany, Italy, Poland, Portugal, and Spain). The research plan can be found in Schroots, Fernández-Ballesteros, and Rudinger (1999a, b), Rudinger and Rietz (1999), and Fernández-Ballesteros, Hambleton, and Van de Vijver (1999), and a first report has already been published (Fernández-Ballesteros et al., 2003).

The research objectives were as follows: (1) to test the impact of age and other sociodemographic variables (education, gender, and rural-urban environment) on the selected variables, (2) to assess the internal structure of our research protocol in an effort to reach an empirical definition of competence, and (3) to explore the potential determinants of competence.

As a first step, after the review of all longitudinal studies on successful aging (for an updated review, see Depp & Jeste, 2006) the European Survey on Ageing Protocol (ESAP) was developed. The ESAP contains items, measures, or instruments for assessing the following variables: health (subjective health as well as health problems, chronic problems, number of aids, sleep problems, hearing, and vision), behavioral lifestyles (physical exercise, smoking, and alcohol consumption), mental abilities (working memory and learning), personality (neuroticism, extraversion, and openness, and sense of coherence) mastery and personal control (internal and external control), subjective competence (appraisal of fitness, strength, flexibility, endurance, and speed), anthropometric measures, biobehavioral measures (pulmonary function, speed, and strength), social relationships (family and friends, and care-giving) and sociodemographic variables. The ESAP was administered through a 90 min (approx.) standardized interview to 672 Europeans aged 30 to 85. They were selected through quota sampling (by age, gender, education, and rural-urban living conditions), with 96 participants from each of the seven countries.

After assessing the equivalence across countries for items, measures, and instruments, psychometric analyses for each instrument or scale were performed, including internal consistency, test-retest reliability, and internal validity. Finally, our cross-sectional data set was examined in an effort to answer our research questions. We shall now briefly describe the most important results.

Regarding age differences, significant differences for age were found in 84% of our measures when ANOVA comparisons were performed; intelligence (digit backwards and digit symbol) and physical measures (peak flow, tapping, and strength) were highly sensitive to age in all age-group comparisons (30–49, 50–64, 65–74, and 75–85). With regard to health, the oldest individuals reported greater numbers of chronic problems and more aids required, as well as perceiving poorer health, and reported more vision problems than the other three groups; there were significant differences between the two younger groups and the two older groups in hearing problems. Also, differences were found between the oldest group and the three younger groups in lifestyles: the older people were less physically active and smoked and drank less than the other three groups. Similar results were obtained in subjective competence: the oldest group perceived significantly less fitness, strength, flexibility, endurance, and speed than the younger groups. As regards anthropometric measures, the younger subjects were significantly taller than the other three groups, but only the middle age-group significantly differed in weight from the oldest group. With respect to personality, as expected, no differences were found in sense of coherence and neuroticism, but the youngest group were significantly more extraverted and more open to experience than the other three age groups. Regarding perceived control, the two younger groups perceived less external control than the two oldest groups, while the oldest group perceived less internal control than the other three age groups. Comparisons in social relationships yielded the following results: in comparison with younger participants, the oldest group had significantly fewer friends, fewer close relationships, less general intimacy and caregiving, and fewer social relationships. Nevertheless, family relationships were not affected by age. Finally, regarding well-being, no differences were found in any of the comparisons performed. In other words, as was found in our study on QoL, there were no differences in well-being resulting from age, gender, education, or living conditions.

Exploratory factor analysis (principal components, varimax rotation) yielded 10 factors (variance explained: 67.85%) corresponding to the following psychosocial conditions: subjective competence, personality, cognitive and physical competence, anthropometry, social relationships, sociodemographic, health, activity, and lifestyles. We also examined the concordance of this factorial structure for the seven countries. Most of the factors show high concordance coefficients in most of the countries (only one country showed low concordance coefficients for most of the factors).

From our exploratory factor analysis two competence factors emerge: subjective competence (loaded by all subjective appraisals referring to competence: fitness, strength, flexibility, endurance, and speed) and objective competence (loaded by intelligence measures of working memory and learning, and by biophysical measures, speed, and vital capacity). Objective (physical and cognitive) competence was selected as dependent variable and, in order to explore the role played by sociodemographic, psychosocial, health, and lifestyle conditions in cognitive and physical competence (after testing several submodels step-by-step), we arrived at the final structural model shown in Figure 3, which accounted for 87% of the variance explained with a reasonable fit of the model to the data.

Summarizing, four latent variables have a direct effect on objective competence (measured by digit symbol and digit span, peak-flow and tapping): age (years); SES (education and income); subjective capacity and health (subject's appraisal of his/her fitness, strength, flexibility, endurance, and speed, and subjective health); and lifestyles (physical activity, smoking, and alcohol consumption). Subjective capacity and health is a buffer that mediates the influence of social network (relationships with family and friends, and caregiving), and of internal control and illness (chronic health problems and sleep disturbances).

Our results were consistent with other cross-sectional and longitudinal studies on aging. The ESAP was highly sensitive to age, but most of the significant differences were found between the younger groups and the oldest group (75–85-year-olds). Also, our final model is in line with other theoretical assumptions in the field of positive aging and competence. Education and income can be considered as the best measures of SES, and are historical or distal determinants of successful aging, as well as of health throughout the life cycle (Adler & Snibbe, 2003). This important, almost nonmodifiable condition expresses the social inequality of successful aging, and the importance of its external socioeconomic determinants. Behavioral lifestyle is also an important factor influencing physical and cognitive competence, both directly, and indirectly through health and chronic problems. Family and friends relationships, and care-giving

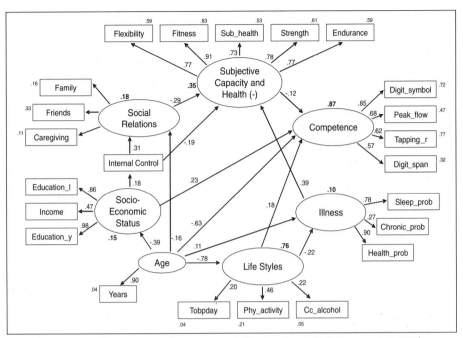

Figure 3. Confirmatory factor analysis of competence (adapted from Fernández-Ballesteros et al., 2003)

and internal control (which we consider an emotional regulation indicator) both influence competence indirectly through subjective capacity and health.

An important inconsistency with theories on positive aging is that well-being or LS are not posited in our model. As we have stressed, our well-being measures did not significantly differ in relation to groups for age, gender, educational background, or rural/urban conditions; therefore, well-being could not be present. In any case, it should be emphasized that the EXCELSA-Pilot is a preliminary study conducted in small samples from seven European countries, and we are waiting to continue our project under the auspices of the PF-7. Even so, four main domains emerged from this research: physical and cognitive fitness, health and behavioral lifestyles, internal control, and social functioning.

Promoting Positive Aging

Promoting healthy or positive aging constitutes the core of the II International Plan of Action on Ageing (UN, 2002). Nevertheless, as has been discussed, although there are preventive programs and European initiatives mainly devoted to increasing physical exercise or reducing risk factors (e.g., the EU program "Ageing Well"), there is no consensus on what would be considered a program for promoting positive aging. Let us briefly introduce our effort to develop a program for the effective promotion of aging well.

On the basis of the scientific literature on successful aging, on the Spanish course "Vivir con Vitalidad" (Fernández-Ballesteros, 2002b), and on the EXCELSA-Pilot, a project for promoting positive aging, the "Vital Ageing-Multimedia Course" was developed under the auspices of the EU. Vital Ageing (VA-M) is a multimedia course supported by the Socrates-Minerva Program ("Vitalgell-C") and produced by a consortium made up of Nettuno (Italy), the Autónoma University of Madrid (Spain), and the Gerontology Institute of the University of Heidelberg (Germany), and with the cooperation of the Open University (UK).

VA-M has a general objective "To promote well-being and quality of life in older Europeans" and the following specific objectives: "To transmit basic knowledge on how to age actively and competently"; "To promote healthy lifestyles"; "To provide strategies for compensating cognitive, memory and functional decline"; "To provide strategies for optimizing affective/emotional, motivational, and social competencies"; and "To promote personal development and social participation"[2].

VA-M ("Vivere con Vitalitá" in Italian or "Vivir con Vitalidad-M" in Spanish) is a video course with supporting materials on the Internet. The course has been taught by European experts from Germany, Italy, and Spain, respectively, in English, Italian, and Spanish, though so far it is generally available only in Spanish. VA-M is a multidimensional program and addresses four behavioral/psychological domains: promotion of healthy habits, cognitive fitness; affect, coping, and control, and social participation. These modules are developed through five units each, and each unit takes 2 to 4 h. There are also presentation and conclusion units. In total the multimedia course contains 50 video-lesson hours.

All units have a similar structure: (1) the trainer makes a general presentation, and talks about supporting evidence for a given topic; (2) a pretest of the particular behavioral or psychological characteristic (diet, physical exercise, self-efficacy, pleasant activities, etc.) is administered; (3) identified competences are trained and the trainer suggests practice and exercises; (4) a posttest is suggested; and (5) the trainer makes some concluding remarks. All recommended materials can be found on the Internet at www.uninettunoit/Vitalagell/frameset.htm.

Several internal and external evaluations of the VA-M course have been carried out. First of all, an external evaluation of the materials of the course was made by the Institute of Gerontology at the University of Heidelberg (Kruse, 2003). Second, formative evaluations were performed assessing intermediate outcomes of the program (lessons' achievements, students' opinions about lessons, etc.). Furthermore, summative evaluations were performed through pre-post quasiexperimental designs measuring objectives of the programs (exercise, nutrition, self-efficacy for aging, level of activity, subjective health, social network and social support, and well-being). Finally, comparisons between the VA-M program and the *in vivo* Vivir con Vitalidad course were conducted with similar designs. In total, 82 volunteers over age 55 (final age range = 59 to 79) living in the community and in residences received the course, and 31 other individuals, registered for other activities in the same settings, were used as controls. These evaluations were reported elsewhere (Fernández-Ballesteros, Caprara, & Garcia, 2004; Fernández-Ballesteros, 2005).

---

2 We also aim to promote knowledge and use of new technologies.

In summary, the evaluation of the VA-M attained most of its objectives: (1) after each lesson, the experimental participants had improved their knowledge in all the issues taught; (2) with the exception of those subjects living in residences, participants improved their lifestyles, increased their physical exercise, and improved their diet; (3) after the course, and in comparison to controls, participants increased their activity level, increased frequencies of cultural, intellectual, affective, and social activities; (4) they perceived an enhancement of their memory; (5) they significantly increased their self-competence for aging and their feeling of control; (6) in pre-post and experimental-control comparisons, participants significantly increased their LS and well-being; (7) contrary to our expectations, experimental subjects did not increase their social relationships (perhaps because they had a very high level of social relationships before the course), and finally, (8) in the follow-up (after 6 months) conducted only in the first evaluation study, all pre-post differences in the experimental group were maintained though, as predicted, positive changes were found in health for the community group.

In summary, although the Vital Ageing Program is in an experimental phase, it can be considered as a first step in the effort to promote positive aging. The program (both *in vivo* and the multimedia versions) continues to be administered (using quasiexperimental designs) in other settings in Spain and Mexico, and will shortly be adapted to Portuguese so that it can be administered in Portugal and Brazil. New evaluation research, as well as efficiency studies, will further assist the promotion of positive aging.

Epilog: The Elderly as Human Capital for Society

As has been stressed throughout this chapter, most of the concepts used here as equivalent to successful aging (active, adaptive, optimal, productive, competent, or positive aging) arise from Western culture, in which "success" is synonymous with fortunate, prosperous, victorious, capable, adequate, or qualified. In a recent study by Matsubayashi et al. (2006) on the views of the elderly on successful aging, conducted in Japan, the authors made comparisons between the views of Japanese (in several cities in Japan) and Americans (in two samples of Japanese Americans and white Americans). The same questionnaire was used in the two countries, and participants were asked to indicate among 20 attributes (present in the scientific literature) those that defined successful aging. While Japanese elderly people indicated just one in three of these attributes, both Japanese Americans and white Americans indicated two in three. More important, 75% of the attributes rated by American respondents (both Japanese and whites) as important were not rated as important by 75% of the Japanese respondents. In short, positive, productive, or successful aging is a cultural concept and different cultures have different understandings of positive aging.

Vaillant and Mukamal (2001) claimed that in order to avoid successful aging being seen as an oxymoron, the concept of aging should be taken not only to connote decline but also to involve change and development. In our view – without neglecting decline – the study of positive aging has the main purpose of identifying those aspects associated with aging that change positively, representing human development and, therefore, human capital. Thus, in this last section, we endorse a reconceptualization of one of the terms in this field: productive aging.

Productivity as a Multifaceted Concept

Productivity in our culture is commonly associated with the making of things (production) and material values, so that speaking of a productive life in old age generally refers to societal productivity, i.e., enrichment, promotion, maintenance, and relief of social systems; however the term productivity is neither restricted to participation in the labor market or voluntary activities nor confined to manual expression (Baltes & Montada, 1996). Rather, an adequate definition of productivity must also consider intellectual, emotional, and motivational expressions of productivity (Kruse, 2002a,b; Staudinger, 1996).

Using an extended definition of productivity, several possibilities for leading a productive life in old age can be distinguished: Being interested in the development, living conditions, and vital interests of younger people, the transmission of information to younger generations, and self-responsible reflection on the experiences and knowledge systems of younger generations are examples of intellectual and emotional productivity in old age, since intergenerational discourse can initiate emotional and intellectual differentiation in older and younger participants. Moreover, by leading an independent and responsible life, even when confronted with serious problems or borderline situations, older people can give a good example to younger people of how to cope with problems and difficulties.

A good example for a productive intergenerational dialog initiated from older people's coping processes can be found in a study by Kruse and Schmitt (1999, 2000) on identity and life review in Jewish emigrants and extermination camp survivors. In this study, one principal way of coping with stressful reminiscence – whereby stressful memories generally became more intense with older age – was based on an individual need to commit to others as well as to society as a whole. This form of coping reflected an intense preoccupation with the future time perspective of younger people, and a commitment to the development of the younger generation as well as to sociocultural and political issues, with the aim of engaging social as well as personal responsibility to the maintenance of democracy and the avoidance of fascism and antisemitism. The people involved in these coping processes took part in history or ethics lessons in schools as "contemporary witnesses of history" and, thus, contributed to a responsible handling of history.

Productivity in the Context of Occupational Activities

The traditional research on human intelligence refers to abilities and skills that are acquired through education in adolescence and early adulthood, whereas abilities and skills required in later years, e.g., for successful occupational development, are regularly neglected in operational definitions of this construct. Only since the mid-1980s has psychological research on the development of human intelligence begun to discover and conceptualize the acquisition of area-specific skills and practical intelligence (Kruse & Schmitt, 2001a, b). The latter can be defined as the ability to solve practical everyday problems and to cope effectively with everyday tasks. Practical intelligence subsumes area-specific skills as well as more general abilities, essential for effective coping with problems and tasks, e.g., overall perspective on a work field, competence in preparation and execution of decisions, or development and further improvement of effective strategies.

Various studies on working expertise in older workers show that continuous occupational activity may be associated with the development of specific skills and knowledge, which can be used to compensate for age-related losses, especially in the fluid component of intelligence. In fact, meta-analyses suggest that there are no significant differences in the performance of younger and older workers (see Kruse & Packebusch, 2006; Kruse & Schmitt, 2006a). Moreover, empirical data show that there is more variance in performance within than between age-groups, i.e., age-related losses are a poor predictor of job performance (Kruse & Schmitt, 2004). However, age-related decline in biological and physiological processes may have an impact on performance in specific professions, e.g., occupational activities that are associated with severe and unbalanced strain of the motor system, or with outside work in poor climatic conditions.

The principal findings of international studies on working performance and possible training gains in older workers can be summarized in the following nine points (see also Kruse & Packebusch, 2006; Kruse & Schmitt, 2006a):
1. Most studies find an inverted U-relationship between chronological age and working performance.
2. Admittedly, age differences in occupational performance are small. Training measures can compensate for age-related slowing.
3. Age-differences can be observed particularly in the less experienced. If any age-differences are found between experienced employees, they are only of a small magnitude.
4. However, in the most cognitively challenging professions experience cannot compensate for age-related deficits. Complex tasks that require extended information processing capacity regularly show some age-related deficits.
5. Previous knowledge can effectively compensate for losses in working memory.
6. The performance of older experts regularly reflects a successful compensation for age-related decline in some components through improvement in other components (knowledge, strategies). Exercise is an essential precondition for development and maintenance of expertise over the whole life span. For a supreme performance musicians need at least 10 years or 10,000 hours of practice.
7. Transfer of training gains depends on task-specific requirements. High specificity in content, personal relevance, and long-term time investment are general conditions of a successful training program.
8. The relationship between chronological age and performance follows different developmental paths; some kinds of performance even improve with age (see Warr, 1995).
9. High levels of performance can be maintained when occupational tasks are adapted to the employees' individual preferences and working rhythms. As a consequence, changes in job placement and job profiles are promising strategies for companies to ensure individual employability of their employees.

The principal points in relation to training in the context of occupational activities and from a life-long learning perspective can be summarized as follows: (1) It has been shown that expertise in the field of work is to be regarded as a potential age-related gain, which can be used to compensate for age-related losses: job performance of older people is not necessarily lower than job performance in younger people. Therefore, older people should have the opportunity to participate in occupational training programs to a greater extent. (2) Poor working conditions do have a greater impact on the job performance of older workers than on the job performance of younger workers. However, age-related losses in performance can be compensated through changes in job profiles, which take into account the specific job-related skills and experience of older people. The skills and experiences of older workers can be used effectively for increasing job performance in younger workers. (3) Learning is life-long; retraining and up-date learning should be opportunities provided in an aging society.

Research on the productivity of older workers in the context of occupational activities supports voluntary retirement as it is recommended in Priority Direction I of the II International Plan of Action on Ageing (United Nations, 2002, see Chapter 1).

Life Competencies of the Old as Human Capital for Society

By the term life competencies we refer to experiences, strategies, and knowledge systems that people have acquired in earlier phases of the life span (Kruse & Schmitt, 2001a,b, 2006b) and through the life-long learning process. Life competencies are built up in the context of effective coping, and enable people to maintain or reestablish a personally satisfying perspective on their life when confronted with serious problems, tasks, and challenges in later years. Building up life competencies in earlier years is a basic requirement for successful development in advanced age, i.e., effective coping with the demands of life in old age. Such demands include practical and psychological demands, as well as interpersonal and ethical ones. Consequently, our understanding of life competencies is not limited to physical and cognitive strategies and knowledge systems acquired in the context of educational and occupational activities. Life competencies are also reflected in ethical judgments, voluntary activities for other people, and the willingness and readiness to take responsibility for oneself, for others, or for society. In this context we should mention that empirical findings show how active coping with developmental tasks and the "ups-and-downs" and limits of life can lead to the establishment of "expert knowledge" or wisdom with respect to life issues (see Baltes & Kunzmann, 2004). Expert knowledge or wisdom is not limited to old age, but can also be developed in earlier years. The only prerequisite for the development of expert knowledge or wisdom is a conscious and responsible preoccupation with a multitude of problems, tasks, and challenges in different periods of life and different contexts of development. Thus, empirical findings support a perspective on life-long educational processes that accentuates the development of the person rather than the cultivation of specific knowledge and skills.

By the term human capital we refer to the significance of life competencies for society and culture, in relation to processes of initiating societal and cultural change and the extent to which societal and cultural change is determined by the life competencies of the elderly. Societal and cultural development depends on the possibility of using individual life competencies. It is necessary here to establish the respective infrastructural conditions: voluntary retirement, availability of life-long learning institutes, and opportunities for volunteers to qualify and to use their experiences, strategies, and knowledge systems effectively.

Ageism, Cognitive Representations of Aging, and Productivity

Robert Butler (1969, 1980) coined the term ageism to refer to a global phenomenon with three distinguishable but interrelated aspects: prejudicial attitudes toward the aged, toward old age, and toward the aging process; discriminatory practices against the elderly; and institutional practices and policies that, often without malice, perpetuate stereotypical beliefs. Butler's ageism hypothesis has stimulated much research because of its obvious political and societal implications: Given that empirical studies support the notion of older people being discriminated against in Western societies, there is an onus on the representatives of these societies to counteract and prevent the manifestation of such tendencies. Likewise, the central concept of the Madrid International Plan of Action on Ageing is *A Society for All Ages*, which was developed from the concept of *A Society for All* (Sidorenko & Walker, 2004).

The results of Kruse and Schmitt (2006b), in a stratified sample of 1275 participants (age range 45–70 years), show that the framework of ageism is too narrow for comprehensive research on the topic of cognitive representations of aging and productivity. Since individual judgments about old age and aging reflect (at least in some ways) independent and, therefore, irreducible dimensions, researchers must not remain satisfied with the search for negative stereotypes. From a closer look at the structure of cognitive representations of aging it follows that we need to know more about the preconditions of and reasons for pessimistic and optimistic beliefs, about the social contexts that contribute to an improved salience of these beliefs in situation-specific categorization processes and about how some images predict healthy aging and survival (see also Levy & Banaji, 2002; McHugh, 2003).

From the perspective of individual development, the realization of productive potential requires a continuous accumulation, elaboration, and integration of personal experiences; from the perspective of societal preconditions, the realization of productive potential requires accessibility to social roles that allow for the training, use, and extension of individual competences after retirement. The aforementioned results imply that the strengths and potentials of old age are still not perceived and used adequately in our society. More specifically, we found that a lack of financial resources and, particularly, perceived deficits in the possibility to use one's competences after early retirement or in cases of unemployment were associated with a one-sided accentuation of decreases and losses in old age. This finding has direct political implications: First, initiatives promoting productive or active aging (Walker, 2002a,b; Kruse, 2002a) should be supported wherever possible – older people's strengths and competences must become obvious to everyone. In this context, improving intergenerational relationships might be a good strategy (Staudinger, 2002). Moreover, older peoples' strengths and potential must become an integral part of political discussion; demographic changes not only endanger the financial basis of social security systems, but on the positive side imply important opportunities for society – increases in life expectancy must not be equated with more years in need of care, and older peoples' health status depends on a concern with lifelong prevention (Kruse, 2002b). However, it is of equal importance that old age is recognized not only as a topic but also as a policy target. Here, it is not enough to hold the right positions. Moreover, these positions must be held by the right people. In several European countries political parties still focus on the needs and preferences of younger voters. Political programs still ignore many older people's needs and interests for leading an active and productive life, and intergenerational relationships are still not recognized as processes of social exchange that imply benefits for both younger and older persons.

Concluding Remarks and Future Perspectives

QoL, well-being, and LS, and successful or positive aging are all major issues in European research supported by several European Commission Framework Programs.

QoL has been defined as a multidimensional and multilevel concept involving personal and environmental as well as subjective and objective approaches. Successful aging is also a multidimensional and multilevel concept empirically defined through biophysical and psycho-social components. There is some confusion between the two because they have common ingredients and multidisciplinary approaches. Nevertheless, while QoL inevitably considers environmental circumstances, positive aging is a person-oriented concept. Finally, subjective well-being and LS are psychological characteristics traditionally considered as individual constructs. More attention should be paid to distinguishing among all of these targets, as well as to harmonizing measures for scientific study in this field throughout Europe.

The implicit concept of QoL assessed in elderly Spaniards is close to the concept held within the scientific field in general, and is in accordance with the factorial structure arising from our independent data. Moreover, it coincides with the QoL concept as defined in other European countries. In sum, health, independence, wealth, and social relationships are the four essential constituents of QoL. Other aspects, such as being active, availability of health and social services, environmental quality, feeling satisfied with life, and opportunities for learning are also ingredients for QoL in old age. Our empirical QoL concept for the elderly (implicitly defined and explicitly considered) was sensitive both to personal variables (age and gender) and to contextual or external conditions.

Older Spaniards (compared to younger ones), men (compared to women), those living in the community (compared to those living in residences), and those from the upper and middle classes (compared to those from the lower classes) all reported higher levels in a range of QoL aspects.

In our attempt to arrive at an empirical concept of competence in the process of aging, based on the results of administering the ESAP (European Survey on Ageing Protocol) to people in seven European countries we defined objective competence through two physical and two cognitive measures (peak-flow and tapping; digit symbol and digit span). SES (education and income) and age are distal factors posited as explanatory factors, while subjective capacity, health, and lifestyles directly influence competence. Finally, social network, internal control, and illness have an indirect influence on objective competence through subjective capacity and health.

On the basis of this model, a European project for promoting positive aging, the "Vital Ageing" multimedia course, was developed by a consortium of four European countries and tested through quasiexperimental designs. Over-65s improved their diet, physical exercise, activity level, and perception of self-efficacy, and finally reported higher levels of LS. Follow-up is required in order to draw conclusions about the long-term efficacy of the project.

Finally, it has been emphasized that elders' strengths and potentialities must be reinforced and promoted, as well as being recognized as social resources. Although there are national, regional, and international plans of action on aging, political programs still ignore many qualities of older people, their needs and their interest in leading an active and productive life. This is a matter that must be urgently addressed, and psychologists should play an active role, disseminating research results on these issues and helping to fight against stereotypes and "reductionist" or negative views of old age.

References

Adler, N.E., & Snibbe, A.C. (2003). The role of psychosocial processes in explaining the gradient between SES and health. *Current Directions in Psychological Science, 12,* 119–123.

Albert, S.M., & Logsdon, R.G. (Eds.). (2000). *Assessing quality of life in Alzheimer's disease.* New York: Springer Publishing.

Baltes, M., & Montada, L. (Eds.). (1996). *Produktives Leben im Alter* [A productive life in old age]. Frankfurt, Germany: Campus.

Baltes, P.B., & Baltes, M.M. (1990). Successful aging: A psychological model. In P.B Baltes & M.M. Baltes (Eds.), *Successful aging. Perspectives from the behavioral sciences.* Cambridge, UK: Cambridge University Press.

Baltes, P.B., & Kunzmann, U. (2004). The two faces of wisdom: Wisdom as a general theory of knowledge and judgment about excellence in mind and virtue vs. wisdom as everyday realization in people and products. *Human Development, 47,* 290–299.

Becker, S., Kaspar, R., & Kruse, A. (2006). Die Bedeutung unterschiedlicher Referenzgruppen für die Beurteilung der Lebensqualität demenzkranker Menschen – Kompetenzgruppenbestimmung mit HILDE [The impact of different reference groups for the assessment of quality of life in people suffering from dementia – Determination of competence groups with HILDE]. *Zeitschrift für Gerontologie und Geriatrie, 39,* 350–357.

Butler, R.N. (1969). Age-ism: Another form of bigotry. *Gerontologist, 9,* 243–246.

Birren, J.E. (Ed.). (1996). *Encyclopedia of Gerontology.* San Diego, CA: Academic Press.

Butler, R.N. (1980). Ageism: A foreword. *Journal of Social Issues, 36,* 8–11.

Carstensen, L.L. (1993). Motivation for social contact and life span: A theory of socioemotional selectivity. In J. Jacobs (Ed.). *Nebraska Symposium on Motivation Developmental Perspectives on Motivation.* Lincoln, NE: University Nebraska Press.

D'Allessandro, M.J., & Peña Torbay, G. (2004). *Calidad de vida en la vejez. Descripción y modelo de ruta* [Quality of life in the elderly. Description and planning]. Master thesis, Simon Bolivar University, Caracas.

Depp, C.A., & Jeste, D.V. (2006). Definitions and predictors of successful aging: A comprehensive review of larger quantitative studies. *American Journal of Geriatric Psychiatry, 14,* 6–20.

Diehl, M. (1998). Everyday competence in later life: Current status and future directions. *The Gerontologist, 38,* 422–433.

Diener, E., & Lucas, R.E. (1999). Personality and subjective well-being. In D. Kahneman, E. Diener, & N. Schwarz (Eds.), *Well-being. The foundation of hedonic psychology* (pp. 213–229). New York: Russell Sage Foundation.

Eisenberg, N., & Fabes, R.A. (1992). Emotion, regulation, and the development of social competence. In M.C. Clark (Ed.), *Review of personality and social psychology, Vol. 14: Emotion and social behavior.* Newbury Park, CA: Sage.

Fernández-Ballesteros, R. (1993). The construct of "quality of life" among the elderly. In E. Beregi, I.A. Gergeli, & K. Rajzi (Eds.), *Recent advances in aging and science* (pp. 1627–1630). Milan, Italy: Moruzzi.

Fernández-Ballesteros, R. (1998a). Quality of life: Concept and assessment. In J.G. Adair, D. Bélanger, & K.L. Dion (Eds.), *Advances in psychological science* (pp. 387–428). East Sussex, UK: Psychology Press.

Fernández-Ballesteros, R. (1998b). Quality of life: The differential conditions. *Psychology in Spain, 2,* 57–66.

Fernández-Ballesteros, R. (2002a). Social support and quality of life among older people in Spain. *Journal of Social Issues, 58,* 645–661.

Fernández-Ballesteros, R. (2002b). *Vivir con vitalidad* [Living with vitality] (5 Vols.). Madrid, Spain: Pirámide.

Fernández-Ballesteros, R. (2002c). Light and dark in the psychology of human strengths: The example of psychogerontology. In K.G. Aspinwal & U.M. Staudinger (Eds.), *A psychology of human strength: Perspectives on an emerging field* (pp. 131–147). Washington, DC: APA Book.

Fernández-Ballesteros, R. (2005). Evaluation of "VITAL AGEING-M": A psychosocial program for promoting optimal aging. *European Psychologist, 10,* 136–145.

Fernández-Ballesteros, R., Caprara, M.G., & García, L.F. (2004). Vivir con Vitalidad-M: Un Programa Europeo Multimedia [Vital aging-M. A European Multimedia Program]. *Intervención Social, 13,* 63–84.

Fernández-Ballesteros, R., Hambleton, R.K., & Van de Vijver, F. (1999). Protocol adaptation procedures. In J.J.F. Schroots, R. Fernández-Ballesteros, & G. Rudinger (Eds.), *Ageing in Europe.* Amsterdam: IOS Press.

Fernández-Ballesteros, R., & Maciá, A. (1993). Calidad de vida en la vejez [Quality of life in the elderly]. *Intervención Social, 5,* 77–94.

Fernández-Ballesteros, R., & Zamarrón, M.D. (1996). New findings on social desirability and faking. *Psychological Reports, 78,* 1–3.

Fernández-Ballesteros, R., & Zamarrón, M.D. (2007). *Cuestionario Breve de Calidad de Vida (CUBRECAVI)* [Short Quality of Life Questionnaire]. Madrid, Spain: TEA Ediciones.

Fernández-Ballesteros, R., Zamarrón, M.D., & Maciá, A. (1996). *Calidad de vida en la vejez en distintos contextos* [Quality of life in the elderly in a different context]. Madrid, Spain: IMSERSO.

Fernández-Ballesteros, R., Zamarrón, M.D., Rudinger, G., Schroots, F.J., Heikkinen, E., Drusini, A. et al. (2003). Assessing competence: The European survey on aging protocol (ESAP). *Gerontology, 50,* 330–347.

Fernández-Ballesteros, R., Zamarrón, M.D., & Ruíz, M.A. (2001). The contribution of sociodemographic and psychosocial factors to life satisfaction. *Ageing and Society, 21,* 1–28.

Ferring, D., Balducci, C., Burholt, V., Wenger, C., Thissen, F., Weber, G. et al. (2004). Life satisfaction of older people in six European countries: Findings from the European study on adult well-being. *European Journal of Ageing, 1,* 15–25.

Fries, J.F., & Crapo, L.M. (1981). *Vitality and aging.* San Francisco, CA: Freeman and Company.

Heckhausen, H., & Schultz, B. (1993). A psychological theory of control. *Psychological Review, 102,* 284–304.

Higgins, E.T., Grant, H., & Shah, J. (1999). Self-regulation and quality of life: Emotional and nonemotional life experiences. In D. Kahneman, E. Diener, & N. Schwarz (Eds.), *Well-being. The foundation of hedonic psychology* (pp. 244–266). New York: Russell Sage Foundation.

Iwarsson, S., Whal, H.-W., & Nygren, C. (2004). Challenges of cross-national housing research with older persons: Lessons from ENABLE-AGE Project. *European Journal of Ageing, 1,* 79–88.

Lawton, M.P. (1975). The Philadelphia Geriatric Center Morale Scale (PGCMS). *Journal of Gerontology, 30,* 85–89.

Lawton, M.P. (1983). Environment and other determinants of well-being in older people. *Gerontologist, 23:*349–357.

Lawton, M.P. (2001). Quality of life at the end of life. In R.H. Binstock & L-K. George (Eds.), *Handbook of aging and the social sciences.* San Diego, CA: Academic Press.

Kahneman, D., Diener,E., & Schwarz, N. (Eds.). (1999). *Well-being. The foundation of hedonic psychology.* New York: Russell Sage Foundation.

Korotky, S. (2003). *Los adultos mayores voluntarios en Uruguay: descripción y perfiles* [Older volunteers in Uruguay: Descriptions and profiles]. Master thesis, Universidad Autónoma de Madrid.

Kruse, A. (2002a). A lifespan perspective on prevention. In S. Pohlmann (Ed.), *Facing an aging world – Recommendations and perspectives* (pp. 69–76). Regensburg, Germany: Transfer Verlag.

Kruse, A. (2002b). Productivity and modes of human activity. In S. Pohlmann (Ed.), *Facing an aging world – recommendations and perspectives* (pp. 107–112). Regensburg, Germany: Transfer Verlag.

Kruse, A. (2003). *Vital-Agell-Course. Evaluation of didactic materials.* Report, Heidelberg: Institute of Gerontology, University of Heidelberg.

Kruse, A., & Packebusch, R. (2006). Alter(n)sgerechte Arbeitsgestaltung [Age-based work structuring]. In B. Zimolong & U. Konradt (Eds.), *Enzyklopädie der Psychologie – Ingenieurpsychologie* [Encyclopediy of psychology – Engineering psychology] (pp. 425–458). Göttingen, Germany: Hogrefe.

Kruse, A., & Schmitt, E. (1999). Reminiscence of traumatic experiences in (former) Jewish emigrants and extermination camp survivors. In A. Maercker, M. Schützwohl, & Z. Solomon (Eds.), *Post-traumatic stress disorder. A lifespan developmental perspective* (pp. 155–176). Seattle, WA: Hogrefe & Huber Publishers.

Kruse, A., & Schmitt, E. (2000). *Wir haben uns als Deutsche gefühlt. Lebensrückblick und Lebenssituation jüdischer Emigranten und Lagerhäftlinge* [We felt like Germans. A review of the life and situation of Jewish emigrants an concentration camp detainees]. Darmstadt, Germany: Steinkopff.

Kruse, A., & Schmitt, E. (2001a). Psychology of education in old age. In N.J. Smelser & P.B. Baltes (Eds.), *International encyclopedia of the social and behavioral sciences* (pp. 4223–4227). Oxford, UK: Pergamon.

Kruse, A., & Schmitt, E. (2001b). Adult education and training: Cognitive aspects. In N.J. Smelser & P.B. Baltes (Eds.), *International encyclopedia of the social and behavioral sciences* (pp. 139–142). Oxford, UK: Pergamon.

Kruse, A., & Schmitt, E. (2004). Differenzielle Psychologie des Alterns [Differential psychology of aging]. In K. Pawlik (Ed.), *Enzyklopädie der Psychologie – Angewandte Differenzielle Psychologie* [Encyclopedia of psychology – Applied differential psychology] (pp. 533–571). Göttingen, Germany: Hogrefe.

Kruse, A., & Schmitt, E. (2006a). Adult education. In J.E. Birren (Ed.), *Encyclopedia of gerontology* (2nd ed.). Oxford, UK: Elsevier.

Kruse, A., & Schmitt, E. (2006b). A multidimensional scale for the measurement of agreement with age stereotypes and the salience of age in social interaction. *Ageing and Society, 26,* 393–411.

Levy, B.R., & Banaji, M.R. (2002). Implicit ageism. In T. Nelson (Ed.), *Ageism: Stereotypes and prejudice against older persons* (pp. 49–75). Cambridge, MA: MIT Press.

Albert, S.M., & Logsdon, R.G. (2000). *Assessing quality of life in Alzheimer's disease.* New York: Springer Pub. Co.

Masterpasqua, F. (1989). A competence paradigm for psychological practice. *American Psychologist, 44,* 1366–1371.

Matsubayashi, K., Masayuki, I., Wada, T., & Okumiya, K. (2006). Older adults' views of "successful aging": Comparison of older Japanese and Americans. *Journal of the American Geriatrics Society, 54,* 184–187.

McHugh, K.E. (2003). Three faces of ageism: Society, image, and place. *Ageing and Society, 23,* 165–185.

Rowe, J.W., & Khan, R.L. (1998). *Successful aging.* New York: Random House.

Rudinger, G., & Rietz, C. (1999a). Methodological issues in a cross-European study. In J.J.F. Schroots, R. Fernández-Ballesteros, & G. Rudinger (Eds.), *Ageing in Europe.* Amsterdam: IOS Press.

Schroots, J.J.F., Fernández-Ballesteros, R., & Rudinger, G. (Eds.). (1999a). *Ageing in Europe.* Amsterdam: IOS Press.

Schroots, J.J.F., Fernández-Ballesteros, R., & Rudinger, G. (1999b). From Eugeron to EXCEL-SA. In J.J.F. Schroots, R. Fernández-Ballesteros, & G. Rudinger (Eds.), *Ageing in Europe* (pp. 143–156). Amsterdam: IOS Press.

Sidorenko, A., & Walker, A. (2004). The Madrid International Plan of Action on Ageing: From conception to implementation. *Ageing and Society, 24,* 147–166.

Staudinger, U. (1996). Psychologische Produktivität und Selbstentfaltung im Alter [Psychologiacal productivity and self-development in old age]. In M.M. Baltes & L. Montada (Eds.), *Produktives Leben im Alter* [Living productively in old age] (pp. 344–373). Frankfurt, Germany: Campus.

Staudinger, U. (2002). Intergenerational relations. In S. Pohlmann (Ed.), *Facing an aging world – Recommendations and perspectives* (pp. 47–52). Regensburg, Germany: Transfer Verlag.

Sternberg, R.J. (1990). *Metaphors of mind.* New York: Cambridge University Press.

Steverink, N., Lindenberg, S., & Slaets, J.P.J. (2005). How to understand and improve older people's self-management of well-being. *European Journal of Ageing, 2,* 235–245.

Tesch-Römer, C. von Kindratowitz, H.J., & Motel-Klingebiel, A. (2001). Quality of life in the context of intergenerational solidarity. In S.O. Daatland & K. Herlofson (Eds.), *Ageing, intergenerational relations, care systems, and quality of life* (pp. 63–73). Oslo, Norway: Nova.

United Nations. (2002). *II Madrid international plan of action on ageing (MIPAA).* New York: Author.

Vaillant, G.E., & Mukamal, K. (2001). Successful aging. *American Journal of Psychiatry, 158,* 839–847.

Venhooven, R. (2000). The four qualities of life. Ordering concepts and measures of the good life. *Journal of Happiness Studies, 1*, 1–39.

Wahrendorf, M., von Knesebeck, O., & Siegrist, J. (2006). Social productivity and well-being of older people: Base line results from SHARE. *European Journal of Ageing, 3:* 67–73.

Walker, A. (2002a). The principals and potential of active aging. In S. Pohlmann (Ed.), *Facing an aging world – Recommendations and perspectives* (pp. 113–118). Regensburg, Germany: Transfer Verlag.

Walker, A. (2002b). The politics of intergenerational relations. *Zeitschrift für Gerontologie und Geriatrie, 35,* 297–303.

Walker, A. (Ed.). (2005a). *Growing older in Europe.* London: Open University Press.

Walker, A. (2005b). A European perspective on quality of life in old age. *European Journal of Ageing, 2,* 2–12.

Warr, P. (1995). Age and job performance. In J. Snel & R. Cremer (Eds.), *Work and aging: A European perspective* (pp. 309–322). London: Taylor & Francis.

WHO. (2002). *Active aging.* Geneva: WHO.

Zamarrón, M.D., & Fernández-Ballesteros, R. (2000). Satisfacción con la vida en personas mayores que viven en sus domicilios y en residencias. Factores determinantes [Life satisfaction in older persons living at home or in residences]. *Revista Española de Geriatría y Gerontología, 35,* 17–29.

13. Wisdom

Adult Development and Emotional-Motivational Dynamics

Ute Kunzmann

Many aging researchers value the investigation of individual characteristics and processes that have the potential for growth during adulthood and old age (e.g., Baltes, Lindenberger, & Staudinger, 2006; Carstensen & Turk-Charles, 1998; Freund & Baltes, 1998; Kunzmann & Grühn, 2005). In this chapter, I consider a human strength that has been thought to be an ideal endpoint of human development, namely, wisdom (e.g., Baltes & Smith, 1990; Erikson, 1959; Staudinger, 1999). At the core of this concept is the notion of a perfect, perhaps utopian, integration of knowledge and character, mind and virtue (e.g., Baltes & Kunzmann, 2003; Baltes & Staudinger, 2000).

Although the psychology of wisdom is a relatively new field, several promising theoretical and operational definitions of wisdom have been developed during the last years (for reviews see Baltes & Staudinger, 2000; Kramer, 2000; Kunzmann & Baltes, 2005; Sternberg, 1998). In these definitions, wisdom is thought to be different from other human strengths in that it facilitates an integrative and holistic approach toward life's challenges and problems – an approach that embraces past, present, and future dimensions of phenomena, values different points of views, considers contextual variations, and acknowledges the uncertainties inherent in any sense-making of the past, present, and future.

A second important feature of wisdom is that it involves an awareness that individual and collective well-being are tied together so that one cannot exist without the other. In this sense, wisdom has been said to refer to time-tested knowledge that guides our behavior in ways that simultaneously optimize productivity on the level of individuals, groups, and even society (e.g., Kramer, 2000; Sternberg, 1998).

Finally, wisdom has been linked to the ancient idea of a good life suggesting that its acquisition during ontogenesis may be incompatible with a hedonic life orientation and a predominantly pleasurable, passive, and sheltered life. Given their interest in maximizing a common good, for example, wiser people are likely to partake in behaviors that contribute, rather than consume, resources (Kunzmann & Baltes, 2003a,b; Sternberg, 1998). Also, an interest in understanding the significance and deeper meaning of phenomena, including the blending of developmental gains and losses, most likely is linked to emotional complexity (Labouvie-Vief, 1990) and to what has been called "constructivistic" melancholy (Baltes, 1997a).

In this chapter, I shall first give an overview of psychological approaches to the definition and assessment of wisdom. In this overview, I will focus on one particular approach, the Berlin wisdom paradigm, which has instigated the most systematic research program on wisdom to date. In the second part of the chapter, I will discuss theoretical and empirical work on the development of wisdom-related knowledge during ontogenesis and on the affective structure and the motivational orientation that go hand in hand with wisdom as it is defined and operationalized in the Berlin wisdom paradigm.

Ways of Conceptualizing Wisdom in Psychological Research

While there appears to be considerable agreement on several important ideas about the definition, development, and functions of wisdom, all existing psychological wisdom models encompass their unique features. On an abstract level of description, there are two ways of studying wisdom in psychological research (see also Baltes & Kunzmann, 2004). A first is to focus on the nature of wise persons, that is, their intellectual, motivational, and emotional characteristics. This work is grounded in research on social and personality psychology (e.g., Ardelt, 2004; Erikson, 1959; Wink & Helson, 1997). A second approach has been to define wisdom as a body of highly developed knowledge a priori and on the basis of relevant cultural and psychological work (e.g., Baltes & Smith, 1990; Baltes & Staudinger, 2000; Baltes, 2004). This second approach proceeds from the idea that a comprehensive definition of wisdom requires going beyond the knowledge and behavior of an individual considered to be wise – simply because wisdom is a conceptual ideal, rather than a state of behavioral expression.

Personality-Based Approaches to Wisdom

In this tradition, wisdom has been conceptualized as a mature part of the individual's personality (e.g., Erikson, 1959). One promising example for this approach is work conducted by Ravenna Helson and her colleagues (Helson & Srivastava, 2002; Wink & Helson, 1997). Consistent with Achenbaum and Orwoll (1991), the authors have distinguished two components of the wise personality, namely, practical and transcendent wisdom. According to Helson, practical and transcendent wisdom both reflect interpersonal development (empathy, understanding, maturity in relationships). In addition, practical but not transcendent wisdom is thought to reflect intrapersonal development (mature affective responses, self knowledge, integrity), whereas transcendent but not practical wisdom reflects interest and skill in the transpersonal domain (self-transcendence, recognition of the limits of knowledge, philosophical/spiritual commitments).

To assess practical wisdom, the authors created an eighteen-item scale consisting of adjectives from the Adjective Check List (ACL; Gough & Heilbrun, 1983). The adjectives were chosen by judges to be indicative (i.e., clear thinking, fair-minded, insightful, intelligent, interest wide, mature, realistic, reasonable, reflective, thoughtful, tolerant, understanding, wise) and contra indicative (i.e., immature, intolerant, reckless, shallow) of a wise person. This scale has been employed as a self-report and an observer-report measure. Transcendent wisdom has been assessed with an open-ended question, namely, "Would you give an example of wisdom you have acquired and how you came by it?" Four judges rate self-descriptive statements in response to this question on a 5-point scale. A statement receives a high score if it is abstract, insightful, and reflects philosophical or spiritual depth, an integration of thought and affect, as well as an awareness of the complexity and limits of knowledge. Both measures of wisdom, practical and transcendence, have been shown to demonstrate satisfactory psychometric characteristics (Wink & Helson, 1997; Helson & Srivastava, 2002).

Another approach to defining the wise personality has been proposed by Ardelt (2003, 2004). Proceeding from work conducted by Clayton and Birren (1980), Ardelt has defined wisdom as an integration of reflective, cognitive, and affective characteristics. Ardelt views the reflective dimension as a prerequisite for the acquisition of the cognitive and emotional elements. Reflection primarily refers to a person's willingness and ability to overcome subjectivity and projections by looking at phenomena and events from different perspectives. The cognitive element is defined as a person's ability to understand life, that is, to comprehend the significance and deeper meaning of phenomena. The affective dimension of wisdom is reflected in the presence of positive emotions toward others (e.g., sympathy, compassion) and the absence of indifferent or negative emotions. To assess the three dimensions of her wisdom model in a sample of older adults, Ardelt (2003) developed a self-report questionnaire on the basis of existing personality inventories. She has provided initial evidence that her questionnaire demonstrates satisfactory psychometric characteristics, at least in a sample of older adults.

Taken together, research in the tradition of personality research has made valuable contributions to our understanding of the wise personality. As the two examples reviewed above indicate, however, different approaches in this tradition have focused on different components of the wise personality making it difficult to make firm conclusions about the exact nature and structure of the wise personality. Furthermore, given the lack of a generally accepted theoretical model of the development and functions of the wise personality, it remains unclear whether certain personality traits (e.g., affect sensitivity) represent an antecedent, constituent, or consequence of the wise personality. Clarifying the structure and content of the wise personality based on rigorous and systematic questionnaire development and multitrait-multimethod factor-analytic work is an important direction for future research in this area (for further details see Kunzmann & Stange, 2006).

Wisdom as a Highly Developed Body of Knowledge

In this tradition, wisdom has been conceptualized in the context of psychometric models of intelligence (e.g., Baltes & Smith, 1990; Baltes & Staudinger, 2000; Sternberg, 1998). Robert Sternberg's wisdom model represents one example. Proceeding from his triarchic theory of intelligence, Sternberg (1998) considers tacit knowledge, a component of practical intelligence, as a core feature of wisdom. According to Sternberg

(1998), tacit knowledge is action oriented, it helps individuals to achieve goals they personally value, and it can be acquired only through learning from one's own experiences, not "vicariously" through reading books or through others' instructions. Sternberg (1998) states that wisdom is not tacit knowledge per se, but rather wisdom is involved when people apply their tacit knowledge in order to maximize a balance of various self-interests (intrapersonal) with other people's interests (interpersonal) and aspects of the context in which they live (extrapersonal). Therefore, what sets wisdom apart from practical intelligence is its orientation toward the maximization of a common good, rather than individual well-being. Sternberg and his colleagues are currently developing open-ended tasks and coding schemes to operationalize their theoretical definition of wisdom. The tasks are complex conflict-resolution problems involving the formation of judgments, given multiple competing interests and no clear resolution of how these interests could be reconciled. Wisdom, assessed by these tasks, refers to a person's ability to identify whose interests are at stake and what the contextual factors are under which one is operating (Sternberg, 1998). A task designed for middle-school students illustrates the tasks used in Sternberg's research lab: "Mary is fighting with her parents over a sleep-over she wants to got to at her friend Lisa's house. Her parents have told her that they are worried about the lack of supervision at the sleep-over and are worried about whether the children's behavior will get out of hand. Mary has had a number of problems with her classmates in the past and sees this sleep-over as an opportunity to strengthen friendships she has made or would like to make. What should Mary do?" (Sternberg, 2001, p. 241). Answers to tasks such as this one will be rated by trained raters according to several dimensions, including demonstration of attempt to reach a common good, balancing on intrapersonal, interpersonal, and extrapersonal interests, and taking into account short- and long-term factors. It will be interesting to see how this measure relates to personality-based wisdom questionnaires and the performance-based wisdom test developed in the context of the Berlin wisdom paradigm which I will discuss next.

The Berlin Wisdom Paradigm

The Berlin wisdom model, which has been proposed by Paul Baltes and his colleagues, is another example of work that conceptualized wisdom as a highly valued form of pragmatic intelligence (e.g., Dixon & Baltes, 1986; Baltes & Smith, 1990; Dittmann-Kohli & Baltes, 1990; Baltes & Staudinger, 2000; Baltes & Kunzmann, 2003). This model has been developed during the last two decades and resulted in the most systematic research program on wisdom to date.

Theoretical Definition and Assessment of Wisdom

Integrating work on the aging mind and personality, life-span developmental theory, and cultural-historical work on wisdom, in the Berlin paradigm, wisdom has been defined as highly valued and outstanding expert knowledge about dealing with fundamental, that is existential, problems related to the meaning and conduct of life (e.g., Baltes & Kunzmann, 2003; Baltes & Smith, 1990; Baltes & Staudinger, 2000). These problems are typically complex and poorly defined, and have multiple, yet unknown, solutions. Deciding on a particular career path, accepting the death of a loved one, dealing with personal mortality, or solving long-lasting conflicts among family members exemplify the type of problem that calls for wisdom-related expertise. In contrast, more circumscribed everyday problems can be effectively handled by using more limited abilities. To solve a math problem, for example, wisdom-related expertise usually is not particularly helpful.

Five criteria were developed to describe this body of knowledge in more detail. Expert knowledge about the meaning and conduct of life is thought to approach wisdom if it meets *all* five criteria. Two criteria are labeled basic because they are characteristic of all types of expertise; these are: (1) rich factual knowledge about human nature and the life course; and (2) rich procedural knowledge about ways of dealing with life problems. The three other criteria are labeled meta-criteria because they are thought to be unique to wisdom and, in addition, carry the notion of being universal: (3) lifespan contextualism, that is, an awareness and understanding of the many contexts of life, how they relate to each other and change over the lifespan; (4) value relativism and tolerance, that is, an acknowledgment of individual, social, and cultural differences in values and life priorities; and (5) knowledge about handling uncertainty, including the limits of one's own knowledge.

To test for wisdom, participants are instructed to think aloud about hypothetical life problems. One might be: "Imagine that someone gets a call from a good friend who says that he or she cannot go on anymore and wants to commit suicide." Another problem reads: "A 15-year-old girl wants to get married right away. What could one consider and do?" Trained raters evaluate responses to those problems by using the five criteria that were specified as defining wisdom-related knowledge. The assessment of wisdom-related knowledge on the basis of these criteria exhibits satisfactory reliability and validity. For example, middle-aged and older public figures from Berlin nominated as life experienced or wise by a panel of journalists – independently of the Berlin definition of wisdom – were among the top performers in laboratory wisdom tasks and outperformed same-aged adults that were not nominated (Baltes, Staudinger, Maerker, & Smith, 1995).

The Development of Wisdom Across the Life-Span: A Theoretical Model

Conceptualizing wisdom as expert knowledge and linking it to lifespan psychology (Baltes, 1987, 1997b; Baltes, Lindenberger, & Staudinger, 2006) suggest a number of conditions under which wisdom is likely to develop. First, as is typical for the development of any expertise, wisdom is thought to be acquired through an extended and intensive process of learning and practice. This process clearly requires a high degree of motivation to strive for excellence as well as supportive environmental conditions. Second, because wisdom is different from other more circumscribed positive characteristics in that it involves an integration of intellect and character, its development and refinement require multiple factors and processes, including certain intellectual abilities, the availability of mentors, mastery of critical life experiences, openness to new experiences, and values referring to personal growth, benevolence, and tolerance. Third, there are most likely several paths leading to wisdom, rather than only one. Put differently, similar levels of wisdom may result from different combinations of facilitative factors and processes. Factors such as a certain family background, critical life events, professional practice, or societal transitions, such as the still increasing trend toward globalization, technological progress, or the demographical changes in western industrial nations may interact in complex additive, compensatory, or time-lagged ways.

These general theoretical perspectives are summarized in the theoretical model of wisdom depicted in **Figure 1**. This model states that three types of factors are influential for the development of wisdom-related knowledge, namely, *facilitative contexts*, as determined for example by a person's gender, social context, or culture; *expertise-specific factors* such as life experience, professional practice, or receiving and providing mentorship; and finally, *person-related factors* such as certain intellectual capacities, personality traits, or emotional dispositions. These three types of factors are thought to have an influence on the development of wisdom-related knowledge because they determine people's lifestyle, that is, the ways in which they plan, manage, and make sense out of their lives. All relations among the three components of our model – facilitative factors, lifestyle, and wisdom-related knowledge – are meant to be bidirectional. As described in the following sections of this chapter, past theoretical research in the context of the Berlin wisdom paradigm has focused on the antecedents of the development of wisdom-related knowledge, whereas more recent research has begun to address the consequences of wisdom-related knowledge for people's lifestyle and living conditions.

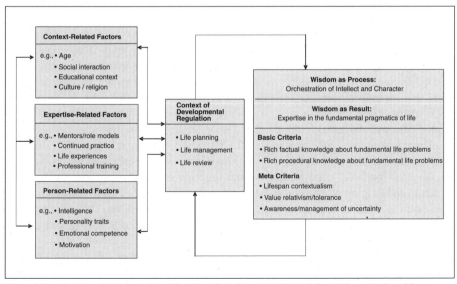

Figure 1 The structure, development, and function of wisdom-related knowledge: A theoretical model

The Berlin Wisdom Model: Past Empirical Evidence

The Berlin research program on wisdom has addressed a broad range of questions concerning the development of wisdom, including individual and social factors that facilitate or hinder its acquisition and refinement (e.g., professional specialization, life experience, academic intelligence, or personality profile). The program also includes laboratory experiments studying ways of activating and improving adults' wisdom-related performance in a given situation. As described in more detail elsewhere (e.g., Baltes & Staudinger, 2000; Kunzmann & Baltes, 2005), the major findings are the following.

First, and consistent with the idea that wisdom is an ideal, rather than a state of being, high levels of wisdom-related knowledge are rare. Many adults are on the way to wisdom, but very few people approach a high level of wisdom-related knowledge as measured by the Berlin wisdom tasks.

Second, wisdom-related knowledge seems to begin develop during the age period of late adolescence to young adulthood. Investigating a sample of 14- to 20-year-olds, Pasupathi, Staudinger, and Baltes (2001) reported that wisdom-related knowledge considerably increased in this life period. Studying older adults, however, did not evince marked further changes for the average case. Specifically, in four studies with a total sample size of 533 individuals ranging in age from 20 to 89 years, the relationship between wisdom-related knowledge and chronological age was virtually zero and nonsignificant (Smith & Baltes, 1990; Staudinger, 1999). Within the limitations of cross-sectional data, this evidence suggests that, on a group-level of analysis, wisdom-related knowledge remains stable over the adult years into the 60s and 70s. Although age-comparative studies on wisdom have been limited to what has been called the third age (i.e., young old adults), the evidence suggests that, given the absence of pathology such as dementia, some older adults will continue to perform well on wisdom tasks beyond their 70s.

Third, for wisdom-related knowledge and judgment to develop during the second half of life, other factors than age become critical. Consistent with the theoretical model depicted in **Figure 1**, the evidence suggests that it takes a complex coalition of expertise-enhancing factors from different domains, ranging from a person's social-cognitive style (e.g., social intelligence, openness to experience) over this person's immediate social context (e.g., presence of role models) to societal and cultural conditions (e.g., exposure to societal transitions). Past prediction studies of wisdom suggest that neither academic intelligence nor basic personality traits play a major role in the development of wisdom-related knowledge during adulthood. General life experiences, professional training and practice, certain motivational preferences such as an interest in understanding and helping others, and social-emotional competencies such as empathic concern seem to be more important (e.g., Staudinger, Smith, & Baltes, 1992; Smith, Staudinger, & Baltes, 1994; Staudinger, Lopez, & Baltes, 1997). If such a coalition of facilitating factors is present, some individuals may continue a developmental trajectory toward higher levels wisdom-related knowledge. Therefore, simply getting older is not a sufficient condition for the development of higher levels of wisdom-related knowledge, and yet, older adults are among the top performers in wisdom-related tasks.

Fourth, the expression of wisdom-related performance, as measured by the Berlin tasks, can be enhanced by relative simple social and cognitive interventions. Boehmig-Krumhaar, Staudinger, and Baltes (2002) demonstrated how a memory strategy, namely, a version of the method of loci, in which participants were instructed to travel on a cloud around the world can be used to focus people's attention on cultural relativism and tolerance. Staudinger and Baltes (1996) conducted an experiment in which participants were asked to think aloud about a wisdom problem under several experimental conditions involving imagined and actual social interactions. For example, before responding individually, some participants had the opportunity to discuss the problem with a person they brought into the laboratory and with whom they usually discuss difficult life problems. This and similar experimental conditions increased performance levels by almost one standard deviation. One important implication of these two studies is that many adults have the latent potential to perform better on wisdom tasks than they actually often do.

The Emotional-Motivational Dynamics of Wisdom

The definition of wisdom as an expert knowledge system about the meaning and conduct of life may suggest to some that the Berlin approach to studying wisdom is purely cognitive and ignores emotional and motivational factors that are also central elements of wisdom. Especially recent theoretical and empirical work in the context of the Berlin wisdom model, however, has discussed emotional and motivational dispositions as antecedent factors in the development of wisdom-related knowledge during ontogenesis and as factors that moderate the expression of wisdom-related knowledge in a given situation (e.g., Baltes & Staudinger, 2000; Kunzmann, 2004; Kunzmann & Baltes, 2003a, 2003b, 2005). In the remainder of this chapter, I will review this work.

Emotional Dynamics of Wisdom

From a developmental point of view, certain emotional experiences and dispositions can be considered as fundamental to the acquisition of wisdom as an expert knowledge system about the meaning and conduct of life. As described above, stimulating social environments, the availability of good educational systems, or a supporting family potentially contribute to the development of wisdom-related knowledge. All else begin equal, however, the effectiveness of these environmental factors depends on a person's affective dispositions and experiences such as his or her level of emotional balance, impulsivity, neuroticism, or sympathy for others.

It is also likely that the expression of wisdom-related knowledge in a particular situation is moderated by certain emotional dispositions and competencies. An advice-giver who is not able or willing to empathize with a needy person, for example, may be less likely to make an effort and engage in wisdom-related thinking which would involve careful and detailed analysis of the advice seeker's problem, the weighting and moderation of different parts of the situation, and the consideration of multiple views. Similarly, during a mutual conflict with another person, being able to imagine how this person feels or how one would feel in the other's place may be one stepping-stone to value tolerance and a cooperative approach typical of wisdom.

At the same time, however, one can easily think of emotional reactions to difficult and potentially stressful situations that are likely to hinder a wisdom-like approach. Examples are self-centered feelings that indicate personal distress, especially if these negative feelings are intense and long lasting. Two examples: If people are not able or willing to control their feelings of anger, contempt, or jealousy, they are likely to hurt or enrage others rather than come up with a wise solution to the problem at hand. Strong and chronic feelings of anxiety might inhibit wisdom-related thinking, which requires distance to the immediate situation, balance, and elaboration. It is in this sense that "cold" cognition and "hot" emotion have been described as two forces that antagonize one another (cf. Keltner & Gross, 1999).

Certainly, the links between other-oriented feelings such as empathy or sympathy and self-centered feelings such as personal distress and anger on the one hand and wisdom-related knowledge on the other can take any direction. The idea that certain emotions hinder or facilitate the activation of wisdom-related knowledge and behavior may be less popular in the literature than the notion that it is wisdom that regulates a person's emotional experiences and reactions. In this vein, wisdom researchers have conceptualized wisdom as a resource or personal characteristic that encourages the experiencing of certain positive emotions such as sympathy and compassionate love, and decreases the experiencing of others (e.g., feelings of hostility, contempt, or personal distress; e.g., Ardelt, 2003; Clayton & Birren, 1980; Kramer, 1990; Labouvie-Vief, 1990).

Although empirical research supporting this claim is sparse, it is reasonable to assume that people with high levels of wisdom-related knowledge experience potentially emotion-evoking events in quite different ways than people with low levels of wisdom-related knowledge. Wisdom, as defined in the Berlin wisdom paradigm, refers to contextual, historical, dialectical, and holistic knowledge that represents events and phenomena on various levels of abstraction and in different time frames. As a consequence, people with high levels of wisdom-related knowledge should be better able to regard phenomena from a broader viewpoint, to put their emotional implications into perspective, and to adopt a detached and less emotional attitude than do people with low levels of wisdom-related knowledge.

This is not to say that wise people do not experience emotions at all or that their emotional life is reduced and flat. To the contrary, people with higher levels of wisdom-related knowledge may even spontaneously react more strongly to certain events because of their deeper understanding of its significance. Seen over time, however, wisdom-related knowledge should facilitate the down-regulation of emotions so that they do not become dysfunctional. Being able to "work" with emotions, to understand emotions, modify them, and use the information they provide to deal with the environment, may be a prerequisite, concomitant, and consequence of wisdom-related knowledge.

A first experimental study that we recently completed in our laboratory addressed this proposal. In this laboratory study we exposed people with different levels of wisdom-related knowledge (high vs. low) to three fundamental life problems, each presented in a short film clip of about ten minutes duration. The problems dealt with an older woman who learns that she has Alzheimer's disease (Alzheimer's film), a young woman who mourns for her husband and little daughter who were killed in a car accident (family-loss film), and a middle-aged woman who escapes her frustrating family life to travel and find herself (personal growth film). We know from previous studies that these films evoke strong emotional reactions, especially sympathy with the main protagonists, feelings of sadness in response to the family-loss and Alzheimer's films, and feelings of happiness in response to the personal growth film (Kunzmann & Grühn, 2005).

The major goal of this study was to provide first empirical support for the notion that people's wisdom-related knowledge influences their inner feelings and experiences in response to fundamental and existential life problems. We had the following more specific predictions for people with high levels of wisdom-related knowledge: (1) Because they are likely to recognize the significance and deeper meaning of events and phenomena, people with high levels of wisdom-related knowledge should first show a salient emotional response when confronted with another person's serious life problem (empathy hypothesis). (2) After further processing of the information, however, people with high levels of wisdom-related knowledge will exhibit effective down-regulation of their emotional responses to distance themselves and to bring their wisdom-related knowledge into foreground (regulation hypothesis).

Our initial findings are consistent with both hypotheses (empathy and regulation). As predicted, people with higher levels of wisdom-related knowledge showed greater emotional reactions to two fundamental life scenarios. They experienced greater pleasantness in response to the personal-growth film, and they experienced greater sadness in response to the film dealing with Alzheimer's. After they had time to reflect upon the emotion-arousing life scenario, however, people with higher levels of wisdom-related knowledge down-regulated their first emotional response.

Together, this initial evidence supports the idea that wisdom, as defined and measured in the Berlin wisdom paradigm, influences people's emotional reactions to fundamental life problems in theory-consistent ways. The evidence opposes the view that people with high levels of wisdom-related knowledge generally are emotionally distant and detached (e.g., Erikson, 1959). Rather, people with higher levels of wisdom appear to sympathize with their fellow mortals, regardless of whether they are experiencing life transitions that potentially lead to personal growth or are going through existential problems dealing with their own death and dying.

Motivational Dynamics of Wisdom

Does wisdom-related knowledge guide a person's behaviors in grappling with difficult problems and interacting with others? How do people use their wisdom-related knowledge in everyday life; and what is the motivational orientation that goes hand in hand with this type of knowledge?

The question of whether wisdom includes the application of knowledge in everyday life has provoked considerable division within both the humanities and the social sciences. On one hand, wisdom has been seen as being quite remote from manifest behavior. Particularly in Eastern philosophical traditions, truly wise persons are thought to deal in essences, to avoid immediate action, and to sometimes demonstrate their competence by refraining from any action at all (Assmann, 1994). On the other hand, several modern philosophers influenced by the tradition of early Greek philosophy have proposed that wisdom is closely linked to our everyday behaviors. In this tradition, wisdom has been thought to be a resource that facilitates a good life both on an individual and a societal level. For example, Ryan (1996) defined a wise person as "person S is wise if and only if (1) S is a free agent, (2) S knows how to live well, (3) S lives well, and (4) S's living well is caused by S's knowledge of how to live well" (p. 241). Kekes (1983) wrote: "wisdom is a character trait intimately connected with self-direction. The more wisdom a person has the more likely it is he will succeed in living a good life" (p. 277).

Notably, a good life is not linked exclusively to self-realization and personal happiness but encompasses more, namely, the well-being of others. In this sense, Kekes (1996) has stressed that wisdom is knowledge about ways of developing oneself not only without violating others' rights but also with coproducing resources for others to develop. Thus, in these philosophical conceptualizations, a central characteristic of a wise person is the ability to translate knowledge into action geared toward the development of oneself and others.

If one accepts the general proposal that, in principle, wisdom-related knowledge does have an effect on our everyday behavior, the question arises: what kind of effect? Put differently, what is the motivational orientation that goes hand in hand with wisdom? On the basis of philosophical work in the early Greek tradition and our own theoretical work in this area, we have predicted that the values and behaviors of people with high levels of wisdom-related knowledge will indicate a striving for a good life. One aspect of a good life in the early Greek tradition refers to the balancing of personal and common interests (see also Sternberg, 1998). A second aspect refers to the preference for personal growth and self-actualization – even if this preference opposes happiness in a hedonistic and materialistic sense (Baltes et al., 2002; Kunzmann & Baltes, 2003a).

To begin to investigate this prediction, we conducted a questionnaire study with an age-heterogeneous sample of young, middle-aged, and older adults (Kunzmann & Baltes, 2003a). In this study, we assessed wisdom-related knowledge by our standard procedure in individual interviews and, in addition, employed questionnaires that measured motivational and emotional dispositions, namely, general value orientations (preference for a pleasurable life, personal growth, insight, well-being of friends, environmental protection, societal engagement); preferred modes of conflict management (dominance, submission, avoidance, cooperation); and affective experiences (pleasant affect and feelings of positive involvement).

As expected, adults with higher levels of wisdom-related knowledge reported less preference for values revolving around a pleasurable and comfortable life. Instead, they reported preferring self-oriented values such as personal growth and insight, as well as a preference for other-oriented values related to environmental protection, societal engagement, and the well-being of friends. People with high levels of wisdom-related knowledge also showed less preference for conflict management strategies that reflect either a one-sided concern with one's own interests (i.e., dominance), a one-sided concern with others' interests (i.e., submission), or no concern at all (i.e., avoidance). As predicted, they preferred a cooperative approach reflecting a joint concern for one's own and the opponent's interests (i.e., cooperation). Finally, people with high levels of wisdom-related knowledge reported that they experience self-centered pleasant feelings less frequently (e.g., happiness, amusement) but process-oriented and environment-centered positive emotions more frequently (e.g., interest, inspiration).

These findings are promising in that they clearly oppose the view that wisdom-related knowledge, as assessed in the Berlin wisdom paradigm, is an abstract body of theoretical knowledge that may only be relevant for philosophical discourse about hypothetical problems. According to the evidence reviewed above, wisdom-related knowledge makes a difference for people's affective experiences, values, and behavioral choices in everyday life. More generally speaking, wisdom-related knowledge seems to go hand in hand with a joint concern for developing one's own and others' potential.

The evidence also points to the complexity of developmental processes, especially the proposition that developmental outcomes are multifunctional and, at the same time, involve gains and losses (e.g., Baltes, 1987, 1997; Baltes et al., 2006). Even striving for a highly priced attribute such as wisdom involves both gains and costs. According to our findings, wisdom is incompatible with a hedonistic lifestyle that prioritizes pleasure and comfort.

Of course, given that the study reviewed above was cross-sectional and correlational, it can be considered only a first step toward understanding how people with different degrees of wisdom-related knowledge differ in their behaviors in everyday life. In addition, we chose a measurement approach that was domain-general and time-enduring; that is, we investigated affective experiences, values, and strategies of conflict management from a dispositional rather than a contextual or state-like perspective. In our ongoing "wisdom-in-action" research we study adults with different levels of wisdom-related knowledge in the laboratory and try to more objectively assess behavioral outcomes.

Concluding Remarks and Future Perspectives

Wisdom is a topic that holds much promise as aging researchers turn their attention to the positive aspects and potential gains of aging and old age. As reviewed above, the evidence suggests that wisdom may be spared from the losses that often accompany age. The majority of adults experience stability in wisdom-related knowledge, at least up to the 1960s and 70s. What's more, there is evidence that most adults have the potential to activate formerly deactivated and hidden bodies of wisdom-related knowledge by applying relatively simple strategies and scripts (e.g., a script about how to imagine a conversation with a person whom one considers close to wisdom). Perhaps even more important, given certain individual resources and favorable life circumstances, some adults manage to experience long-term growth in wisdom well into very old age. Importantly, most of these facilitative resources and conditions are not beyond an individual's control, but are related to a person's life style and preferences (e.g., interest in other people's well-being, pursuit of personal growth values, or a cooperative interpersonal style). Finally, although the way toward wisdom may be cumbersome at times, striving for wisdom is valuable not only for the individual but also for his or her environment. First evidence suggests that people with higher levels of wisdom-related knowledge are affective sensitive and highly empathic with their fellow mortals. Higher levels of wisdom-related knowledge facilitate a growth-related value orientation and the awareness that individual and collective well-being are tied together. Considering the intricate problems of our lives in a society that is often driven by individualistic and materialistic motives, wisdom points to another set of avenues for satisfaction and happiness. Its very foundation lies in the orchestration of mind and virtue toward a common good.

References

Achenbaum, W.A., & Orwoll, L. (1991). Becoming wise: A psycho-gerontological interpretation of the Book of Job. *International Journal of Aging and Human Development, 32,* 21–39.

Ardelt, M. (2003). Empirical assessment of a three-dimensional wisdom scale. *Research on Aging, 25,* 275–324.

Ardelt, M. (2004). Wisdom as expert knowledge system: A critical review of a contemporary operationalization of an ancient concept. *Human Development, 47,* 257–285.

Assmann, A. (1994). Wholesome knowledge: Concepts of wisdom in a historical and cross-cultural perspective. In D.L. Featherman, R.M. Lerner, & M. Perlmutter (Eds.), *Life-span development and behavior* (Vol. 12, pp. 187–224). Hillsdale, NJ: Erlbaum.

Baltes, P.B. (1987). Theoretical propositions of life-span developmental psychology: On the dynamics between growth and decline. *Developmental Psychology, 23,* 611–626.

Baltes, P.B. (1997a). Wolfgang Edelstein: Über ein Wissenschaftlerleben in konstruktivistischer Melancholie [Wolfgang Edelstein: A scientific life in constructive melancholy]. *Reden zur Emeritierung von Wolfgang Edelstein* [Papers on the occasion of Wolfgang Edelstein's rrtirement festivities]. Berlin, Germany: Max Planck Institute for Human Development.

Baltes, P.B. (1997b). On the incomplete architecture of human ontogeny: Selection, optimization, and compensation as foundation of developmental theory. *American Psychologist, 52,* 366–380.

Baltes, P.B. (2004). *Wisdom: The orchestration of mind and virtue.* Unfinished Book. Available at http//www.mpib-berlin.mpg.de/dok/full/baltes/orchestr/index.htm.

Baltes, P.B., & Kunzmann, U. (2003). Wisdom: The peak of human excellence in the orchestration of mind and virtue. *The Psychologist, 16,* 131–133.

Baltes, P.B., & Kunzmann, U. (2004). Two faces of wisdom: Wisdom as a general theory of knowledge and judgment about excellence in mind and virtue vs. wisdom as everyday realization in people and products. *Human Development, 47,* 290–299.

Baltes, P.B., Lindenberger, U., & Staudinger, U.M. (2006). Lifespan theory in developmental psychology. In W. Damon (Series Ed.) & R.M. Lerner (Volume Ed.), *Handbook of child psychology* (6th ed., Vol. 1, pp. 569–664). New York: Wiley.

Baltes, P.B., & Smith, J. (1990). The psychology of wisdom and its ontogenesis. In R.J. Sternberg

(Ed.), *Wisdom: Its nature, origins, and development* (pp. 87–120). New York: Cambridge University Press.

Baltes, P.B., & Staudinger, U.M. (2000). Wisdom: A metaheuristic (pragmatic) to orchestrate mind and virtue toward excellence. *American Psychologist, 55*, 122–136.

Baltes, P.B., Staudinger, U.M., Maerker, A., & Smith, J. (1995). People nominated as wise: A comparative study of wisdom-related knowledge. *Psychology and Aging, 10*, 155–166.

Boehmig-Krumhaar, S.A., Staudinger, U.M., & Baltes, P.B. (2002). Mehr Toleranz tut Not: Lässt sich wert-relativierendes Wissen und Urteilen mit Hilfe einer wissensaktivierenden Gedächtnisstrategie verbessern [In need of more tolerance: Is possible to improve value-relativistic knowledge and judgment]? *Zeitschrift für Entwicklungspsychologie und Pädagogische Psychologie, 34*, 30–43.

Carstensen, L.L., & Turk-Charles, S. (1998). Emotion in the second half of life. *Current Directions in Psychological Science, 7*, 144–149.

Clayton, V.P., & Birren, J.E. (1980). The development of wisdom across the lifespan: A reexamination of an ancient topic. In P.B. Baltes & O.G. Brim, Jr. (Eds.), *Life-span development and behavior* (Vol. 3, pp. 103–135). New York: Academic Press.

Dittmann-Kohli, F., & Baltes, P.B. (1990). Toward a neofunctionalist conception of adult intellectual development: wisdom as a prototypical case of intellectual growth. In C.N. Alexander & E.J. Langer, *Higher stages of human development* (pp. 54–78). New York: Oxford University Press.

Dixon, R.A., & Baltes, P.B. (1986). Toward life-span research on the functions and pragmatics of intelligence. In R.J. Sternberg & R.K. Wagner (Eds.), *Practical intelligence: Nature and origins of competence in the everyday world* (pp. 203–235). Cambridge, UK: Cambridge University Press.

Erikson, E.H. (1959). *Identity and the life cycle*. New York: International University Press.

Freund, A.M., & Baltes, P.B. (1998). Selection, optimization, and compensation as strategies of life-management: Correlations with subjective indicators of successful aging. *Psychology and Aging, 13*, 531–543.

Gough, H.G., & Heilbrun, A.B. (1983). *The Adjective Check List manual*. Palo Alto, CA: Consulting Psychologist's Press.

Helson, R., & Srivastava, S. (2002). Creative and wise people: Similarities, differences, and how they develop. *Personality and Social Psychology Bulletin, 28*, 1430–1440.

Kekes, J. (1983). Wisdom. *American Philosophical Quarterly, 20*, 277–286.

Kekes, J. (1996). *Moral wisdom and good lives*. Ithaca, NY: Cornell University Press.

Keltner, D., & Gross, J.J. (1999). Functional accounts of emotions. *Cognition and Emotion, 13*, 467–480.

Kramer, D.A. (2000). Wisdom as a classical source of human strength: Conceptualizing and empirical inquiry. *Journal of Social and Clinical Psychology, 19*, 83–101.

Kunzmann, U. (2004). Approaches to a good life: The emotional-motivational side to wisdom. In P.A. Linley & S. Joseph (Eds.), *Positive psychology in practice* (pp. 504–517). Hoboken, NJ: Wiley.

Kunzmann, U., & Baltes, P.B. (2005). The psychology of wisdom: Theoretical and empirical challenges. In R.J. Sternberg & J. Jordan (Eds.), *Handbook of wisdom* (pp. 110–135). New York: Cambridge University Press.

Kunzmann, U., & Baltes, P.B. (2003a). Wisdom-related knowledge: Affective, motivational, and interpersonal correlates. *Personality and Social Psychology Bulletin, 29*, 1104–1119.

Kunzmann, U., & Baltes, P.B. (2003b). Beyond the traditional scope of intelligence: Wisdom in action. In R.J. Sternberg, J. Lautry, & T.I. Lubart (Eds.), *Models of intelligence for the next millennium* (pp. 329–343). Washington, DC: American Psychological Association.

Kunzmann, U., & Grühn, D. (2005). Age differences in emotional reactivity: The sample case of sadness. *Psychology and Aging, 20*, 47–59

Kunzmann, U., & Stange, J. (2006). Wisdom as a classical human strength: Psychological conceptualizations and empirical inquiry. In A.D. Ong & M. Van Dulmen (Eds.), *Varieties of positive experience: Structure, variability, and change* (pp. 306–322). New York: Oxford University Press.

Labouvie-Vief, G. (1990). Wisdom as integrated thought: historical and developmental perspectives. In R.J. Sternberg (Ed.), *Wisdom: Its nature, origins, and development* (pp. 52–83). Cambridge, MA: Cambridge University Press.

Pasupathi, M., Staudinger, U.M., & Baltes, P.B. (2001). Seeds of wisdom: Adolescents' knowledge and judgment about difficult life problems. *Developmental Psychology, 37*, 351–361.

Ryan, S. (1996). Wisdom. In K. Lehrer, B.J. Lum, B.A. Slichta, & N.D. Smith (Eds.), *Knowledge, teaching, and wisdom* (pp. 233–242). Dordrecht, The Netherlands: Kluwer.

Smith, J., Staudinger, U.M., & Baltes, P.B. (1994). Occupational settings facilitating wisdom-related knowledge: The sample case of clinical psychologists. *Journal of Consulting and Clinical Psychology, 62*, 989–999.

Staudinger, U.M. (1999). Older and wiser? Integrating results on the relationship between age and wisdom-related performance. *International Journal of Behavioral Development, 23*, 641–664.

Staudinger, U.M., & Baltes, P.B. (1996). Interactive minds: A facilitative setting for wisdom-related performance? *Journal of Personality and Social Psychology, 71*, 746–762.

Staudinger, U.M., Lopez, D.F., & Baltes, P.B. (1997). The psychometric location of wisdom-related performance: Intelligence, personality, and more? *Personality and Social Psychology Bulletin, 23*, 1200–1214.

Staudinger, U.M., Smith, J., & Baltes, P.B. (1992). Wisdom-related knowledge in a life review task: Age differences and the role of professional specialization. *Psychology and Aging, 7*, 271–281.

Sternberg, R.J. (Ed.). (1990). *Wisdom: Its nature, origins, and development.* New York: Cambridge University Press.

Sternberg, R.J. (1998). A balance theory of wisdom. *Review of General Psychology, 2*, 347–365.

Sternberg, R.J. (2001). Why schools should teach for wisdom: The balance theory of wisdom in educational settings. *Educational Psychologist, 36*, 227–245.

Wink, P., & Helson, R. (1997). Practical and transcendent wisdom: Their nature and some longitudinal findings. *Journal of Adult Development, 4*, 1–15.

14. Toward a Theory of Successful Aging

Selection, Optimization, and Compensation

Alexandra M. Freund and Paul B. Baltes

Introduction

Many might consider the very term "successful aging" an oxymoron. After all, doesn't aging primarily entail loss, the experience of cognitive and physical decline, and a confrontation with our own mortality? Is it even possible to age successfully? Of course, there are aspects of aging related to loss and decline, particularly in very old age (Baltes & Smith, 2003), and managing losses can be seen as one of the key tasks of successful aging. Aging, however, also entails plasticity and even the potential for growth. A comprehensive understanding of successful aging, then, necessitates addressing how older people can promote gains as well as prevent losses. Our approach posits that three distinct but interrelated processes are vital for successful aging: selection, optimization, and compensation. In this chapter, we will provide an overview and empirical evidence of the theory of selection, optimization, and compensation (SOC).

Defining Successful Aging

There is currently no generally agreed upon definition of "successful aging." This is probably due to both components of the term: (1) What is *aging* and when does it start? The notion of *successful aging* seems to imply discontinuity in developmental processes when people enter old age. Assuming continuity, many researchers prefer the more general term *successful development*. (2) What could be general criteria for *success*? Criteria for success are necessarily relative to social and cultural values. Whereas for certain cultures, accumulation of material possessions might seem a valid indicator of success, wisdom might constitute the highpoint of successful development in others.

Not astonishingly, then, there is no generally accepted definition of successful aging available. On a very abstract level, however, there is agreement that successful development is best conceptualized as a process encompassing the simultaneous maximization of gains and minimization of losses (M.M. Baltes, 1987; Brandtstädter, 1998; Labouvie-Vief, 1981). The dynamic of gains and losses will be elaborated in more detail in the following section.

Aging: A Changing Dynamic of Gains and Losses

Childhood-based conceptions define development primarily as a process of increasing level of functioning, one of specification and differentiation. In contrast, aging, until fairly recently, was seen as the reverse trajectory of losses in functioning and dedifferentiation. Theoretically and empirically, these were two entirely distinct areas of theorizing and empirical research. Only the advent of lifespan psychology, with its view of development spanning the entire life from conception to death, allowed a more comprehensive view of development as encompassing gains *and* losses, stability *and* change, differentiation *and* dedifferentiation (e.g., Baltes, 1987; Thomae, 1979). One domain of functioning in which multidimensionality, multidirectionality, and multifunctionality have been found is cognitive functioning. The mechanics and pragmatics of intelligence show different trajectories with respect to directions, onsets, and rates of change across adulthood. Whereas the mechanics (e.g., speed of information processing) reach their peak in early adulthood and decline already in early mid-age, cognitive pragmatics (e.g., vocabulary) peak in middle adulthood and show high stability up into the *1970s* (for an overview, see Baltes, Lindenberger, & Staudinger, 2006). In addition, losses can even be a source of gains as is the case when acquiring new, compensatory skills in response to losses. Similarly, gains can involve losses when optimizing one domain of functioning hinders improvement in others due to interference or resource constraints (e.g., Baltes, 1987; Freund, Li, & Baltes, 1999; Riediger, Freund, & Baltes, 2005).

Taking a lifespan approach, then, development across the lifespan – including old age – entails both gains *and* losses (Baltes, 1987; Labouvie-Vief, 1981). The ratio of gains to losses, however, changes with age (e.g., Baltes et al., 2006; Baltes & Smith, 2003; Brandtstädter, 1999; Freund & Ebner, 2005; Heckhausen, Dixon, & Baltes, 1989; Staudinger, Marsiske, & Baltes, 1995). There are multiple sources of losses in old age. For instance, M. Baltes and colleagues (Baltes, Maas, Wilms, Borchelt, & Little, 1999) found that the level of expanded everyday competence (i.e., the degree of engagement in activities other than self-care and resting) was negatively related to chronological age, mostly due to health-related decline and psychosocial factors. Most older people experience a decline in physical capacity and health (e.g., Steinhagen-Thiessen & Borchelt, 1999). Moreover, older people are also likely to lose close social partners (e.g., Lang & Carstensen, 1994). One of the central questions concerning successful aging, then, is how people manage the changing ratio of gains to losses in resources. In our view, there are currently three main theories addressing this question: The model of primary and secondary control by Heckhausen and Schulz (1995), the model of assimilative and accommodative coping (Brandtstädter & Renner, 1990), and the model of selection, optimization, and compensation (Baltes & Baltes, 1990). These theories both emphasize the role of proactive and motivational processes in shaping and adapting to age-related changes in resources. In the remainder of this chapter, we review one of these theories in more detail, the theory of selection, optimization, and compensation (SOC).

Processes of Successful Aging: Selection, Optimization, and Compensation

In 1987, Paul B. Baltes laid out seven propositions of life-span developmental psychology. These propositions served as the foundation of a theory of successful aging – the theory of selection, optimization, and compensation (SOC):

1. *Distinguishing normal, optimal, and pathological aging.* The concept of optimal aging denotes the specification of age-friendly environments that allow optimal functioning well into old age. Normal aging subsumes developmental processes that are not due to (biological-medical) diseases such as Alzheimer's disease. Pathological aging refers to trajectories that are characterized by illness and disease.

2. *Aging as heterogeneous process.* Aging is not a general and uniform process but is characterized by large interindividual variability regarding size, direction, and speed of change.

3. *Latent reserve capacity.* Results of intervention studies show that cognitive abilities in old age are to some degree malleable and can be enhanced by training. These results imply a latent reserve capacity that, under normal circumstances, is not used.

4. *Age-related losses at limits of reserve capacity.* Studies training younger and older adults until they have reached their personal asymptote show that older adults profit from training but do not reach the level of performance of younger adults after training.

5. *Age-related losses in fluid intelligence can be compensated by crystallized intelligence.* As research in the domain of cognitive aging shows, the differential trajectories of fluid (mechanic aspects of intelligence) and crystallized (knowledge-based aspects) intelligence help to counteract age-related losses. This highlights two things: (a) the importance of experience and knowledge in the process of aging, and (b) the importance of compensation for maintenance of functioning.

6. *The balance of gains to losses becomes increasingly negative in old age.* Whereas childhood is characterized by rapid gains in functional levels and resources, losses become increasingly prevalent across adulthood and particularly in old age.

7. *The self maintains its elasticity in old age.* The maintenance of self-esteem, personal control, and subjective well-being in old age is based on three factors: (a) A rich self-definition allows flexibility and adaptivity in the face of change; (b) adjusting personal goals to losses in resources increases the likelihood of actually reaching them; (c) adapting social comparison standards to match one's level of functioning leads to positive self-evaluation.

These seven propositions are the basis of the theory of selection, optimization, and compensation (Baltes & Baltes, 1980; 1990; Freund et al., 1999; Freund & Baltes, 2000). This theory describes general processes of developmental regulation throughout the lifespan. Because of lower reserve capacity (proposition 4) and increasing losses (proposition 6), selection, optimization, and compensation are assumed to be of particular relevance for successful aging.

Selection, optimization, and compensation are proposed to be universal processes of developmental regulation that can vary in phenotypic expression depending on sociohistorical and cultural context, domain of functioning, as on the unit of analysis (Baltes, 1997). Therefore, SOC theory does not assign specific content or mechanisms to its proposed developmental regulatory processes but outlines general purpose processes of specification by selection of developmental pathways, preferences, or goals, optimization of functioning through acquisition and refinement of resources and skills, and maintenance of functioning in the face of loss or decline through compensation.

More specifically, *selection* refers to specifying a particular pathway or set of pathways of development. This selective specification includes the narrowing down of a range of alternatives within the scope of plasticity, as delineated by biological and cultural constraints. Selection also addresses the fact that resources such as time and energy are limited throughout the lifespan as resources are concentrated on a limited set of functional domains. Selection thereby serves to provide constraints that allow specification and differentiation. In this way, selection is a basis for the acquisition of new resources.

Optimization refers to the acquisition, application, and integration of resources involved in attaining higher levels of functioning. Such resources range from internal (e.g., intelligence) to external personal means (e.g., social support) and sociocultural conditions (e.g., health care system). Resources signify potential, and only translate into actual improvement of functioning when invested into selected pathways of development.

Compensation addresses the management of impending or actual losses in function by substituting available resources. Compensation is often overlooked as a key process of developmental regulation. This might be the case because, traditionally, development was primarily seen as related to growth or gains, and the multidirectionality of development has only been recognized since the advance of lifespan theory and aging research (Baltes, 1987).

The orchestration of selection, optimization, and compensation refers not only to their interactions, but also to their coordination over time (Baltes, 1997; Baltes & Carstensen, 1996; Marsiske, Lang, Baltes, & Baltes, 1995). We submit that developmental processes typically entail all three components to varying degrees. Selection, optimization, and compensation are proposed to be universal processes of developmental regulation in that they contribute to adaptive functioning across domains of functioning, age groups, and cultures. The behavioral expressions, however, can vary greatly depending on domain, age, and individual skills and preferences. For instance, in an observational study by Gignac, Cott, and Badley (2002), almost all of the older osteoarthritis patients in their study showed behavior reflecting selection (e.g., restricting activity), optimization (e.g., practicing movements), or compensation (e.g., using a walking aid). At the same time, however, Gignac et al. observed substantial interindividual variability in the expression of specific SOC behaviors, underscoring the individual specificity of the expression of SOC.

SOC can be applied within different theoretical perspectives, to a variety of domains of functioning (e.g., social, cognitive, physical), and to different levels of analysis. For instance, the focus can be on a specific behavioral or functional domain (such as working memory) or on personal functioning in a more general sense (such as subjective well-being or longevity). In the remainder of this chapter, we will elaborate on one application of SOC that uses an action-theoretical framework focusing on the role of goals for successful aging (Freund, 2007; Freund & Baltes, 2000; Freund et al., 1999).

Embedding SOC in an Action-Theoretical Framework

Within an action theoretical framework, the focus is on motivational processes and goals, stressing the importance of the dynamic interplay of proactively creating as well as reacting to one's environment (Baltes, 1997; Brandtstädter, 1998; Freund & Baltes, 2000; Freund et al., 1999). The role of a person in his or her development is not only seen in reacting to a changing environment and opportunity structures. Instead, a person also proactively shapes and selects his or her environment. From this perspective, a person is neither seen as only reacting to external stimuli, nor as a closed, self-sufficient system. A person creates an environment in a way that best fits the given social, cultural, and biological constraints, on the one hand, and his or her goals, on the other (Lawton, 1989; Lerner & Busch-Rossnagel, 1981). Thus, an adequate description of development must take the social (and physical) environment as well as the active role of the person into account. Proactive choices (e.g., such as moving to a ground floor apartment) can have long-term consequences in their effect on how well the environment fits personal demands (e.g., when mobility decreases). One of the results of a good person-environment fit, according to Lawton (1989), is subjective well-being and life satisfaction.

One of the central assumptions in psychological action theories is that goals are the building blocks of development as they organize and structure behavior over time and across situations into hierarchical action sequences of setting and pursuing goals (for an overview of this approach, see Freund & Riediger, 2006). Embedding SOC in an action-theoretical framework, the theory of SOC posits that developing and committing to a set and hierarchy of personal goals (elective selection) and engaging in goal-directed actions and means (optimization) contribute to achieving higher levels of functioning. In order to maintain a given level of functioning in the face of loss and decline in goal-relevant means, people need to invest in compensatory, substitutive means. When the costs for goal achievement or maintenance outweigh their expected gains, it is adaptive to reconstruct one's goal hierarchy by focusing exclusively on the most

Table 1. Selection, optimization, compensation: Action-theoretical definition and functions

Process	Definition	Functions
Selection	Delineating (a set of) goals	Specification; directionality; focuses limited resources
Elective	Developing and committing to a subset of possible options; building a clear goal hierarchy	Organizes and structures behavior over time
Loss-based	Restructuring goal hierarchy; reformulation of goals	Managing blocked goals
Optimization	Acquisition, refinement, coordination, and investment of goal-relevant means	Promoting gains in functional capacity
Compensation	Acquisition, refinement, coordination, and investment of substitutive means	Counteracting losses; maintenance of functional capacity

important goals, developing new goals, or adapting goal standards (loss-based selection). Thus, the SOC model conceptualizes processes that promote gains (primarily through elective selection and optimization), but also processes that counteract losses, which inevitably occur in life (compensation, loss-based selection). **Table 1** summarizes an action-theoretical definition of SOC.

Together, selection, optimization, and compensation are proposed to advance adaptive mastery across the life span and into old age. These processes can be active or passive, conscious or nonconscious, and external or internal (Freund et al., 1999). As development occurs in interaction between a person and his or her sociocultural as well as physical environment, we assume that SOC processes always entail to some degree active *and* passive, internal *and* external, as well as conscious *and* nonconscious aspects. In the following, this is exemplified by Freund's (2003, 2007) heuristic framework of goals.

A Developmental Framework of Goals

Goals, the central construct within an action-theoretical framework, are states that a person, group, or society regards as either desirable or undesirable. Developmental goals can be located on different levels of analyses, namely on the level of age-related expectations or on the level of personal goals. Age-related expectations are reflected in social norms (e.g., mandatory retirement age) that inform about age-related constraints and opportunity structures. Age-related norms can be reflected in laws or institutions as well as general cultural beliefs about what kind of behavior is expected of and appropriate for a specific age group. Such general age-related beliefs can influence individual development by sanctioning the appropriate timing of developmental transitions. Moreover, social expectations about the age at which a person ought or ought not do something can serve as orientation for the development, selection, pursuit, and maintenance of personal goals (e.g., Cantor, 1994; Heckhausen, 1999). Personal beliefs about the appropriate timing and sequencing of goals are informed but not entirely determined by social norms and expectations. They also reflect individual values and experiences.

Age-related beliefs can operate both on the conscious and nonconscious level. People might consciously seek out age-related social expectations as a standard of comparison to guide and evaluate their behavior (Heckhausen, 1999). As research on the perception-action link shows, behaviors conforming with age-related beliefs can also be activated automatically. In the seminal study by Bargh, Chen, and Burrows (1996), young participants walked more slowly after being primed with the concept of old age, a time in life that is commonly associated with walking more slowly. These findings suggest that information about the age of a person leads to the activation of age-related beliefs that are then translated into behavior.

The influence of social expectations is not restricted to the content of behavior or goals; it extends to the processes of goal selection and goal pursuit. In research on naive theory or folk psychology, proverbs are viewed as a body of folk knowledge or social expectations about human life. Proverbs are short statements summarizing advice on how to deal effectively or in morally correct ways with everyday life situations. If sociocultural expectations about SOC as fundamental processes of development exist, it should also be possible to identify proverbs reflecting such processes. Consistent with this expectation, we (Freund & Baltes, 2002a) found that a substantial number of proverbs contain statements about behaviors reflecting selection, optimization, and compensation. An example of a proverb reflecting selection is "Jack of all trades is master of none," one reflecting optimization is "Practice makes perfect," and one reflecting compensation is "When there's no wind, grab the oars." On the level of personal beliefs, we found that young and older adults chose SOC-related proverbs more frequently than alternative proverbs as adaptive strategies of life mastery.

Together, social and personal expectations can directly influence behavior as well as the personal goals a person selects and pursues. In addition to consciously represented personal goals, nonconscious (automatized) goals and motives influence behavior and development. According to the automotive model by Bargh and Gollwitzer (1994), the repeated activation of a goal in a certain situation leads to an association of the respective goal and situational cues. Such situational features can then automatically trigger a goal and activate goal-relevant actions without conscious awareness of the respective goal (e.g., Bargh, 1990).

Taken together, goals can be defined socioculturally or by the individual him- or herself, or, as is probably true in most cases, by a combination of both. The pursuit of these goals might draw on an individual's internal resources (e.g., intelligence), external resources (e.g., social support), or a combination of both. And finally, goals can involve conscious, nonconscious processes, or, again most likely, a combination of both. This perspective integrates motivational processes of goal selection and goal pursuit into a lifespan perspective by taking a long-term temporal dimension and the individual's developmental context into account.

Most of the current empirical research directly addressing the processes of selection, optimization, and compensation and their association with successful aging investigates SOC on the level of conscious, intentional, active expressions. We will provide an overview of this research in the following section. We will also review a different research approach that sheds light on managing limited resources in older age using a dual-task paradigm.

Empirical Evidence for the Usefulness of SOC for Understanding Successful Aging

There is a large body of research that is compatible with and supportive of the SOC theory in general and successful aging in particular (see Staudinger & Lindenberger, 2003, for applications of SOC to different fields within psychology as well as different disciplines such as economy or neurosciences; for an excellent overview of SOC-related developmental research, see Baltes et al., 2006). There are also a growing number of studies directly investigating the role of SOC in successful aging using personal goals as the main level of analysis or using dual-task paradigms in cognitive and sensorimotor functioning. Taken together, this research provides evidence that SOC is related to successful aging as indexed by indicators of subjective well-being and that the relative focus on optimization and compensation changes when resources decline. Methods include self-report, observation, and experiments.

Self-Reported SOC Strategies and Successful Aging

As a first approach to assessing SOC, Baltes, Baltes, Freund, and Lang (1999) developed a self-report instrument. **Table 2** shows sample items for each of the SOC processes. A number of studies using samples of different ages from young to very old adulthood attest to the usefulness of this self-report instrument for assessing SOC. For instance, a set of studies (Baltes & Heydens-Gahir, 2003; Freund & Baltes, 1998, 2002b; Wiese, Freund, & Baltes, 2000, 2001) show that SOC is associated with higher levels of subjective indicators of successful development such as subjective well-being, positive emotional experience, loneliness, and satisfaction with aging. The pattern of correlations is stable across adulthood into old and very old age, and is robust when controlling for other personality and motivational constructs. In other words, adults who report that they develop a clear set of goals, build a goal hierarchy, and focus on their most important goals (selection), who report that they invest time, effort, and other necessary goal-relevant means into the pursuit of the selected goals (optimization), and who report using compensatory strategies in order to maintain functioning when encountering a loss or decline in resources (compensation) also show higher levels of subjective developmental success. Recently, Jopp and Smith (2006) have shown that particularly in very old age the self-reported use of SOC strategies buffers against negative effects of restricted resources. Moreover, comparing resource-rich and resource-poor older adults longitudinally replicated the results that SOC has a protective effect against a decline of resources in old age (for similar results, see also Baltes & Lang, 1997; Lang, Rieckmann, & Baltes, 2002).

Taken together, then, these studies show that the self-reported engagement in SOC-related behaviors contributes to successful aging and declining resources. Interestingly, however, the very engagement in these strategies – and particularly in such resource-intense strategies as optimization and compensation – consumes resources. Pursuing higher levels of functioning and maintaining them against increasing losses takes time, energy, and other goal-relevant resources. Therefore, it is not surprising that we observe the highest level of self-reported SOC in adults. In old age, when resources decline, optimization and compensation become less prevalent strategies of life management, while elective selection continues to be prominent (Freund & Baltes, 1998, 2002b). By being highly selective, older adults might focus their fewer resources on optimizing and compensating in their most important goals only. This interpretation is consistent with the finding by Jopp and Smith (2006) that shows negative correlations of resources and self-reported SOC. In the group of the very old adults, optimization in particular was affected by the availability of resources.

Table 2. Sample items of the SOC questionnaire by Baltes, Baltes, Freund, and Lang (1999): Each item consists of the description of behavior indicative of selection, optimization, or compensation paired with a description of an alternative, non-SOC behavior. Participants are asked to choose between these two options. Research has shown that this particular format decreases the effects of social desirability and contributes to more balanced item difficulty (see Freund & Baltes, 2002b, for more information on the questionnaire)

SOC-related ("target") behavior	Alternative behavior
Elective Selection	
I always pursue goals one after the other.	I always pursue many goals at once, so I easily get bogged down.
I know exactly what I want and what I don't want.	I often only know what I want as the result of a situation.
When I decide on a goal, I stick to it.	I can change a goal again at any time.
Loss-based Selection	
When things don't go as well as before, I drop some goals to concentrate on the more important ones.	When things don't go as well as before, I wait for better times.
When something gets increasingly difficult for me, I define my goals more precisely.	When something gets increasingly difficult for me, I try to distract myself.
When something gets increasingly difficult for me, I consider which goals I could achieve under the circumstances.	When something gets increasingly difficult for me, I accept it.
Optimization	
I think about exactly how I can best realize my plans.	I don't think long about how to realize my plans, I just try to.
When something is important to me, I don't let setbacks discourage me.	Setbacks show me that I should turn to something else.
I make every effort to achieve a given goal.	I prefer to wait for a while and see if things will work out by themselves.
Compensation	
When things don't go as well as they used to, I keep trying other ways until I can achieve the same result I used to.	When things don't go as well as they used to, I accept it.
When something in my life isn't working as well as it used to, I ask others for help or advice.	When something in my life isn't working as well as it used to, I decide what to do about it myself, without involving other people.
When it gets harder for me to get the same results I used to, I keep trying harder until I can do it as well as before.	When it gets harder for me to get the same results I used to, it is time to let go of that expectation.

Investigating the role of selection for successful aging, Riediger and Freund (2006) distinguished between two facets of selectivity: (1) restricting oneself to fewer goals and (2) focusing on central and similar goals. A longitudinal study showed differential results for these two facets of selection. Whereas focusing was associated with an increase in goal involvement (i.e., optimization) over time, restricting was not. Focusing was positively associated with selection of goals that facilitate each other. Consistent with other studies (Riediger & Freund, 2004; Riediger, Freund, & Baltes, 2005), facilitation between goals predicted optimization. Selectivity in terms of focusing increases from middle to older adulthood, as does a goal system characterized by higher facilitation among goals. Higher selectivity, then, might contribute to the maintenance of high goal involvement into later adulthood despite aging-related increases in resource limitations.

Changing Adaptivity of Focus on Gains (Optimization) and Losses (Compensation)

Given the shifting ratio of gains to losses in resources over the lifespan toward a more negative ratio in older adulthood, one could argue that goals focused on enhancing one's functioning (optimization goals) should be less prevalent as compared to goals aimed at the maintenance of functioning in the face of losses (compensation goals) (Freund & Ebner, 2005; Staudinger et al., 1995). Consistent with this assumption, Heckhausen (1999) found that middle-aged and older adults, as compared to younger adults, reported fewer personal goals associated with gains and more goals in domains reflecting the avoidance of losses. Similarly, Ebner, Freund, and Baltes (2006) showed that younger adults reported a stronger focus on growth, and older adults a stronger focus on maintenance and prevention of loss, in their personal goals. This shift in goal focus also proved adaptive. In contrast to younger adults, a goal focus on maintenance and loss avoidance was positively related to subjective well-being in older adults. Moreover, a direct link between resource availability and goal focus was observed in an experimental study: When they were experimentally induced to perceive their resources as being limited, both younger and older adults increasingly selected goals that were geared toward maintaining instead of improving functioning.

Does goal focus also differentially affect the actual pursuit of a goal in younger and older adults? This question was addressed in a set of behavioral studies by Freund (2006). As expected, younger adults showed more persistence in pursuing a goal that offered the possibility of achieving a better outcome (i.e., optimization), while older adults were more persistent when working on goals aimed at counteracting losses (i.e., compensation). These effects were robust against instructional variations and when controlling for differences in achievement motivation and instead seemed to depend crucially on the actual experience of a loss.

Taken together, these studies show that goal focus shifts with age. Younger adults, who typically have room for improvement and gains in many domains of functioning, more often select and are more motivated to pursue optimization goals. In contrast, older adults, who typically experience more losses, more often select and are more motivated to pursue compensation goals aimed at counteracting losses. This shift in goal focus might help prevent declines in functioning in the face of losses, thereby contributing to the maintenance of functioning in old age.

SOC in Dual-Task Paradigms

Another line of inquiry into the usefulness of SOC for successful aging takes advantage of the dual-task paradigm. This paradigm assesses how people manage to perform more than one task at a time. A comparison of performance on one task with performance on two simultaneous tasks (i.e., dual-task costs) provides insights into how people allocate limited resources. Moreover, the dual-task paradigm has high ecological validity as performing more than one task at a time is typical for everyday life (e.g., walking while talking, driving while listening to the radio). Dual- or multitasking becomes more difficult, i.e., dual-task costs become larger, the fewer (cognitive, physical) resources a person has. Therefore, not surprisingly, older adults generally show greater dual task costs than younger adults (Craik & Salthouse, 2000). One of the interesting questions of successful aging, then, is how older people adaptively allocate their resources in multiple-task situations.

The theory of SOC offers a framework concerning how older adults manage to carry out multiple tasks. Here, selection refers to a primary focus on vital or essential goals that have high functional significance. In other words, the SOC model emphasizes the need to prioritize tasks of higher immediate importance when resources are limited. An example is a situation involving keeping one's balance when walking on difficult terrain while memorizing a word list. According to SOC, older adults should focus more on keeping their balance while walking than on memorizing because, at their age, losing their balance and falling might cause serious health-related problems threatening their mobility (Lindenberger, Marsiske, & Baltes, 2000).

A number of studies combining a cognitive and a motor balance task empirically support this prediction (Li, Lindenberger, Freund, & Baltes, 2001; Rapp, Krampe, & Baltes, 2006). Replicating other studies, older adults showed greater dual-tasks costs. These dual-tasks costs, however, were not equal for the two tasks. The relative dual-task costs were higher for older adults in the cognitive task. This means that older adults allocated more resources to keeping their balance than to performing a relatively unimportant cognitive task (i.e., memorizing word lists, keeping track of numbers). Moreover, attesting to the effectiveness of the use of compensatory strategies, older adults invested more compensatory means into the maintenance of keeping their balance and they profited more from them than younger adults.

Regarding compensation in a dual-task situation involving walking while talking, Kemper, Herman, and Lian (2003) found that older and younger adults use different compensatory strategies when the task demands exceeded their resources. While walking, younger adults reduced the length and grammatical complexity of sentences, while older adults spoke more slowly. Simplifying their sentences or reducing their rate of speech, respectively, helped younger and older adults to preserve speaking when the walking task required resources that had previously been used for talking.

A study by Rapp et al. (2006) investigated the robustness of the prioritization of motor over cognitive functioning using a group of patients with Alzheimer's disease (AD), a group of healthy older adults of the same age, and a group of younger adults. Including patients with Alzheimer's disease allowed them to test the limits of the ability to prioritize a vital domain (maintaining balance) over a less vital one (cognitive performance) as resources in AD patients are severely limited and, accordingly, dual-task performance decrements go beyond those found due to normal aging (e.g., Baddeley, Baddeley, Bucks, & Wilcock, 2001). Again, using a dual-task paradigm, cognitive and balance performance were measured while task difficulty with respect to balancing was manipulated (standing on a stable vs. moving platform). As expected, large dual-task performance deficits emerged in older adults, and more so in Alzheimer patients. However, when balancing was made more difficult, older adults prioritized balancing over cognition. This pattern was more pronounced in Alzheimer patients, indicating the preservation of adaptive prioritization in the face of significant biological decrements.

Taken together, these studies show that in times or situations of limited resources, adults focus on the task that is more important and vital for overall functioning, and are able to use efficient compensatory means. However, in many everyday situations, adaptive resource allocation does not lie in consistently focusing one's resources on one function over another. Instead, it is often important to flexibly allocate resources to the optimization or compensation of tasks depending on situational demands. Bondar, Krampe, and Baltes (2003) found that both younger and older adults can learn to allocate resources to different task requirements. When a vital functional domain is threatened, however, older adults focus their resources on that domain (e.g., to prevent falling), regardless of the task instructions. It seems, then, that flexibility of resource allocation is constrained by threats to important functional capacity, such as motor functions and balance. Taken together, studies using the dual-task paradigm support the SOC theory. Older people direct their resources toward functional domains of high vital priority.

Summary and Conclusions

Successful aging can be defined as the process of promoting gains and preventing losses. Our approach posits that the three processes of selection, optimization, and compensation (SOC) are central for managing the changing balance of gains and losses in old age. Adopting an action-theoretical perspective, processes promoting gains develop and commit to a set of personal goals (i.e., elective selection) as well as acquire and invest new skills and resources into achieving the selected goals (i.e., optimization). The theory of SOC places equal emphasis on processes counteracting losses in resources that inevitably occur, particularly in old age. Processes aimed at minimizing losses restructure and adjust one's goals (i.e., loss-based selection) as well as acquire and invest remaining resources into the maintenance of functioning (i.e., compensation).

Empirical evidence supports SOC as a theory of successful aging. A number of studies have consistently shown that self-reported SOC is related to subjective indicators of aging well, such as subjective well-being, positive emotions, or satisfaction with aging. Consistent with the notion of an increase in losses in old age, compared to younger adults, older adults focus more on compensation and the maintenance of functioning. This shift in goal focus appears to be adaptive, both for subjective well-being and goal pursuit. More generally, research using the dual-task paradigm shows that older people primarily allocate their resources to functional domains of high importance when resources are limited. Taken together, there is compelling evidence that selection, optimization, and compensation can be viewed as processes of successful aging.

To our knowledge, there do not yet exist intervention studies training older people to increase their use of SOC. Such intervention studies could focus on implementing strategies of selection, optimization, and compensation in their everyday lives. For instance, as it appears to be adaptive to select personal goals that are mutually facilitative and that focus on the same overarching themes, it might be helpful to encourage older people to review their goal system as a whole and specify interrelations among goals. In addition, on the basis of studies on the adaptive shift of goal focus, encouraging older people to focus on compensation and maintenance of functioning, rather than primarily aspiring for new gains and growth, might help them to invest their resources wisely. Such intervention programs might also be directed at rehabilitation patients who have difficulty allocating their resources to their most important goals and acquiring goal-relevant means for compensation. Another interesting line of inquiry is the use of technology to make environments more elderly-friendly and providing assistance in areas where older people typically experience losses (e.g., navigation systems to help older people find their way). It is our hope that, in the long run, our research on SOC will contribute to understanding as well as improving successful aging.

References

Baddeley, A.D., Baddeley, H.A., Bucks, R.S., & Wilcock, G.K. (2001). Attentional control in Alzheimer's disease. *Brain, 124*, 241–256.

Baltes, B.B., & Heydens-Gahir, H.A. (2003). Reduction of work-family conflict through the use of selection. *Journal of Applied Psychology, 88*, 1005–1018.

Baltes, M.M., & Carstensen, L.L. (1996). The process of successful aging. *Ageing and Society, 16*, 397–422.

Baltes, M.M., & Lang, F.R. (1997). Everyday functioning and successful aging: The impact of resources. *Psychology and Aging, 12*, 433–443.

Baltes, M.M., Maas, I., Wilms, H.-U., Borchelt, M., & Little, T.D. (1999). Everyday competence in old and very old age: Theoretical considerations and empirical findings. In P.B. Baltes & K.U. Mayer (Eds.), *The Berlin Aging Study: Aging from 70 to 100* (pp. 384–402). New York: Cambridge University Press.

Baltes, P.B. (1987). Theoretical propositions of lifespan developmental psychology: On the dynamics between growth and decline. *Developmental Psychology, 23*, 611–626.

Baltes, P.B. (1997). On the incomplete architecture of human ontogeny: Selection, optimization, and compensation as foundation of developmental theory. *American Psychologist, 52,* 366–380.

Baltes, P.B., & Baltes, M.M. (1980). Plasticity and variability in psychological aging: Methodological and theoretical issues. In G.E. Gurski (Ed.), *Determining the effects of aging on the central nervous system* (pp. 41–66). Berlin, Germany: Schering.

Baltes, P.B., & Baltes, M.M. (1990). Psychological perspectives on successful aging: The model of selective optimization with compensation. In P.B. Baltes & M.M. Baltes (Eds.), *Successful aging: Perspectives from the behavioral sciences* (pp. 1–34). New York: Cambridge University Press.

Baltes, P.B., Baltes, M.M., Freund, A.M., & Lang, F. (1999). *The measurement of selection, optimization, and compensation (SOC) by self report: Technical report 1999.* Berlin, Germany: Max Planck Institute for Human Development.

Baltes, P.B., Lindenberger, U., & Staudinger, U.M. (2006). Lifespan theory in developmental psychology. In R.M. Lerner (Ed.), *Handbook of child psychology. Vol. 1: Theoretical models of human development* (6th ed., pp. 569–664). New York: Wiley.

Baltes, P.B., & Smith, J. (2003). New frontiers in the future of aging: From successful aging of the young old to the dilemmas of the fourth age. *Gerontology, 49,* 123–135.

Bargh, J.A. (1990). Goal ≠ intent: Goal-directed thought and behavior are often unintentional. *Psychological Inquiry, 1,* 248–277.

Bargh, J.A., Chen, M., & Burrows, L. (1996). Automaticity of social behavior: Direct effects of trait constructs and stereotype activation on action. *Journal of Personality and Social Psychology, 71,* 230–244.

Bargh, J.A., & Gollwitzer, P.M. (1994). Environmental control of goal-directed action: Automatic and strategic contingencies between situations and behavior. *Nebraska Symposium on Motivation, 41,* 71–124.

Bondar, A., Krampe, R. Th., & Baltes, P.B. (2003). *Balance takes priority over cognition: Can young and older adults deliberately control resource allocation?* Unpublished manuscript, Max Planck Institute for Human Development, Berlin.

Brandtstädter, J. (1998). Action theory in developmental psychology. In R.M. Lerner (Ed.), *Handbook of child psychology: Vol. 1. Theoretical models of human development* (pp. 807–866). New York: Wiley.

Brandtstädter, J. (1999). The self in action and development: Cultural, biosocial, and ontogenetic bases of intentional self-development. In J. Brandtstädter & R.M. Lerner (Eds.), *Action and self-development: Theory and research through the life span* (pp. 37–65). Thousand Oaks, CA: Sage.

Brandtstädter, J., & Renner, G. (1990). Tenacious goal pursuit and flexible goal adjustment: Explication and age-related analysis of assimilative and accommodative strategies of coping. *Psychology and Aging, 5,* 58–67.

Cantor, N. (1994). Life task problem solving: Situational affordances and personal needs. *Personality and Social Psychology Bulletin, 20,* 235–243.

Craik, F.I.M., & Salthouse, T.A. (Eds.). (2000). *The handbook of aging and cognition* (2nd ed.). Hillsdale, NJ: Erlbaum.

Ebner, N.C., Freund, A.M., & Baltes, P.B. (2006). Developmental changes in personal goal orientation from young to late adulthood: From striving for gains to maintenance and prevention of losses. *Psychology and Aging, 21,* 664–678.

Freund, A.M. (2003). Die Rolle von Zielen für die Entwicklung [The role of goals for development]. *Psychologische Rundschau, 54,* 233–242.

Freund, A.M. (2006). Differential motivational consequences of goal focus in younger and older adults. *Psychology and Aging, 21,* 240–252.

Freund, A.M. (2007). Levels of goals: Understanding motivational processes across adulthood.

In B.R. Little, K. Salmela-Aro & S.D. Phillips (Eds.), *Personal project pursuit: Goals, action and human flourishing* (pp. 247–270). Mahwah, NJ: Erlbaum.

Freund, A.M., & Baltes, P.B. (1998). Selection, optimization, and compensation as strategies of life-management: Correlations with subjective indicators of successful aging. *Psychology and Aging, 13*, 531–543.

Freund, A.M., & Baltes, P.B. (2000). The orchestration of selection, optimization, and compensation: An action-theoretical conceptualization of a theory of developmental regulation. In W.J. Perrig & A. Grob (Eds.), *Control of human behavior, mental processes, and consciousness* (pp. 35–58). Mahwah, NJ: Erlbaum.

Freund, A.M., & Baltes, P.B. (2002a). The adaptiveness of selection, optimization, and compensation as strategies of life management: Evidence from a preference study on proverbs. *The Journals of Gerontology Series B: Psychological Sciences and Social Sciences, 57*, P426–P434.

Freund, A.M., & Baltes, P.B. (2002b). Life-management strategies of selection, optimization, and compensation: Measurement by self-report and construct validity. *Journal of Personality and Social Psychology, 82*, 642–662.

Freund, A.M., & Ebner, N.C. (2005). The aging self: Shifting from promoting gains to balancing losses. In W. Greve, K. Rothermund, & D. Wentura (Eds), *The adaptive self: Personal continuity and intentional self-development* (pp. 185–202). Cambridge, MA: Hogrefe & Huber Publishers.

Freund, A.M., Li, K.Z.H., & Baltes, P.B. (1999). Successful development and aging: The role of selection, optimization, and compensation. In J. Brandtstädter & R.M. Lerner (Eds.), *Action and self-development: Theory and research through the life span* (pp. 401–434). Thousand Oaks, CA: Sage.

Freund, A.M., & Riediger, M. (2006). Goals as building blocks of personality and development in adulthood. In D.K. Mroczek & T.D. Little (Eds), *Handbook of personality development.* (pp. 353–372). Mahwah, NJ: Erlbaum.

Gignac, M., Cott, C., & Badley, E. (2002). Adaptation to disability: Applying selective optimization with compensation to the behaviors of older adults with osteoarthritis. *Psychology and Aging, 17*, 520–524.

Heckhausen, J. (1999). *Developmental regulation in adulthood: Age-normative and sociostructural constraints as adaptive challenges.* New York: Cambridge University Press.

Heckhausen, J., Dixon, R.A., & Baltes, P.B. (1989). Gains and losses in development throughout adulthood as perceived by different adult age groups. *Developmental Psychology, 25*, 109–121.

Heckhausen, J., & Schulz, R. (1995). A lifespan theory of control. *Psychological Review, 102*, 284–304.

Kemper, S., Herman, R.E., & Lian, C.H.T. (2003). The costs of doing two things at once for young and older adults: Talking while walking, finger tapping, and ignoring speech or noise. *Psychology and Aging, 18*, 181–192.

Jopp, D., & Smith, J. (2006). Resources and life-management strategies as determinants of successful aging: On the protective effect of selection, optimization, and compensation. *Psychology and Aging, 21*, 253–265.

Labouvie-Vief, G. (1981). Proactive and reactive aspects of constructivism: Growth and aging in life-span perspective. In R.M. Lerner & N.A. Busch-Rossnagel (Eds.), *Individuals as producers of their development* (pp. 197–230). New York: Academic Press.

Lang, F.R., & Carstensen, L.L. (1994). Close emotional relationships in late life: Further support for proactive aging in the social domain. *Psychology and Aging, 2*, 315–324.

Lang, F.R., Rieckmann, N., & Baltes, M.M. (2002). Adapting to aging losses: Do resources facilitate strategies of selection, compensation, and optimization in everyday functioning? *The Journals of Gerontology Series B: Psychological Sciences and Social Sciences, 57*, P501-P509.

Lawton, M.P. (1989). Environmental proactivity in older people. In V.L. Bengston & K.W. Schaie (Eds.), *The course of later life: Research and reflections* (pp. 15–23). New York: Springer Verlag.

Lerner, R.M., & Busch-Rossnagel, N.A. (1981). *Individuals as producers of their development.* New York: Academic Press.

Li, K.Z.H., Lindenberger, U., Freund, A.M., & Baltes, P.B. (2001). Walking while memorizing: Age-related differences in compensatory behavior. *Psychological Science, 12,* 230–237.

Lindenberger, U., Marsiske, M., & Baltes, P.B. (2000). Memorizing while walking: Increase in dual-task costs from young adulthood to old age. *Psychology and Aging, 15,* 417–436.

Marsiske, M., Lang, F.R., Baltes, P.B., & Baltes, M.M. (1995). Selective optimization with compensation: Life-span perspectives on successful human development. In R.A. Dixon & L. Bäckman (Eds.), *Compensating for psychological deficits and declines: Managing losses and promoting gains* (pp. 35–79). Mahwah, NJ: Erlbaum.

Rapp, M.A., Krampe, R. Th., & Baltes, P.B. (2006). Adaptive task prioritization in aging: Selective resource allocation to postural control is preserved in Alzheimer disease. *American Journal of Geriatric Psychiatry, 14,* 52–61.

Riediger, M., & Freund, A.M. (2004). Interference and facilitation among personal goals: Differential association with subjective well-being and persistent goal pursuit. *Personality and Social Psychology Bulletin, 30,* 1511–1523.

Riediger, M., & Freund, A.M. (2006). Focusing and restricting: Two aspects of motivational selectivity in adulthood. *Psychology and Aging, 21,* 173–185.

Riediger, M., Freund, A.M., & Baltes, P.B. (2005). Managing life through personal goals: Intergoal facilitation and intensity of goal pursuit in younger and older adulthood. *The Journals of Gerontology Series B: Psychological Sciences and Social Sciences, 60B,* P84–P91.

Staudinger, U.M., & Lindenberger, U. (Eds.). (2003). *Understanding human development: Dialogs with lifespan psychology.* Amsterdam: Kluwer.

Staudinger, U.M., Marsiske, M., & Baltes, P.B. (1995). Resilience and reserve capacity in later adulthood: Potentials and limits of development across the life span. In D. Cicchetti & D. Cohen (Eds.), *Developmental psychopathology. Vol. 2: Risk, disorder, and adaptation* (pp. 801–847). New York: Wiley.

Steinhagen-Thiessen, E., & Borchelt, M. (1999). Morbidity, medication, and functional limitations in very old age. In P.B. Baltes & K.U. Mayer (Eds.), *The Berlin Aging Study: Aging from 70 to 100* (pp. 131–166). New York: Cambridge University Press.

Thomae, H. (Ed.). (1979). *The concept of development and life-span developmental psychology* (Vol. 2). New York: Academic Press.

Wiese, B.S., Freund, A.M., & Baltes, P.B. (2000). Selection, optimization, and compensation: An action-related approach to work and partnership. *Journal of Vocational Behavior, 57,* 273–300.

Wiese, B.S., Freund, A.M., & Baltes, P.B. (2001). Longitudinal predictions of selection, optimization, and compensation. *Journal of Vocational Behavior, 59,* 1–15.